Edited by

GLENN V. DALRYMPLE, M.D.

Professor of Radiology (Nuclear Medicine), Biometry,
and Physiology-Biophysics; Chairman, Division of Nuclear
Medicine and Radiation Biology, University of Arkansas
Medical Center, Little Rock, Arkansas; Chief, Nuclear
Medicine Service, Veterans Administration Hospital,
Little Rock, Arkansas

MARY ESTHER GAULDEN, Ph.D.

Emma Freeman Associate Professor of Radiology;
Chief, Radiation Biology Section, Radiology Department,
The University of Texas Southwestern Medical
School, Dallas, Texas

G. M. KOLLMORGEN, Ph.D.

Associate Professor, Department of Radiological Sciences,
The University of Oklahoma School of Medicine; Associate
Member, Cancer Section, Oklahoma Medical Research Foundation,
Oklahoma City, Oklahoma

HOWARD H. VOGEL, Jr., Ph.D.

Professor and Head, Section of Radiation Biology,
Department of Radiology, and Professor of Physiology, The
University of Tennessee School of Medicine, Memphis, Tennessee

Medical
Radiation
Biology

1973

W. B. SAUNDERS COMPANY • Philadelphia • London • Toronto

W. B. Saunders Company: West Washington Square
Philadelphia, Pa. 19105

12 Dyott Street
London, WC1A   1DB

833 Oxford Street
Toronto 18, Ontario

R M 847
m 39

Medical Radiation Biology   ISBN   0-7216-2865-6

Print No.:   9   8   7   6   5   4   3   2   1

Contributors

GAIL D. ADAMS, Ph.D., Professor and Vice Chairman, Radiological Sciences; Professor, Radiation Physics; Vice Chairman, Graduate Affairs; and Radiation Safety Officer, University of Oklahoma Health Sciences Center, Oklahoma City. Consultant, Oklahoma City Veterans Administration Hospital, Oklahoma City, Oklahoma.

KURT I. ALTMAN, Ph.D., Associate Professor of Experimental Radiology, Radiation Biology and Biophysics, and Biochemistry, University of Rochester School of Medicine and Dentistry, Rochester, New York.

MAX LESLIE BAKER, Ph.D., Assistant Professor of Nuclear Medicine-Radiation Biology and of Physiology-Biophysics, University of Arkansas Medical Center, Little Rock, Arkansas.

HOWARD J. BARNHARD, M.D., Professor and Chairman, Department of Radiology, University of Arkansas School of Medicine, Little Rock. Chief of Radiology, University Hospital, Little Rock. Chief of Radiology, Little Rock Veterans Administration Hospital, Little Rock, Arkansas.

JOEL S. BEDFORD, D.Phil., Associate Professor, Department of Radiology, Vanderbilt University Medical School, Nashville, Tennessee.

MICHAEL A. BENDER, Ph.D., Associate Professor of Radiology, Vanderbilt University School of Medicine, Nashville, Tennessee.

L. H. BLACKWELL, Ph.D., Associate Professor of Radiation Biology; Assistant Professor of Physiology and Biophysics, University of Tennessee Medical Units, Memphis, Tennessee.

CARL ROBERT BOGARDUS, JR., M.D., Professor of Radiology, University of Oklahoma School of Medicine, Oklahoma City. Director of Radiation Therapy, University of Oklahoma Health Sciences Center, Oklahoma City, Oklahoma.

GEORGE W. CASARETT, Ph.D., Professor of Radiation Biology and Biophysics; Professor of Radiology, University of Rochester School of Medicine, Rochester, New York.

VINCENT P. COLLINS, M.D., Professor of Radiology, University of Texas Medical Branch, Galveston. Director of Radiotherapy, Rosewood General Hospital, Houston, Texas.

GEORGE COOPER, JR., M.D., Professor and Chairman, Department of Radiology, University of Tennessee School of Medicine, Memphis. Visiting Professor of Radiology, University of Virginia School of Medicine, Charlottesville, Virginia.

GLENN VOGT DALRYMPLE, M.D., Professor of Radiology, Biometry, Physiology and Biophysics, University of Arkansas School of Medicine, Little Rock. Head, Division of Nuclear Medicine and Radiation Biology, University of Arkansas Medical Center, Little Rock. Acting Chief, Nuclear Medicine Service, Little Rock Veterans Administration Hospital, Little Rock, Arkansas.

MARY ESTHER GAULDEN, Ph.D., Emma Freeman Associate Professor of Radiology, University of Texas Southwestern Medical School, Dallas. Radiation Biologist, Parkland Memorial Hospital, Dallas, Texas.

MELVIN L. GRIEM, M.D., Professor of Radiology; Director, Chicago Tumor Institute, University of Chicago Hospitals and Clinics, Chicago, Illinois.

GERALD EUGENE HANKS, M.D., Associate Clinical Professor, University of California, Davis. Assistant Clinical Professor, Stanford University, Palo Alto. Staff, Radiation Therapy Center, Sutter General Hospital, Sacramento, California.

JOHN JAGGER, Ph.D., Professor of Biology, University of Texas, Dallas. Adjunct Professor, Department of Radiology, University of Texas Southwestern Medical School, Dallas, Texas.

BERNARD N. JAROSLOW, Ph.D., Associate Immunologist, Biology Division, Argonne National Laboratory, Argonne, Illinois.

DONALD J. KIMELDORF, Ph.D., Professor of Radiation Biology, Oregon State University, Corvallis, Oregon.

GEORGE JOHN KOLLMANN, Ph.D., Associate, Bioscience Staff, Department of Nuclear Medicine, Albert Einstein Medical Center, Philadelphia, Pennsylvania.

G. MARK KOLLMORGEN, Ph.D., Associate Professor, Department of Radiological Sciences, University of Oklahoma Health Sciences Center, Oklahoma City. Associate Member, Cancer Section, Oklahoma Medical Research Foundation, Oklahoma City, Oklahoma.

G. DAVID LEDNEY, Ph.D., Associate Professor of Radiation Biology, University of Tennessee Medical Units, Memphis, Tennessee.

WILLIAM S. MAXFIELD, M.D., Formerly Professor and Chairman, Department of Radiology, Louisiana State University Medical School, New Orleans, Louisiana. Head of Radiation Therapy, University Community Hospital, Tampa, Florida.

ALFRED JEFFERSON MOSS, JR., Ph.D., Assistant Professor of Physiology-Biophysics and of Nuclear Medicine-Radiation Biology, University of Arkansas Medical Center, Little Rock. General Physical Scientist (Research), Little Rock Veterans Administration Hospital, Little Rock, Arkansas.

DONALD J. PIZZARELLO, Ph.D., Associate Professor of Radiology, New York University Medical Center, New York. Consultant, Bronx Veterans Administration Hospital, New York. Consultant, Montefiore Hospital and Medical Center, New York, New York.

PHILIP RUBIN, M.D., Chief and Professor, Division of Therapeutic Radiology, University of Rochester School of Medicine and Dentistry, Strong Memorial Hospital, Rochester, New York.

ROBERTS RUGH, Ph.D., Professor of Radiology, Columbia University, New York, New York.

AARON P. SANDERS, Ph.D., Professor of Radiology, Duke University School of Medicine, Durham, Director, Division of Radiobiology, Duke University Medical Center, Durham, North Carolina.

ARTHUR C. UPTON, M.D., Professor of Pathology and Dean of the School of Basic Health Sciences, State University of New York, Stony Brook. Attending Pathologist, Brookhaven National Laboratory Hospital, Long Island, New York.

JAMES F. VANDERGRIFT, M.S., Assistant Professor of Radiology, University of Arkansas School of Medicine, Little Rock. Radiation Safety Officer, University Hospital, Little Rock, Arkansas.

HOWARD H. VOGEL, JR., Ph.D., Professor and Head, Section of Radiation Biology, Department of Radiology, and Professor of Physiology, University of Tennessee School of Medicine, Memphis. Staff, City of Memphis Hospital, Memphis, Tennessee.

RICHARD L. WITCOFSKI, Ph.D., Associate Professor of Radiology, and Associate in Neurology, Bowman Gray School of Medicine of Wake Forest University, Winston-Salem, North Carolina.

JOHN P. WITHERSPOON, Ph.D., Ecologist, Environmental Sciences Division, Oak Ridge National Laboratory, Oak Ridge, Tennessee.

Editors' Preface

We believe this to be the first textbook in radiation biology specifically directed to the student of human health sciences. Consequently, the title *Medical Radiation Biology* indicates the scope and purpose, as well as the introductory nature, of the effort. Wherever possible, we have stressed man—human data, human pathology, and human experience. We believe the book will serve well as a text for teaching radiation biology to students at several levels: Residents, undergraduate medical students, other college and graduate students, and students in radiologic and nuclear technology. We specifically hope it will be of value to radiology residents and physicians in other specialties who do not have access to a formal course in radiation biology.

In the past, teachers of radiation biology in health science areas have been forced to develop their own teaching materials. The unpredictable responses of students so taught is not surprising. Therefore, all those involved in this present effort have tried to define and develop those topics which constitute the "core" of basic medical radiation biology. Reluctantly we performed necessary paring and condensing of material in certain areas to make the book teachable in a one-semester course. Nothing was abridged or altered, however, without prolonged deliberation.

All royalties resulting from sales of this book are to be used for the improvement of the teaching of radiation biology. The American College of Radiology has kindly agreed to serve as a depository for the royalties. The funds will be used to develop teaching materials such as slide sets, film strips, movies, and videotapes. As these materials are developed, they will be made available to individuals who need them.

Although we have made strenuous efforts to obtain broad and comprehensive reviews, the possibility exists that errors and omissions have occurred. As editors, we must take full responsibility for the final version. We strongly encourage readers of this book to communicate to us any errors or omissions they may find. We will attempt to include these corrections in the second edition of the book.

Finally, the editors are particularly grateful to Mrs. Lillian M. Worthington for her extraordinary work in organizing, retyping, and handling of manuscripts.

GLENN V. DALRYMPLE
MARY ESTHER GAULDEN
G. MARK KOLLMORGEN
HOWARD H. VOGEL, JR.

Contents

1 THE DEVELOPMENT OF RADIATION SCIENCE

George Cooper, Jr., M.D.

Frustrating mists of time obscure people and events involved in the beginnings of civilization, but it is, nevertheless, clear that a historical review of almost every intellectual effort must commence with the recording of contributions made by people who lived within an amazingly small area and within an amazingly brief period. The area comprises the islands and lands whose shores are washed by the Aegean Sea, and the period is that during which Greek city-states dominated the region, roughly 700 to 300 B.C., from the rise of the poleis to their submission to the Macedonian father-son team of Philip and Alexander. If the obscuration of the centuries could be cleared a bit, we might see that the Greeks owed more than we can know to their predecessors; but, whatever their debt, the fact remains that mankind's longest intellectual strides were taken by the classical Greeks, the most magnificent hybrids yet to emerge from the human amalgam.

It is not surprising, therefore, to find the development of radiation science commencing in Miletus, a Greek polis in Asia Minor, during the sixth century B.C. To one of the Seven Wise Men of ancient Greek philosophy, Thales of Miletus, is attributed the observation that when amber (Greek: *elektron*) is rubbed with wool, it attracts light objects. From a modern perspective it is impossible to be certain that Thales really deserves sole credit, but it is clear that Thales and those around him engaged in the first significant consideration of the phenomenon and related it to the capacity of lodestone (Greek: *magnetis*) to attract iron.

From Thales to the Abbé Nollet, a seventeenth century Frenchman, is an enormous jump in time, but, insofar as our subject is concerned, the events of those 2200 years can be summarized by recording that many men in many countries produced a body of knowledge which placed electrostatics and magnetostatics upon firm foundations and brought them together under electromagnetism. However, since the medical profession has benefited so tremendously from radiation science, we should pause long enough to note that a physician made one of the landmark contributions. In 1600, William Gilbert, whose patients included Queen Elizabeth I of England, published the important work *De Magnete* in which he advanced the concept that electrical phenomena are due to the liberation of some material when bodies are electrified by friction, without an accompanying change of form or loss of weight. In the mid-seventeenth century, the Abbé Nollet commenced studies which were to culminate in the explosive events of 1895 that precipitated the great expansion of radiation science through which we are now living. The Abbé Nollet and his successors, through Roentgen, had no objective other than to

1

satisfy their curiosity concerning the consequences of passing a high potential current through a glass bulb containing separated terminals as the atmospheric pressure within the bulb was progressively lowered. Surely one can cite a no more startling illustration of serendipity than the by-product of that curiosity. Nollet reported that at unaltered pressure, a stream of sparks jumped the gap, and as he lowered the pressure as much as his glass could tolerate, the stream of sparks became wider and confluent, finally changing into a luminous band.

During the next several hundred years there was great progress in the understanding of electricity, magnetism, and electromagnetism, but Nollet's observations received little attention. Then Julius Plucker, a professor of physics at the University of Bonn, called on Heinrich Geissler, a glass blower, to help him in his study of light produced by electrical discharges in gases at reduced pressure. Geissler had glass available that permitted him to construct tubes which could withstand much higher vacuums than those with which Nollet experimented. He prepared for Plucker the first gaseous discharge tubes, the prototypes of the helium, neon, mercury, and fluorescent lamps which are such garish features of our times and which are still often called Geissler tubes. Plucker, Geissler, and J. W. Hittorf, a student of Plucker who later became professor of physics and chemistry at the University of Münster, together pursued the observations reported by Nollet. In 1859 Geissler reported that in the higher vacuums attainable in his tubes, Nollet's luminous band faded to a pale delicate glow. In 1860, Hittorf observed that Geissler's glow was deflected by a magnet, a bit of information which was to serve Roentgen extraordinarily well.

During the next several decades, the leading contributor to this field of investigation was the English scientist, William Crookes (he was not knighted until 1897). Crookes had developed a tube in which the anode was in a pocket projecting from a lateral aspect of the tube, leaving the end opposite the cathode consisting of glass only. The glass available to Crookes could withstand almost a total vacuum. He found that as he evacuated the activated tube to below 0.00013 atm, the glow reported by

Geissler disappeared and a bluish beam could be seen extending from the cathode. Largely through Crooke's studies, we now understand that this was a beam of electrons from the cathode, or cathode rays, made visible by excitation of the gas molecules with which the electrons collided. Crookes noted that below 0.0000013 atm the molecular collisions became so few that the blue beam faded out, but the relatively unobstructed bombardment of the anticathode region of the tube heated the glass and caused emission of a brilliant apple-green light. He further reported that a concave cathode, designed to focus the cathode rays on a small portion of the anticathode, increased the heat and the brilliance of the green fluorescence.

In the early 1890's, the scene of major interest shifted back to the University of Bonn where a professor of physics, H. R. Hertz, inserted discs of various substances in the path of the cathode rays. He reported that enough of the rays could penetrate thin discs of a light metal (aluminum) to produce some fluorescence in the portion of the anticathode shadowed by the discs. It did not occur to him that anything other than cathode rays might be involved. Philipp Lenard, at that time an assistant to Hertz, went still further, sealing a piece of aluminum foil in a window in the anticathode region of a Crookes tube and then studying the radiation outside of the tube. He observed that the radiation which penetrated the aluminum window was capable of passing through a variety of light-impermeable substances to reach barium platinocyanide and causing it to fluoresce. He even noted that this filtered radiation fogged a photographic plate. How close he came to discovering the "Lenard ray" and founding the science of "Lenardology"! But, like Hertz, he did not suspect that he was dealing with anything but cathode rays.

The physicists at Bonn and elsewhere continued their studies, but in the fall of 1895, Wilhelm Konrad Roentgen, professor of physics at the University of Würzburg, became interested in the phenomenon and promptly stole the show. Roentgen designed a different series of experiments. He wished to exclude the possibility that light rays were responsible for phenomena reported by Lenard. Instead of sealing an aluminum window in the anticathode region of a Crookes tube, Roentgen enclosed an entire tube in a cardboard box thick enough and so fitted as to be impermeable to light. On November 8, 1895, he was activating the tube while a piece of platinocyanide paper lay on a nearby bench. He noticed that a black line appeared across the paper. Startled and puzzled, he repeatedly activated the tube while concentrating his attention on the paper and in a few minutes satisfied himself that rays originating in the tube were passing through the cardboard and producing fluorescence of the platinocyanide, even at distances of up to two meters. It seemed that the only possible explanation was that some kind of peculiar, hitherto unrecognized, light rays were being produced. Feeling insecure with so shattering a concept, Roentgen kept his observations to himself, locked the door of his small laboratory, and worked day and night to repeat and expand his experiments. By placing various substances between the tube and the platinocyanide, he proved that the degree of penetration of any material by the radiation depended on the material's density. Taking a cue from Hittorf, he explored the effect of a magnet upon the radiation. Finding that he could not deflect it in this manner, he went on to demonstrate that he could neither reflect nor refract it. Having excluded the presence of cathode rays, he apparently had also excluded transversely vibrating light rays. He could only speculate that the radiation represented longitudinal vibrations in the "ether." In any event, it was certain that he had serendipitously stumbled upon radiation, the existence of which had not been suspected and the nature of which was totally unknown. Unconsciously paying a deserved compliment to Thales of Miletus, Roentgen borrowed the Greek symbol for the unknown and called the radiation "X-rays."

His observations to this point were to have a jarring impact upon the physical sciences, an impact which was to be transmitted to the biologic sciences with compounded force when he went on to his next series of observations. While holding a sheet of lead in front of a barium platinocyanide coated screen, thus repeating the demonstration that X-rays could not penetrate lead, he was dumbfounded to see on the fluorescing screen, within the outline of that portion of his thumb and fingers not shielded by the lead, the shadows of the bones within his flesh! The intensity of his experimentation increased, and long hours of sleepless soul-searching ensued. It occurred to him to place his wife's hand on a photographic plate during activation of the tube. Since roentgenograms are now commonplace, it is almost impossible to recreate the overwhelming drama of the first one, but, as we can remember the drama of the first trip to the moon, we can to some degree imagine the Roentgens' feelings when they developed and looked at that plate.

At length, satisfied with his proof that when a multidensity object is placed in an X-ray beam before a fluorescent screen or a photographic plate, a shadowgraph of the sub-surface structures is produced, Roentgen prepared his paper, "A New Kind of Ray," and presented it to the Physical Medical Society of Würzburg on December 28, 1895. It was published at once and electrified the world. Roentgen had feared that his report would so astound that he would be the target of skepticism and ridicule. Instead, he saw his entire work accepted immediately. The medical profession seized the tools which he had presented it and put the fluoroscope and roentgenogram to use within a few days. The time between the announcement of a major medical advance and its use has never been shorter, and the influence of such a breakthrough upon medical practice has never been greater. With the help of contrast media to produce a different density in structures surrounded by other structures of the same density, the physician's capacity to see into the human body was carried to fantastic heights which have not yet been fully scaled. The extension of the physician's sense of vision made possible undreamed of diagnostic accuracy. This, in turn, vastly increased the understanding of disease, the effects of trauma, and how to manage both. Furthermore, the ability to diagnose so accurately inspired surgeons to develop techniques with which to perform procedures that would not have occurred to a medical Jules Verne prior to December 28, 1895. As medical knowledge and skills mushroomed, the area which any one physician could master shrank proportionately. Consequently, the advent of diagnostic roentgenology quickly called into being the specialties and sub-specialties of modern medicine.

Because of the relation between X-rays and fluorescence, naturally fluorescent substances received fresh attention. In February, 1896, Henri Becquerel, Professor of Physics at École Polytechnique in Paris, placed crystals of a uranium compound on a photographic plate wrapped in black paper and demonstrated that the uranium rays which affected the photographic plate possessed the same characteristics as X-rays. Marie and Pierre Curie pursued the subject of radioactivity and in 1898 successively isolated from Bohemian pitchblende ore polonium and radium. In the meantime, exposures to the X-rays produced by the first gas tubes had resulted in varying skin reactions, ranging from a transient erythema to a deep, persistent ulceration. Becquerel carried a glass tube containing a bit of the Curies' radium in his vest pocket and was later surprised to find an underlying skin erythema like that which was produced after exposure to X-rays. Pierre Curie confirmed the observation by deliberately producing a radium erythema on a forearm. With the recognition of essentially identical biologic effects caused by both X-rays and natural radioactivity, the science of radiobiology was born, but the birth passed unnoted for many years. The first concern was to determine whether or not radioactivity possessed therapeutic value, a concern which led to the clinical specialty of therapeutic radiology.

Initially, radiology (diagnostic and therapeutic) was an adjunctive interest of clinicians whose primary training and experience were in other fields of medicine, but within Roentgen's lifetime (he died in 1923) many physicians had chosen to limit their practice to the burgeoning new science. Some of them developed training programs, and medical college graduates began electing the specialty at the commencement of their professional careers. In 1934, Frédéric and Irène (a daughter of the Curies) Joliot-Curie bombarded aluminum with alpha particles and produced artificial radioactivity. From this accomplishment grew yet a third major clinical radiologic science — nuclear medicine. The mass of knowledge and the variety of skills lumped together in radiology grew too great for the average physician to encompass. The three clinical areas began drifting apart, and today we are witnessing not only the full establishment of the three sub-specialties, but also the appearance of sub-specialties in diagnostic radiology.

Clearly physicists, not physicians, made the basic observations responsible for the existence of radiology. Not only did they found the science, but by exploring, expanding, and exploiting the work of Roentgen, the Curies, and the Joliot-Curies, they brought a depth of understanding which could be applied in terms of techniques and equipment to bring about revolutionary innovations in all three of the clinical areas. Radiation physics became an important division of physics and the radiation physicist an essential collaborator and colleague of radiologic clinicians. Because physicians are biologic scientists, there has never been any question about the radiologists' dependence upon the radiation physicists, and the indispensable role of the radiation physicist has always been clear. In contrast, it is only in recent years that the role of the radiobiologist has emerged.

In retrospect, as noted earlier, radiobiology commenced when it was observed that X-rays and the radioactivity of radium produced the same skin reactions. Though the physicians who first used X-rays and radium were primarily interested in their diagnostic and therapeutic application, they inescapably witnessed the sequelae of exposures in themselves, as well as in their patients. As the systematic cataloguing of the sequelae of single large exposures generated a similar appreciation of the sequelae of repeated moderate exposures, and then of repeated small exposures, physicians inevitably sought explanation in an effort to devise treatment and prevention measures. They soon found that their explorations were carrying them deeply into cellular biology and biochemistry, so deeply that the clinicians began calling for investigators in these and other fields to help them out. Many of the investigators became so absorbed in the effort to understand the biologic effects of radiation that they devoted themselves exclusively to the task. They attracted other scientists to do the same and some established laboratories complete with graduate students and trainees, all devoted to trying to answer the unexpectedly complex and basic questions which had arisen. A body of knowledge grew which increasingly determined modifications and innovations in the various divisions of clinical radiology.

It became essential that intelligent radiologic clinicians possess a firm grasp of certain principles of radiobiology, as well as radiation physics. Formal teaching in both subjects became an integral part of the radiologic training programs, and support of radiobiologic investigation became an added function of radiology. Where once the very existence of radiobiology was overlooked, today we recognize that clinical radiology is the practical application of radiation physics and radiobiology, that major clinical advances must await the answering of basic questions, and that instruction in wisely selected portions of the basic sciences is a necessary ingredient of sound radiologic training.

Thales of Miletus initiated the gestation of all the radiologic sciences. Roentgen, the Curies, and the Joliot-Curies precipitated and presided over the delivery. Because the independent life of radiobiology spans only the mid-twentieth century, a history of the toddler is decidedly premature; yet it seems not inappropriate to hazard, in this particular volume, sketchy notes about some contributions which, at this too close range, appear formative.

By the early 1920's, there was a consensus that the biologic effects of particulate and higher energy electromagnetic radiations are a reflection of ionizations in tissue. This implied that investigation must be at the cellular and intracellular levels. It was soon realized that there are two categories of effects—those resulting from ionizations in the direct track of the radiation and those resulting from the secondary reactions of free radical by-products which diffuse away from the radiation track.

From about 1925 to 1945, significant insight was gained into the effects of ionizations in the direct track. Outstanding contributors in this area were F. G. Spear and D. E. Lea of the Strangeways Laboratory, Cambridge; N. Timofeaff-Ressovsky and K. G. Zimmer in Germany; and H. J. Muller who, with characteristic American itchiness, commenced his career at Columbia University, went on to the University of Texas, spent a few years at the Academy of Sciences in Moscow, and then settled down at Indiana University. The first four investigators were chiefly responsible for the development of the "Treffertheorie," or target theory, which permitted a quantitative evaluation of many of the biologic effects of radiation; this approach has been tremendously helpful, especially in an understanding of the genetic effects of radiation. Lea's book, *Action of Radiation on Living Cells*, is a basic tome in the library of every scientist concerned with any biologic aspect of radiations. Muller won the Nobel Prize for Medicine in 1946 for his demonstration of the influence of X-rays on gene mutation rate.

Around 1940, interest shifted from effects in the direct radiation track to the secondary reactions of diffused free radicals. Study of the role of oxygen upon radiation effect had been initiated by the independent efforts of H. Holthusen and E. Petry in the early 1920's. The subject was pursued by J. D. Mottram and L. H. Gray, and in 1947 J. N. Thoday and J. Read, co-workers of Spear and Lea, discovered that the frequency of chromosome breakage increased, independently of the target theory effect, as oxygen tension increased in the irradiated tissue. The clinical applications of the oxygen studies have as yet been disappointing, but their stimulation of radiobiologic investigation has been most productive. For instance, they led directly to the discovery by W. N. Dale that enzymes in solution can be protected from interaction with free radicals produced by irradiation ionization of water by adding to the solution sulfur-containing compounds which attract the free radicals. Perhaps not of major individual import, this and other related observations are adding rapidly to the basic insight so desperately needed to define confidently the safety limits in diagnostic radiologic procedures and to realize completely the potentials of therapeutic radiology and nuclear medicine. The value of these observations has been enhanced and the making of further observations expedited by the work of such men as G. Failla and L. Taylor, who injected the exactness of mathematics and physics into radiobiologic investigations.

Because radiobiology is the most recently developed of the radiation sciences, those designing training programs are uncertain as to just what portion of radiobiologic knowledge should be placed before trainees in the various clinical divisions of radiology. A series of conferences between interested teachers has led to tentative conclusions which are offered in the subsequent chapters of this book.

2 PHYSICAL PRINCIPLES

Gail D. Adams, Ph.D.

2.0 GENERAL COMPOSITION OF MATTER

Occurrences of consequence in radiation biology for the most part may be considered to take place in aqueous solution, that is, they take place in the liquid state. Two other states of matter are normally distinguished from liquids; these are gases and solids. Each of these states has certain distinguishing physical characteristics (color, specific gravity, electrical conductivity, specific heat, and so on) and chemical composition. The smallest unit of a substance, which retains the chemical and physical properties of the substance, is called a molecule. Gases, except at high pressures, may be considered as groups of individual molecules, each separated from neighboring molecules by substantial distances. Consequently, forces which might otherwise operate between molecules have little opportunity to do so.

By contrast, the solid state is highly ordered, the basic units being arranged in a repetitive pattern called a crystal. The basic units may not be molecules in the same sense as found in gases. Molecules are formed from atoms, which are the smallest units entering into chemical reactions. The periodic table is an ordered array of the different kinds of chemical atoms, called elements, with the arrangement determined by chemical reaction characteristics. Atoms and molecules are ordinarily found

to be electrically neutral. Charged forms of either atoms or molecules are called ions. Some crystals — for example, sugar — are ordered arrays of neutral molecules; others, such as salt, are ions. In salt, the ions Na^+ and Cl^- alternate in each of the three principal rectilinear directions. Each sodium ion has six chloride ions for nearest neighbors, and vice versa. The strong force between opposite charges is responsible for the stability of this ionic crystal.

The liquid state may be regarded as intermediate between gases and solids. The molecules are adjacent to each other but do not maintain ordered arrangements for any sustained periods. An object moving through a liquid encounters resistance (viscosity) in making its way through the molecules of the liquid. Glass is a liquid of very high viscosity. One class of electrically neutral molecular fragments is known as the free radical. Their importance is in the transport of energy mainly through liquids by diffusion.

2.1 SUBATOMIC PARTICLES

For some purposes the ultimate construction of matter might be molecules; for others it might be atoms. Early in the twentieth century Niels Bohr proposed a model of the atom which is still useful today. In this model each atom is portrayed with some characteristics of a solar system: a central portion, the nucleus, containing

TABLE 2-1   PROPERTIES TO DISTINGUISH SOME PARTICLES

Name	Symbol	Mass	Charge	Spin
Proton	p	1	+1	$1/2$
Neutron	n	1	0	$1/2$
Electron	e^-, β^-	1/1836	−1	$1/2$
Positron	e^+, β^+	1/1836	+1	$1/2$
Photon	γ	0	0	1
Neutrino	ν	~0	0	$1/2$
Alpha	α	4	+2	0
Deuteron	d	2	+1	0

*Masses are approximate and are given in relation to the proton's mass.

most of the mass is encircled by light particles in specific orbits. The nucleus is formed from protons and neutrons. The exterior particles are electrons. A few properties of some important particles are given in Table 2-1.

What is a particle? Nobody has ever seen one! Consider an analogy: we allege that the physician does not see a disease. In the patient he observes certain signs and symptoms and describes these by the shorthand name agreed upon for the disease. Likewise, a particle's name is a shorthand designation for a collection of properties and characteristics which are observed and measured. Three properties are used here to distinguish these particles: mass, charge, and spin. *Mass* is given in relation to the proton mass; *charge* is found to exist in integral multiples of a least amount, the same magnitude whether positive or negative; *spin* is similar to the rotation of the earth on its axis, but in the spin of a particle the angular momentum occurs in discrete amounts (which are half-integral multiples of $h/2\pi$, h being Planck's constant).

2.2   RADIOACTIVITY

Radioactivity is the spontaneous decay of an atomic nucleus, and energy is released by each decay. There are four common modes of decay, which are described in this section.

It is necessary to understand the shorthand notation used to describe specific atomic nuclei. The numbers of protons and neutrons are of primary concern. The atomic number (Z) of the element is the number of protons; the mass number (A) is the total number of protons plus neutrons and is more commonly used than the neutron number (N). Nuclei having the same number of protons but differing in mass number are chemically the same element but have different physical properties, notably mass. These physically different nuclear species (of the same element) are called isotopes of that element. For example, hydrogen (Z = 1) has three isotopes: A = 1, 2, and 3. These happen to have special names: ordinary hydrogen, deuterium or heavy hydrogen, and tritium or doubly-heavy hydrogen. Ordinary hydrogen and deuterium are stable; tritium is unstable (radioactive). If Ch stands for the chemical symbol for an arbitrary element, then the notation used for an isotope of that element is: ^A_ZCh. Thus, the known isotopes of hydrogen are represented by $^1_1$H, $^2_1$H, $^3_1$H.

The existence of radioactivity has introduced second names for some particles. The nucleus of the common isotope of helium, $^4_2$He, is also known as the alpha (α) particle. The nucleus $^2_1$H is known as the deuteron (d). High-speed positrons (β^+) or electrons (β^-) emitted from nuclei are beta particles. Photons from nuclei are gamma (γ) rays.

Alpha-emitters, with a few exceptions, have an atomic number greater than that of lead, for which Z = 82. Each alpha particle as emitted carries a specific amount of energy. For some alpha-emitters this amount is unique; for others there may be a small number of slightly differing specific amounts. Gamma rays may or may not accompany alpha emission. Alpha particles are very seldom used biomedically, primarily because they are absorbed by very thin layers of material. They cannot penetrate to a useful depth.

Beta-emitters are the most numerous of the radioactive isotopes. In β^- decay the energy released is shared between the electron and neutrino. Of the energy released in β^+ decay, 1.02 MeV is used in the production of the positron, and the remainder is shared between the positron and a neutrino. In either case, the sharing results in a distribution of energies given to the beta particle and the neutrino. This share may be any value between zero and the full energy available (E_{max}). For dosimetry it is useful to characterize the sharing by the average energy ($\overline{E}_\beta$) given to the beta particle. Gamma rays may accompany beta decay.

There is no mode of nuclear disintegration known specifically as gamma decay. The one called isomeric transition would, however, be a suitable candidate. Nuclei have the ability to store excess energy in excitation levels. The de-excitation of this excess energy is usually quite prompt. When the de-excitation is delayed to the point that the isotope demonstrates a measurable half-life, the excited state and the ground state are known as isomers (radionuclides of same Z *and* same A).

The last radioactive decay mode of importance to our discussion is called electron capture. The nucleus is said to capture one of the inner orbital electrons and to release a neutrino. There may also be one or more gamma rays released following the capture, and there will also be characteristic X-rays from the daughter atom. Electron capture competes with β^+ decay for energy release accompanied by reduction of the atomic number by one. Either mode is possible with energies above 1.02 MeV; electron capture alone is possible with energies below 1.02 MeV.

Gamma rays (photons of nuclear origin) are not restricted to any mode of decay. One important characteristic of gamma rays is that each represents a particular release of nuclear energy. Thus, the gamma rays from the disintegration of a particular radionuclide may all have identical energy or may be partitioned into a few groups of identical energies if the nuclide releases its excess energy in steps.

The fate of the positron is also of some consequence. Emitted typically in β^+ decay, this particle loses its energy as it passes through matter and ultimately comes essentially to rest. It forms then a brief partnership with a nearby electron, but shortly both particles completely disappear (i.e., their charges and masses cease to exist). In their place appear two photons, emerging in opposite directions, each of 0.51 MeV. This is annihilation radiation. The 1.02 MeV required for the formation of the positron is liberated as annihilation radiation.

For any radionuclide, each nucleus has a fixed probability for decay per unit of time. This probability is the same for every nucleus of any particular radionuclide, it is independent of the time interval after the radionuclide was formed, and it is measurable. Since a recognizable sample of a radionuclide inevitably contains a large number of atoms, the probability per unit time for decay of an individual nucleus multiplied by the number of such nuclei gives the rate of decay. The rate of decay is clearly proportional to the number of nuclei which at any time are subject to decay. We can express this concept as an equation: the number decaying per unit time = (decay constant) × (number present), where the constant of proportionality is given the name "decay constant" and is frequently represented by λ (lambda). If N_0 is the number present at any arbitrary origin in time, the number N present at any time interval, t, thereafter is $N = N_0 e^{-\lambda t}$ (See the Appendix for more on this equation). Some nuclei among the N_0 decay very soon, some very late; but the average time for a population to decay is $t = 1/\lambda$. This time interval is known as the mean life. In more customary usage are the time intervals for half of a given sample to decay; that is, $N/N_0 = 1/2 = e^{-\lambda T}$. Therefore, $T = 0.693/\lambda$, and is commonly called the physical half-life.

Radionuclides enjoy many uses as tags on molecules of biomedical interest. When the situation involves active physiological processes, the molecule of interest, and hence the tag, may be eliminated from the overall picture. While it is the responsibility of the investigator to show the truth of each situation, frequently the biologic elimination rate appears to be proportional to the number of molecules of that kind present. In this instance physical and biologic processes operate simultaneously to reduce the number of decayable nuclei present; that is, the effective decay constant is the sum of physical and biologic decay constants: $\lambda_e = \lambda_p + \lambda_b$. This expression in terms of half-lives is $1/T_e = (1/T_p) + (1/T_b)$, or $T_b = T_e T_p/(T_p - T_e)$. T_p is known, so if the observed situation gives an apparent half-life T_e which is appreciably less than T_p, then recognizable biologic elimination occurs and the biologic half-life may be calculated.

It is useful to introduce a method to portray radioactive disintegration modes. For this we use the energy level diagram, in which increasing amounts of energy potentially available are plotted upward continuously and atomic numbers in unit steps are plotted sidewise. Kinds of particles emitted, energies, and other relevant data are recorded. Common examples are shown in Figure 2–1.

2.3 GENERATION OF PARTICLES

Practical sources of subatomic particles in some instances result from natural processes and in others from artificial means. The natural processes are called radio-

activity and involve the spontaneous alteration of atomic nuclei; these were discussed early in the chapter. The artificial means include man-made machines which accelerate charged particles to substantial energies. The energetic particles may be brought out of these accelerators for direct use or they may be caused to strike a target for indirect use.

Perhaps the simplest and most common accelerator is the X-ray machine, in which electrons from a hot filament are accelerated across an evacuated space by direct application of a large potential difference be-

ENERGY LEVEL DIAGRAMS

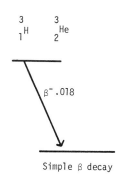

Simple β decay

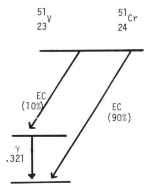

Electron capture with branching

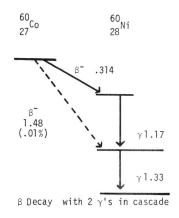

β Decay with 2 γ's in cascade

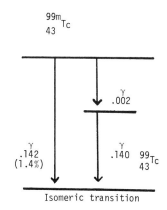

Isomeric transition

FIGURE 2–1 Energy level diagrams for typical decay schemes. Energies associated with the various particle emissions, given in MeV, are near the particle symbol; branching percentages are given in parentheses. For clarity energy spans are indicated but are not to scale.

tween the filament and an anode, or target. These electrons lose their energies in the target, some of which reappear as X-rays. X-rays are photons. Just as γ-ray is the name applied to photons of nuclear origin, so X-ray is the name applied to photons created by electron bombardment. There are two subdivisions of X-rays: characteristic X-rays and bremsstrahlung, or continuous X-rays.

Bremsstrahlung (German for braking radiation) is the natural consequence of a close encounter between the incident high speed electron and an atomic nucleus. The strong attractive force between charged particles deflects the electron, which loses energy. This energy appears as the X-ray, which is considered to arise from the application of brakes; hence the term "bremsstrahlung." The amount of energy given to the X-ray photon depends on the closeness of the encounter and, since all degrees of closeness are possible, the resulting X-rays may have energies from zero to a maximum determined by the energy of the incident electrons. The distribution describing the frequency with which photons do appear across the full range of allowed energies is called the photon spectrum. Since bremmstrahlung appears as a continuous distribution, it is sometimes called continuous X-rays.

Characteristic X-rays arise from transitions of orbital electrons. These electrons are grouped into shells. The shell closest to the nucleus (K-shell) can accommodate at most two electrons. The next shell outward (L) can contain eight. Succeeding shells (M, N, . . .) have limits of 18, 32, . . . electrons. The inner two shells are normally filled for all atoms of atomic number ten or higher. But an incident high speed electron may pass close enough to one of these to exert a sufficient repulsive force (like charges repel each other) to expel an orbital electron from the atom. Such a vacancy is very vulnerable when in an inner orbit. Promptly, the atom undergoes a change (transition) in which an electron from an outer shell fills the inner vacancy. The transition releases potential energy, appearing externally in the form of a photon. In general, this form of photon production is known as fluorescence. Here we are considering a special case of fluorescence in which the inner shells have the initial

vacancy, whence the emerging photons carry relatively high energy. These have been named characteristic X-rays. The energy associated with each electron orbit is highly specific, as are the possible transitions; hence, the energies seen in the emitted characteristic X-rays are also highly specific. The bremsstrahlung spectrum is continuous, but characteristic X-rays (and γ-rays) are a set of discrete lines. It is useful to distinguish among characteristic X-rays according to the element and the shell in which the initial vacancy occurred. Those appearing consequent to the production of a vacancy in the K-shell in molybdenum are Mo K X-rays. The existence of K X-rays implies the existence of L X-rays since a K-shell vacancy may be filled by a transition of an electron from the L-shell. This transposes the vacancy to the L-shell. The X-ray that appears is characteristic of the element (Z) and of the shells involved (L $\rightarrow$ K, for example).

X-ray generators in ordinary use are those in which the full acceleration potential is applied between electron source and target. For potential differences above a few million volts, the difficulty of insulating the potential difference makes this method impractical. High energy devices (linear accelerator, betatron, synchrotron) use indirect means of increasing electron energy far beyond the potential difference which appears at any instant. Nevertheless, if the accelerated electrons are caused to strike a target, X-rays are produced. Both the quantity and quality of the X-radiation increase with increasing energy given to the electrons. On some occasions, the accelerated electrons are brought out of the accelerator through a thin window so that they may be used directly as a particle beam. A particular advantage achieved thereby is that all electrons in such a beam carry substantially equal energy (in contrast to the continuous energy distribution of β-rays).

Beams of other particles may also be produced, and these enjoy some biomedical usage. The cyclotron is usually required to impart to the heavy charged particles (p, d, α) energies above the same potential difference limitation as for electrons. There are some heavy ion linear accelerators, and, of course, the proton synchrotrons, which produce the highest energies. A description of the construction and operation of all these devices is beyond the scope of this presentation.

Neutron beams tend to be classified as fast or slow (thermal), but there are many intermediate categories. Usefully large quantities of slow neutrons are typically available only from a nuclear reactor. Fast neutrons are produced by nuclear transmutation reactions. These require bombardment of a target material with heavy ions, for which purpose various heavy ion accelerators are used. One useful reaction, involving the resonant absorption of 100 KeV deuterons in a tritiated target, gives monoenergetic 14 MeV neutrons: $_1^3H + _1^2H \rightarrow _0^1N + _2^4He$. This reaction is also written $_1^3H$ (d,n) $_2^4He$. Other (d,n) reactions are also used when high energy deuterons are available, as from a cyclotron. When a large neutron flux is needed, $_4^9Be$ (d,n) $_5^{10}B$ is used; when the highest neutron energy is required, $_3^7Li$ (d,n) 2α is used.

2.4 INTERACTION OF PARTICLES WITH MATTER

A. Charged Particles

Charles Coulomb described the force which exists between charges (including charged particles). The force is directly proportional to the product of the charges and inversely proportional to the square of the distance separating them. The force is attractive when the charges are of unlike sign, repulsive when of like sign. This Coulomb force is the principal consideration in mediating energy transfers from a charged particle to the atoms of a medium through which the particle is moving. The primary interaction occurs between the charged particle and one (or more) of the orbital electrons. If any one encounter is sufficiently close and not too brief, an energy transfer is likely. Such a transfer may be energetic enough to remove an electron from the atom (this is called ionization because an ion is produced), or it may only supply enough energy to raise an electron to a higher orbit (excitation). The de-excitation procedure involves many steps with various alternatives. It includes the breaking of molecular bonds, the production of free radicals, the emission of fluorescence photons, and the excitation of vibrational modes in molecules (sometimes rotational modes); but inevitably the degradation endpoint is increased kinetic energy of the molecules of the medium: heat.

Some charged particles expend their energy in other ways. Electrons may be deflected around a nucleus and produce bremsstrahlung (described earlier). If high enough in energy, they may also react with a nucleus, promoting a nuclear transmutation. The heavier charged particles cause nuclear transmutations much more efficiently than do electrons.

Nevertheless, the Coulomb interactions,

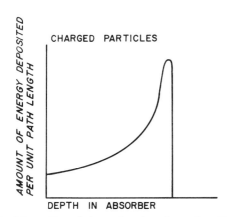
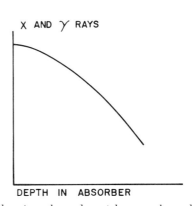

FIGURE 2–2 Attenuation of charged and uncharged particles. As a charged particle nears the end of its range it will have lost most of its energy, will be moving more slowly, will thus spend more time near atoms along its path, and will thereby transfer energy to more of these atoms per unit path length than when energetic. Finally, the last few transfers bring the particle nearly to rest and the transfers cease. In contrast, uncharged particles exhibit quasi-exponential attenuation with a small number penetrating to great depths. The energy transfer events suffered by uncharged particles are rare but catastrophic.

leading to ionizations and excitations, account for the majority of the interactions for photon energies of concern here. For example, the radiative energy loss (bremsstrahlung) for 0.5 MeV electrons is less than 2 per cent of the collision loss (ionizations and excitations). This holds even in the X-ray target, which has a relatively high atomic number (74). As a charged particle transverses matter, it makes many energy transfers, each relatively small. As this particle loses its energy it slows down, thus spending a longer time in the vicinity of any particular atom. Hence, the time interval during which it can exert a force on the atom or any electron is increased. This implies that the probability for an energy transfer is increased as the particle velocity decreases, and we would measure a larger total energy transfer in a micron of path. Bragg first noted this effect in gases. The Bragg curve (Figure 2–2) portrays for a given charged particle the increase in energy transfer rate as the particle nears the end of its range (all energy spent).

B. Uncharged Particles

We are here concerned with neutrons and photons. It is important to comprehend the difference between the interactions with matter of charged and of uncharged particles. Charged particles, because they are charged, are directly responsible for Coulomb forces which mitigate the many small energy transfer events which in turn reduce the kinetic energy of the incident charged particle towards the ambient thermal value. In contrast, uncharged particles offer no counterpart of the Coulomb force. The immediate conclusion is that the probability of interaction with any one atom is drastically smaller for uncharged particles than for charged particles. In fact, an incident uncharged particle will pass by a very large number of atoms and leave no evidence whatever of its path. For perspective, consider that the interatomic distance for typical materials is roughly 2.5×10^{-8} cm. Thus, if the mean interaction distance is 1 cm (a condition easily found), then 4×10^7 atoms have on the average been passed without interaction. To complete the contrast, the smallest rate at which charged

particles impart energy to a tissue-like medium is 0.2 KeV per μm, or 2×10^6 eV per cm. If we take the typical energy transfer event as 10 eV, then some 2×10^5 events occur per centimeter, which involves about one atom in every 200.

We now turn to those interactions which involve neutrons. All neutron interactions involve the nucleus. Some are simple mechanical collisions; others involve nuclear transmutation.

Mechanical collisions of this sort are quite adequately compared to those involving elastic spheres; that is, kinetic energy and linear momentum are conserved. The more energetic incident particle (neutron) loses energy on each encounter. The energy lost is not great if the target nuclei are heavy and hence hard to set in motion, but on the average half of the incident energy is lost if the target nuclei are protons (the masses of a proton and a neutron are about equal). When fast neutrons are incident on tissue, roughly 90 per cent of the energy transferred is by such recoil protons. The mean free path in tissue for neutrons of energy E_n is approximately:

0.7 cm,   Thermal $< E_n \leq 0.1$ MeV

$0.7\sqrt{10E_n}$ cm, $0.1 < E_n < 10$ MeV

Nuclear transmutations may be induced by both fast and slow neutrons. Fast neutrons can induce whole families of transmutations, mainly (n,n'), (n, 2n), and (n,p). However, these are of no particular consequence for tissue-like materials and for neutron energies normally available. A slow neutron may be captured by a nucleus. In tissue, the important capture processes are:

$^1_1H(n, \gamma)\, ^2_1H$ γ energy = 2.2 MeV
$^{14}_7N(n, p)^{14}_6C$ p energy = 0.66 MeV

Fast neutrons pervading tissue are slowed down by elastic collisions and then captured by a proton (hydrogen nucleus). Radiation therapy of cancer has been attempted using slow neutrons and tissue loaded with boron (as borate):

$^{10}_5B(n, \alpha)\, ^7_3Li$ ^7_3Li and α share 2.3 MeV

Neutron counters, usually filled with the gas BF_3, use this reaction. Slow neutrons in a pile, when captured in target nuclei, are used to produce useful isotopes.

We turn now to interaction processes involving photons. For the most part, we will consider processes of practical importance—those which make energy available to the interaction medium. The exception, briefly, is Thomson or coherent scattering, in which an incident photon is scattered from the photon beam, appearing in a new direction without doing work on the medium. This phenomenon is never of principal importance and no energy loss occurs.

Of the photon interactions which deposit energy, the one most important at lower energies (e.g., below .05 MeV for Al, 0.5 MeV for Pb) is called the photoelectric effect. In this process, an orbital electron is expelled from an atom, and the photon disappears entirely. The photon must carry at least the amount of energy needed to remove the particular electron affected (i.e., it must supply its binding energy); any excess is given to the electron as kinetic energy. Thus, for a particular orbital electron, the higher the photon energy (above the binding energy threshold), the greater the kinetic energy of the expelled electron. In ordinary experience more exertion is required to give an object greater kinetic energy. At the atomic level the equivalent statement is that the probability of interaction between a photon and an atom decreases as the energy transfer to the expelled electron is increased; that is, as the photon energy increases. Thus, the importance of the photoelectric effect fades at higher photon energies.

At intermediate energies (to 15 MeV for Al, 5 MeV for Pb) a process known as the Compton effect (also called modified or unelastic scattering) predominates among interactions. In this, the incident photon seems to be scattered by an orbital electron, at which time it loses some energy to the electron, which is then expelled from the atom. The amount of energy transferred to the electron depends on the energy of the incident photon and on the angle through which it is scattered. As the photon energy is increased, the probability of Compton effect also decreases, but not as rapidly as the probability of photoelectric effect.

At highest photon energies, pair production predominates. In this process, as in photoelectric effect, the incident photon entirely disappears. In this instance the disappearance results from an interaction with a charged body, usually the nucleus, but occasionally an orbital electron. After the photon disappears, there exists an electron and a positron. Note that the net charge in the universe is thereby unchanged, but a portion of the energy of the incident photon is transformed into particle masses ($E = mc^2$ for each). The energy equivalent of the mass of the electron-positron pair is 1.02 MeV. Thus, pair production is not possible for photons carrying a charge of less than 1.02 MeV. As the photon energy is increased above this threshold, the probability for this process increases. When the pair is produced near an orbital electron, the threshold is 2.04 MeV, the orbital electron is expelled, and the process then may be called triplet production. This occurs much less often (about $1/Z$) than pair production.

A similarity may be noted between radioactive decay and photon attenuation. In radioactivity a given initial number of decayable nuclei is reduced at a rate proportional to the number present; in other words, the fractional reduction in number per unit time is a constant (λ). The same reasoning applied to photons, with one-dimensional space replacing time, leads to the recognition that the fractional reduction in number per unit thickness of attenuating material is also constant (μ). Further, just as it is convenient in discussing radioactivity to use the half-life ($T = 0.693/\lambda$), so with photon attenuation it is convenient to express penetrating ability in terms of half-value layer ($HVL = 0.693/\mu$). The concept of quality of a photon beam is related to the capability of that beam to penetrate materials; a statement of HVL frequently is given as a shorthand notation to describe quality, large HVL representing X-rays of high quality.

Before concluding this section on the attenuation of uncharged particles we should note again that consequential processes (elastic scattering for fast neutrons, photoelectric effect, Compton effect, and pair production for photons) all result in transferring energy to a charged particle. It is this secondary charged particle which is directly responsible for almost all of the energy deposited in the material, and this by mediation of Coulomb forces.

2.5 SUMMARY

Some general properties of solids, liquids, and gases are presented, followed by a description of subatomic particles. Radioactivity is introduced as the spontaneous decay of the nucleus of the Bohr atom; the four common modes of radioactive decay are described. The major thrust of the section follows and is the discussion of the generation and attenuation of the useful particles, both charged and uncharged.

References

1. Beiser, Arthur: *Concepts of Modern Physics*, rev. ed. New York, McGraw-Hill, 1967.
2. Braestrup, C. B., and Wycoff, H. O.: *Radiation Protection.* Springfield, Ill., Bannerstone House, 1958.
3. Evans, R. D.: *The Atomic Nucleus.* New York, McGraw-Hill, 1955.
4. Hendee, W. R.: *Medical Radiation Physics Year Book.* Chicago, Yearbook Medical Publishers, 1970.
5. Johns, H. E., and Cunningham, J. R.: *Physics of Radiology.* Springfield, Ill., Bannerstone House, 1969.
6. Kemp, L. W., and Oliver, C. R.: *Basic Physics in Radiology,* Springfield, Ill., Bannerstone House, 1959.
7. Lederer, C. M., Hollander, J. M., and Perlman, I.: *Table of Isotopes,* 6th ed. New York, John Wiley, 1967.

3 RADIATION CHEMISTRY[*]

Kurt I. Altman, Ph.D.

3.0 INTRODUCTION

Radiation chemistry as a quantitative science began with the study of radiation-induced chemical changes in gases during the first and second decades of this century. The data obtained with gaseous systems were interpreted on the basis of the concept of "ion cluster formation" due to the ionizing particle. This early notion was replaced in the 1930's by the "free radical hypothesis"; the latter has been superseded by the current view that models designed for the purpose of interpreting and elucidating chemical changes produced by ionizing radiations must take into account the reactions, interactions, and production of radicals, ions and excited molecules.

Fundamental radiation chemistry is concerned primarily with the study of the primary and intermediary species formed as a result of exposing a chemical system to ionizing radiations. Such studies include: (a) elucidation of reaction mechanisms; (b) determination of the chemical nature of the primary and intermediary species; (c) assessment of the reactivities of these species toward other molecular structures; (d) measurement of the yields per unit energy absorbed for each of these species. As the early stages of radiobiologic change involve such radiation chemical processes as ionization and excitation, these radio-biologic changes may be viewed as events of a radiation chemical nature.

Classical radiation chemistry deals with stationary states and relies primarily on the measurement and distribution of yields of stable end products of radiolysis. The nature of the experimental approach in classical radiation chemistry precludes the detection and measurement of intermediate, short-lived chemical species. The experimental approach in classical radiation chemistry is characterized by a very long duration of the period of exposure to radiation relative to the lifetime of the intermediate species produced. Furthermore, the rate of production of short-lived intermediates is very slow so that the equilibrium concentration of these intermediates at any time during irradiation is low.

In recent years pulse radiolysis was added to the armamentarium of the radiation chemist, enabling him to study short-lived intermediate species, mainly those present during the chemical stage, with respect to reaction rates, physical and chemical properties, and quantitative measurements. In order to carry out the latter type of investigation, pulse radiolysis was coupled with optical measurements of absorbency, since many of these intermediate species have distinct spectra in the ultraviolet and visible region. The success of pulse radiolysis in this context may be ascribed in part to the fact that the duration of the irradiation period can be kept short with respect to the lifetime of the intermediate. The dose of

[*]This work performed under contract with U.S. Atomic Energy Commission, University of Rochester Atomic Energy Project.

15

radiation delivered during the short exposure is high enough to ensure the presence of intermediate concentrations which can be detected. Since the detection and measurement of short-lived intermediates has thus become feasible, and resolution of different intermediates with respect to time possible, more complex systems can now be studied than previously.

3.1 INTERACTION OF IONIZING RADIATIONS WITH MATTER

The *physical stage* is characterized by the formation of a variety of activated molecules which are distributed in a spatially nonuniform manner. The formation of these "primary products" is the result of the absorption of energy imparted to these molecules by the incident energetic particle during interactions with the moving field. These interactions constitute the "primary process" of radiation action; the transfer of energy from incident energetic particle to atoms and molecules occurs at the expense of the kinetic energy of the particle.

Although the primary products have, until now, eluded identification, an all-encompassing mechanism for the action of ionizing radiation must take into account the nature and number of the primary products present under the prevailing conditions of irradiation. These primary products are the general agents responsible for the effects of the absorption of radiation, regardless of whether these effects are physical, chemical, or biologic in nature. Because of their extreme instability and very short lifetime, primary products have been explored only by theoretical means. The transient species which have been investigated experimentally should not be confused with the primary products, since the former intermediates are formed during later stages of radiation action.

The *physicochemical stage* includes reactions which lead to the establishment of thermal equilibrium as well as secondary reactions involving primary products. The reactions in which primary products participate occur either spontaneously or in collisions.

During the *chemical stage* free radicals or ions react with each other or with the medium, i.e., the solvent or solute(s) or both. In contrast with gaseous systems, condensed systems (liquids and solids) begin the chemical stage with a period characterized by inhomogenous spatial distribution of reactive species (the so-called "track" period), followed by a period of uniform distribution. Much progress has been made during recent years in the identification, specification, and measurement of the dominant reactive species present during this stage. Certain stable "molecular" products are formed during this stage and represent the result of interactions or recombination reactions of more reactive chemical species.

The *biologic stage* encompasses that phase of the action of radiation during which the multi-faceted response of the irradiated organism occurs.

3.2 TYPES OF PARTICLES PRODUCING RADIATION EFFECTS

One can distinguish two general types of ionizing particles on the basis of their *modi operandi* in producing ionizations in atoms and molecules in their surroundings: *Directly ionizing particles* are particles which carry a charge (e.g., electrons, protons, and α-particles) and which have sufficient kinetic energy to produce ionizations by means of direct interactions with atoms and molecules. *Indirectly ionizing particles* are uncharged particles, e.g., neutrons, photons, and electromagnetic radiations, such as X- and γ-rays; these are also capable of interacting with the medium either through the agency of protons (fast neutrons), nuclear reactions (slow neutrons), or free electrons (X- and γ-rays) and, thus, of producing ionizations or excitations in atoms and molecules.

3.3 MECHANISMS OF INTERACTION OF RADIATIONS WITH MATTER

A. Electromagnetic Radiations

In contrast with energy loss by charged particles, electromagnetic radiations lose energy by way of three processes: production of positron-electron pairs in the medium, Compton scattering, and photoelectric scattering as these radiations traverse matter. Other means of energy dissipation are of minor importance so far as the initiation of chemical changes is concerned. Thus, photonuclear reactions occur at energies above 10 MeV, but these reactions deposit little energy in the medium and contribute only short-lived radioactivity. Low-energy radiations produce some coherent scattering, but the energy imparted to molecules of the medium is insufficient to produce chemical changes.

Pair Production. The electron and positron produced as a result of the interaction of electromagnetic radiations with matter, are sufficiently energetic to induce ionized, excited, or both states in atoms and molecules in their surroundings. The positron eventually combines with an electron to generate, as a rule, two photons, each having an energy of 0.5 MeV. This radiation is generally referred to as "annihilation radiation." This energy loss process is only important with very high-energy gamma rays or electron beams.

Compton Scattering. Electromagnetic radiations may lose their energy by Compton scattering. In this process, which frequently represents the predominant effect of X- or γ-rays (e.g., ^{60}Co effects in water), photons lose a portion of their energy by ejecting electrons from atoms. The ejected electrons, in turn, produce ionization and excitation, whereas the scattered photons lose energy by interacting by way of either Compton scattering or photoelectric absorption. This is the predominant loss process for medium-energy gamma rays or electrons.

Photoelectric Absorption. In this process atomic absorption of a photon causes the ejection (as a rule, from an inner shell) of a fast electron. This electron is endowed with all of the energy carried by the incident photon with the exception of the binding energy. The latter energy may either become manifest as a very soft X-ray or, more probably, effect the ejection of a second electron from the same atom which gave rise to the first electron. The second electron is referred to as the Auger electron. The photoelectric effect predominates with radiation of low energy in a medium of high Z (atomic number).

Effect of Secondary and Primary Electrons. Fast electrons, arising from X- and γ-rays as products of energy-loss processes, are sufficiently energetic to produce appreciable chemical changes. These electrons produce their effects by interacting with outer-shell electrons of atoms or molecules. The result of this interaction may be either excitation of the outer electron to higher energy levels or ejection of this electron, leaving in its wake a positive ion. The ejected electrons may also be energetic enough to interact further with outer-shell electrons. When these electrons represent a substantial fraction of the energy carried by the initial fast electrons, these ejected electrons are called "secondary electrons"; when the fraction of energy distributed among the ejected electrons represents a small fraction of the energy of the fast electrons, these electrons are known as delta-rays ($>10^2$ eV). At even lower energy levels of about 10 eV, these electrons are capable of initiating ionizations and excitations of molecules or atoms within the immediate vicinity.

B. Positively Charged Particles

Positively charged particles, of which the most common examples are the proton, deuteron, and alpha particle, lose energy in passage through a medium partly by inelastic collisions. Secondary phenomena, such as the production of delta-rays, are a consequence of these collisions. Toward the end of their range, when the velocity of the particles approaches that of orbital electrons, the particles become neutralized. The neutral atom then loses energy by "knock-on" collisions with atoms of similar size. Some of these target atoms are ejected from their chemical bonds, resulting in molecular fragmentation.

C. Linear Energy Transfer (LET)

In order to provide information as to the linear density of interactions along the track formed by the incident radiations, the term LET is used; it is defined in terms of radiation energy absorbed per unit track length (KeV/μ). LET increases with the square of the charge on the incident particle and decreases with increasing particle speed. LET varies with different types of ionizing radiations. Frequently used radiation sources can be arranged in decreasing order of LET.: (1) fission fragments; (2)

stripped nuclei of low atomic number; (3) α-particles, protons, and deuterons; (4) low-energy electrons or X-rays; (5) intermediary high-energy electrons or X- or γ-rays. It should also be pointed out that, in reality, there are regions of different LET along tracks. As the incident particle slows down, LET increases. In δ-tracks or clusters produced by fast electrons, LET is higher than the mean value since, as in the case of α-particles, much of the effect (ionization and excitation) takes place in the δ-tracks. The theoretical minimum for any particle of the mean energy absorption per μ of water is about 0.22 KeV/μ. At one extreme of the range of values are the values for uranium fission fragments (4000 KeV/μ), and at the opposite end of the range are found values for ^{60}Co (0.42 KeV/μ) and others.

D. Ionization and Excitation of Atoms and Molecules

Although a great deal of the earlier work on the mechanism of action of ionizing radiations was carried out in the gas phase, more recent efforts have been concerned with events in condensed phases. Since the aqueous phase is of particular interest to the radiobiologist and radiotherapist, the radiation chemistry of water will be emphasized at this point. In liquid media ionizations are of considerable importance because of the large energies involved. The deposition of energy in the materials traversed by the ionizing particle results in the production of ions which, in turn, interact with other products formed during or after exposure to radiation. The ionization process is the ejection of an electron from a molecule in which case a positively charged ion is formed. Negatively charged ions may also be formed in those instances where electrons attach themselves to molecules. Excited molecules result either from neutralization of positively charged ions by an electron or negative ion or from direct excitation effected by high energy particles. The entire molecule enters into the excited state, and the excitation energy of the excited molecule can be transferred to other molecules. Such excited molecules may undergo a number of other reactions, in addition to transferring their energy to other molecules. For example, excited molecules may fluoresce or may lose their energy by non-radiative means, namely, by internal conversion of excitation energy to vibrational energy at a lower electronic state. Excited molecules may also form free radicals,* biradicals, or stable molecular products. Free radicals, as reactive species which have a lone, free electron rather than an electron pair within their structure, may participate in a number of reactions, particularly H-abstractions and additions to unsaturated carbon-carbon bonds. Free radicals are removed by disproportionation, dimerization reactions, or electron transfer reactions.

E. The Radiolysis of Water

The initial products of the radiolytic cleavage of water are due to ionization of water molecules, as shown by Equation 1.

---

*Free radicals are substances which are characterized by an unpaired electron at some locus within the molecular structure. This radical may be either un-ionized or ionized. Radicals are relatively unstable and highly reactive because of the unpaired electron which tends to pair with another electron.

(Eq. 1)

$$H_2O \longrightarrow H_2O^+ + e^-$$

(Eq. 2)

$$H_2O^+ + H_2O \longrightarrow H_3O^+ + OH^{\cdot *}$$

(Eq. 3)

$$e^- + nH_2O \longrightarrow e_{aq}^-$$

---

*Symbols of elements accompanied by dots, e.g., H·, indicate that these atoms or molecules, often represented as R·, are free radicals. "Dot" is accompanied by a charge sign when ion (+ or −) radicals are written.

TABLE 3-1 REACTION RATE CONSTANTS FOR THE INTERACTION OF THE HYDRATED ELECTRON WITH VARIOUS REACTANTS

Reactant	Product	Rate Constant*
$OH \cdot$	OH^-_{aq}	3.0×10^{10}
$H \cdot$	$H^2 + OH^-_{aq}$	3.0×10^{10}
H_3O^+	$H \cdot + H_2O$	2.3×10^{10}
O	$OH \cdot + OH^-_{aq}$	0.6×10^{10}
O_2	O^-_2	2.0×10^{10}
H_2O_2	$OH \cdot + OH^-_{aq}$	1.2×10^{10}
H^+	$0.5 H_2$	2.3×10^{10}
e^-_{aq}	$H_2 + 2 OH^-_{aq}$	1.0×10^{10}
H_2O	$H \cdot + OH^-$	5×10^2

(Hydroxyl Radical with Various Reactants)

$OH \cdot$	H_2O_2	4×10^9
OH^-	$O^- + H_2O$	3×10^8
H_2O_2	$H_2O + HO_2$	4×10^7
H_2	$H_2O + H \cdot$	4×10^7
$(O^- + O_2 \longrightarrow O^-_3$		$2.6 \times 10^9)**$

*Rate constants are expressed as moles^{-1} sec^{-1}.

**Although $OH \cdot$ does not react directly with O_2, the dissociation product O^- does react at a respectable rate in alkaline solutions.

TABLE 3-2 REACTION RATE CONSTANTS FOR THE INTERACTION OF HYDROGEN ATOMS WITH VARIOUS REACTANTS

Reactant	Product	Rate Constant*
O_2	HO_2	2×10^{10}
$H \cdot$	H_2	1×10^{10}
OH^-	$e^-_{aq} + H_2O$	2×10^7
H_2O_2	$H_2O + OH \cdot$	1×10^8

*All rate constants are expressed in units of moles^{-1} sec^{-1}.

These products subsequently undergo further, separate reactions, H_2O^+ reacting with the solvent H_2O and the ejected electron also reacting with solvent molecules, as shown in Equations 2 and 3.

One of the products of the reaction shown by Equation 2 is the oxidizing radical $OH \cdot$; the product of the reaction in Equation 3, a reducing species, is the hydrated electron, e^-_{aq}.

The mechanism of formation and the nature of the hydrated electron requires some comment at this point. In general, one may distinguish two types of ejected electrons depending on their energy, i.e., whether their kinetic energy lies above or below the level of the lowest electronic excitation in the medium. In the former case, energy loss by inelastic collisions takes place until the electron energy is lower than any excited electronic state in the medium molecules. The electron then cannot lose energy to electronic systems of molecules with which it collides; it spends approximately 10^{-11} seconds in this electronic state before attaining thermal equilibrium in the medium. Water molecules at room temperature have a relaxation time of 10^{-11} seconds, at the end of which a region of positively charged polarization will form around the thermalized electron. This is a trap for the electron which initiated the polarization process. The region of the polarized water molecules plus the trapped electron form a "complex" known as the hydrated electron; it is a reducing species.

The electron ejected in ionization (Equation 1) is recaptured by its parent molecule, the ionized water molecule. The recapture of an electron by an ionized water molecule (See Equation 6) results in the formation of an excited water molecule, which can dissociate.

$$e^-_{aq} + H_2O \longrightarrow H \cdot + OH^-_{aq} \qquad \textbf{(Eq. 4)}$$

$$e^-_{aq} + H^+ \longrightarrow 0.5 H_2 \qquad \textbf{(Eq. 5)}$$

$$H_2O^+ + e^- \longrightarrow H_2O^* \longrightarrow H \cdot + OH \cdot \qquad \textbf{(Eq. 6)}$$

*An asterisk designates an activated state (H_2O^*).

The reaction shown in Equation 6 constitutes another major source of H·, the other important reducing species. The reaction rate constants for the interaction between hydrated electrons and H· and various other reactants derived from water, oxygen, or both are shown in Tables 3–1 and 3–2.

Reaction rate constants are of considerable interest in radiation chemistry, particularly if these constants represent absolute rate constants; they shed light upon the reaction kinetics, as well as on the mechanisms underlying the chemical reaction. As can be seen by comparing Tables 3–1 and 3–2, the hydrated electron is somewhat more reactive than H· and, therefore, participates in many more reactions than does H·. It is of particular interest that H· neither reacts with water nor exchanges H with the latter, and yields a hydrated electron when reacting with hydroxyl ions. One property which clearly distinguishes H· from the hydrated electron is the capacity of H· to act as an oxidizing agent as well as a reducing agent.

The hydroxyl radical (OH·) represents the major oxidizing species resulting from the hydrolysis of water. This highly reactive, biologically very important radical is the product of either of two reactions, that shown in Equation 2 or that shown in Equation 5. Although OH· is un-ionized, it may exist in a positively charged form in an acid medium. See Equation 7.

In an alkaline medium, however, OH· dissociates ($pK = 11.9$), as shown by Equation 8.

The uncertainties regarding the existence and chemical nature of hydroxyl and other radicals, which prevailed during the early developmental period of radiation chemistry and which had resulted from inadequate methods of radical production and measurement, are no longer a matter of concern.

Pulse radiolysis, which has supplemented the less adequate technique of "stationary" irradiation in recent years, has made possible the measurement of absolute reaction rates, as well as the detection of discrete spectral absorption peaks associated with different radical intermediates, e.g., transient chemical species arising in the course of radiolysis of water. The optical properties of the short-lived products of the radiolysis of water can be determined when high-energy radiation in the form of pulses is delivered at a rate which reduces the total exposure time to less than the lifetime of the reactive transient under study. Pulse radiolysis as a technique is particularly applicable to solutions in which transients exhibit specific absorption spectra, either in the solvated or free form.

The chemical potentialities of OH· are best reflected by the chemical reactions into which this radical enters. Three general classes of reactions can be delineated: (1) electron transfer reactions-reaction (Equation 9); (2) addition reactions involving hydroxyl radical-reactions (Equations 10 and 11); and (3) hydrogen atom transfer reactions (Equation 12).

A second oxidizing radical, the hydroperoxyl (or perhydroxyl) radical, $HO_2·$, is

(Eq. 7) $\qquad OH· + H_3O^+ \longrightarrow H_2O^+_{aq} + H_2O$

(Eq. 8) $\qquad OH· \longrightarrow O^- + H^+$

(Eq. 9) $\qquad Br^- + OH· \longrightarrow Br· + OH^-; \; Br· + Br^- \longrightarrow Br_2^-$

(Eq. 10)

TABLE 3–3 G-VALUES FOR PRODUCTS OF
THE RADIOLYSIS OF WATER FOR ^{60}Co
GAMMA RAYS

Product	G	Comments
H$^{\cdot}$	0.6	for a pH range from 3 to 10
H$_2$	0.4	for a pH range from 3 to 10
H$_2$O$_2$	0.7	for a pH range from 3 to 10
HO$_2^{\cdot}$	0.02	
e$_{aq}^{-}$	2.6	in acidic solution, G = 3.0
OH$^{\cdot}$	2.6	G increases above pH 10 and at pH 0.0

the product of an interaction of molecular oxygen with H$^{\cdot}$ according to the reaction shown in Equation 13. This radical does not exist above pH 5.0 although its dissociation products are stable above this pH. The reaction in Equation 14 shows the dissociation of this radical. The hydroperoxyl radical is capable of reacting with another molecule of its kind. This radical-radical interaction represents a disproportionation reaction in which one radical is reduced and the other oxidized (Equation 15). The hydroperoxyl radical is a more slowly reacting radical than OH$^{\cdot}$. The G-value* for G$_{HO_2}{}^{\cdot}$ is low (0.02) for low LET ^{60}Co

---

*The G-value is defined as the number of molecules altered (damaged) [G(−M)] or of the product formed per 100 eV of energy absorbed; it is analogous to the term quantum yield used in photochemistry. Both are measures of the rate of a radiation-induced process, G-value is used in radiation chemistry because the concept of quantum has no pertinency.

γ-radiation (Table 3–3), but considerably higher for ^{210}Po α-radiation (0.023). The O$_2^{-}$ anion is unlikely to produce biologic damage since its reactivity is very low.

3.4 THE FORMATION OF MOLECULAR PRODUCTS

The primary species may embark on two courses of action: (a) they may react with solute molecules in the vicinity or (b) they may react with other molecules of their own kind (recombination reactions of radicals). These two types of reactions are in competition with each other, and the level of concentration of radicals will determine which of these possibilities will prevail. If the local concentration of radicals is high, recombination reactions, with formation of molecular products, are favored; radical-solute interactions are predominant at lower concentrations of the radical species. The two competing reactions are not coordinated in time, i.e., the radical-radical interactions are completed by the time radical-solute interactions begin. Some radical-radical interactions are so rapid, however, that the radicals never diffuse out to react with solutes. The reaction rates of radicals with a solute may vary considerably for different radicals. The initial radius of the distribution of radicals within the spur is one of the determining factors as to the fate of the radicals.

$$HO_2^{\cdot} + OH^{\cdot} \longrightarrow H_2O_3^{\cdot} \qquad \textbf{(Eq. 11)}$$

$$RSH + OH^{\cdot} \longrightarrow RS^{\cdot} + H_2O \qquad \textbf{(Eq. 12)}$$

$$H^{\cdot} + O_2 \longrightarrow HO_2^{\cdot} \qquad \textbf{(Eq. 13)}$$

$$HO_2^{\cdot} \longrightarrow O_2^{-} + H^{+} \qquad \textbf{(Eq. 14)}$$

$$HO_2^{\cdot} + HO_2^{\cdot} \longrightarrow H_2O_2 + O_2 \qquad \textbf{(Eq. 15)}$$

The formation of molecular hydrogen in the interactions of hydrated electrons (Table 3–1) proceeds at a slower rate than the formation of hydrogen peroxide from OH· because hydrated electrons are distributed over a wider radius than OH·. The initial radical spur containing an average of 6 radicals per spur (OH·, H·, and O·) has a radius of 6 Å, whereas the radius of the spur containing the hydrated electron is 19 Å. The spatial distribution of the primary species is influenced considerably by the type of radiation. Radiations with high LET, e.g., α-particles, produce very high concentrations of radicals, which is the reason for the predominance of molecular products with this type of radiation and, incidentally, for a negligible oxygen-enhancement effect because H· is mostly consumed in recombination reactions.

Equations for reactions known to occur in the spur follow. OH_{aq}^- and hydrogen peroxide are presumed absent from the spur, whereas H·, OH·, and e_{aq}^- are present in appreciable concentrations and are capable of diffusing away from the spur to react with solute molecules in the immediate environment. The molecular products are generally stable, with the possible exception of hydrogen peroxide. The latter product may act as an oxidizing or reducing agent, may also react with radicals, and may interact with a variety of substances of biologic importance, including catalase or peroxidase, which destroy it.

$$OH· + OH· \longrightarrow H_2O_2$$
$$e_{aq}^- + e_{aq}^- \longrightarrow H_2 + 2\ OH_{aq}^-$$
$$e_{aq}^- + H_3O^+ \longrightarrow H· + H_2O$$
$$e_{aq}^- + H· \longrightarrow H_2 + OH_{aq}^-$$
$$H· + H· \longrightarrow H_2$$
$$e_{aq}^- + H_2O \longrightarrow H· + OH_{aq}^-$$
$$OH· + H· \longrightarrow H_2O$$
$$e_{aq}^- + OH· \longrightarrow OH_{aq}^-$$

The formation of molecular products is also influenced by the concentration of solute in the irradiated solution. At high concentrations (10M) the solute molecules can penetrate the spur and suppress radical-radical interactions for radicals which are the dissociation products of ionized water. However, molecular hydrogen is still formed on a small scale (about 20 per cent of the normally observed amount) by a first-order reaction which may be the

breakdown of excited water molecules. Addition of specific solute molecules which are capable of acting as radical scavengers lowers the yield of molecular products by removing radicals. These scavengers, present as a second solute with a special affinity for particular types of radicals, thus exert a radiation-protection effect. Thus, increasing the concentration of an OH· scavenger in an aqueous solution subjected to irradiation reduces the yield of hydrogen peroxide, decreases the extent of the OH· + e_{aq}^- reaction, and increases the yield of OH^- and H_2.

If the molecular products were formed as the result of second-order reactions of homogenously distributed radicals, a strong dependence of product yield on the dose rate would be expected, as well as the elimination of radical-radical interactions at $10^{-6}M$ solute concentration. However, experimental data show that the yields are independent of dose rate up to 10^5 rads per second. Thus, the molecular products are formed in the reactions of inhomogeneously distributed radicals in the track or spur.

3.5   RADICAL, IONIC, AND MOLECULAR YIELDS AND SOME OF THE FACTORS INFLUENCING THEIR MAGNITUDE

Some of the more important G-values for products of the radiolysis of water are shown in Table 3–3. The effect of the presence of scavengers of radicals or ions has been discussed in preceding sections. Other factors are also known to affect these product G-values. One of these factors is the prevailing temperature. There is a marked change in product G-values over the temperature range from 4° K to 100° K, and a fraction of the effective "cross section" remains constant below 100° K; an Arrhenius plot of the G-values has a slope corresponding to 1 Kcal/mole. At temperatures above 100° K the activation energy is 6.5 Kcal/mole. It appears at the present time that the reactions of H· are the components with the lower energy of activation, although further study of these phenomena is indicated.

Another factor which influences yields of radiolytic products concerns the presence or absence of molecular oxygen during the period of exposure to ionizing radiations. Because of the paramagnetic character of the oxygen molecule, molecular oxygen reacts rapidly with the radicals produced in the radiolysis of water and with the radicals produced from biological molecules by interaction with H·, OH· and HO$_2$. The products of the reaction of O$_2$ with radicals are radicals of the type XO$_2$. In aqueous solution, oxygen is more likely to react with H· to yield HO$_2$, which will be present in biologic systems as the anion of the radical (i.e., O$_2^-$, an ionic radical of low reducing power and low electron affinity). The oxygen enhancement effect is small or absent in aqueous solutions and is marked in the radiolysis of intact cells. The effect appears to be linked to repair phenomena rather than to sensitization effects, since the number of damaged molecules does not increase. The presence of high concentrations of H$^+$ or OH$^-$ has a marked effect on the yield of individual products of radiolysis, as was previously noted.

3.6 RADICAL-SOLUTE INTERACTIONS

A number of reactions take place between the radicals produced as a result of radiolysis of water and various types of solutes. The discussion here is concerned primarily with solutes of an organic nature which have a direct bearing upon radiobiologic problems.

A. Abstraction of Hydrogen Atoms

H· and OH· are capable of abstracting H from the C–H and –OH bonds in organic solutes (R), and e$_{aq}^-$ is unable to abstract hydrogen; as a product of these reactions, solute radicals are formed (See Equations 16 and 17). Certain functional organic groups, –CONH$_2$, –CONH–NH$_2$, –OH, –COOH, react much more slowly than the C–H bond in alkyl groups.

B. Dissociation Reactions

Organically bound functional groups may react with radicals and thus be removed from the parent substance (Equations 18 and 19).

C. Addition Reactions

All three primary radicals can add to centers of unsaturation such as vinyl groups and carbonyl groups (Equation 20).

D. Perhydroxylation Reactions

These reactions are shown in Equation 21.

$$R\text{–}H + H\cdot \longrightarrow R\cdot + H_2 \qquad \textbf{(Eq. 16)}$$

$$R\text{–}H + OH\cdot \longrightarrow R\cdot + H_2O \qquad \textbf{(Eq. 17)}$$

$$R\text{–}NH_3^+ + e_{aq}^- \longrightarrow R\cdot + NH_3 \qquad \textbf{(Eq. 18)}$$

$$R\text{–}NH_2 + H\cdot \longrightarrow R\cdot + NH_3 \qquad \textbf{(Eq. 19)}$$

$$\textbf{(Eq. 20)}$$

$$\textbf{(Eq. 21)}$$

3.7 REACTIONS OF SOLUTE RADICALS IN AQUEOUS SOLUTIONS

Since the interaction between solute molecules and primary radicals always generates solute radicals, it is of interest to summarize the types of reactions which take place and are of particular importance to the radiation biologist.

A. Dimerization Reactions

In these reactions (Equation 22), radical-radical additions take place leading to the formation of stable dimers. An example is the reaction of cysteine radicals (Equation 23).

B. Disproportionation Reactions

These are shown in Equations 24 to 27.

C. Addition of Oxygen and HO_2^- (Equations 28 and 29)

D. Hydrogen Transfer Reactions (Equation 30)

3.8 REACTIONS OF PRIMARY REACTIVE PRODUCTS OF THE RADIOLYSIS OF WATER WITH BIOLOGICALLY IMPORTANT MOLECULES

A. Proteins

This group of biologically important macromolecules includes a multitude of structurally, conformationally, and functionally varied substances ranging from fibrous scleroproteins to globular serum proteins. An individual member of this class may differ widely from all others and thus present a special problem for the radiation chemist as well as for the radiation biologist.

Proteins differ widely from each other with respect to their responses to radia-

(Eq. 22) $$R_1^- + R_1^- \longrightarrow R_1—R_1$$

(Eq. 23) $$2 \, CyS^- \longrightarrow Cy—S—S—Cy$$

(Eq. 24) $$2R—\dot{C}H—CH_3 \longrightarrow R—CH_2CH_3 + R—CH = CH_2$$

(Eq. 25) $$HO^- + RCONHCHR_2 \longrightarrow H_2O + R—CONH\dot{C}R_2$$

(Eq. 26) $$2 \, RCONH\dot{C}R_2 \longrightarrow R—CON = CR_2 + RCONHCHR_2$$

(Eq. 27) $$R—CON = CR_2 + 2H_2O \longrightarrow RCOOH + NH_3 + R_2C = O$$

(Eq. 28) $$R^- + O_2 \longrightarrow RO_2^- \longrightarrow ROOH$$

(Eq. 29) $$R^- + HO_2^- \longrightarrow ROOH$$

(Eq. 30) $$R_1^- + R_2H \longrightarrow R_1H + R_2^-$$

tions. Not all proteins have a biological activity or function which is easily measured and which is sensitive to radiation. Only a few proteins exist for which the structure has been completely described. Therefore, only a very limited number of "ideal" situations exists in which one can take advantage of measurable biologic activity as well as of established structure as aids in the search for sites of radiation damage which are involved in the loss of biologic activity. It seems fair to state that radiation-induced loss of biologic activity is not an all-or-none phenomenon, but often represents a gradual structural breakdown. Irradiation of proteins with enzymatic activity of the radiation-sensitive variety generates (1) fully inactivated enzyme molecules, (2) fully active enzyme molecules, and (3) enzyme molecules with various degrees of enzymatic activity.

Although in a few instances the sensitivity of enzyme molecules toward ionizing radiations represents a weighted summation of the sensitivities [G(–M) values] of the individual constitutive amino acids of the protein, this is not generally true. Thus, while gelatin, a fibrous protein, exhibits reasonably good agreement between sensitivity of total protein and that of amino acid summation, the enzymes lysozyme and ribonuclease show a lower sensitivity than that computed by summing the sensitivities of the constitutive amino acids. Charge distribution effects and peptide chain folding probably account for the observed differences. Radiation-induced enzyme inactivations which are the result simply of alterations in the folding of the enzyme can be reversed by denaturing and then restructuring the enzyme. Enzyme inactiva-

TABLE 3–4   REACTIONS WITH AMINO ACIDS

Amino Acids	e_{aq}^-	OH·
Cysteine, cystine°	most reactive	highly reactive
Histidine (protonated)	most reactive	
Aromatic amino acids	moderately reactive	highly reactive
Glutamic acid	moderately reactive	
Arginine	moderately reactive	
Glycine	unreactive	
Alanine	unreactive	
Methionine	unreactive	highly reactive
Glutathione°	most reactive	highly reactive

°These amino acids react also with H·.

tions which are the result of the reaction of the enzyme with O_2 or NO are usually irreversible, since these radical reactions are not reversible (See Equations 31 to 33). The reactivation process shown in Equation 33 depends on the availability of a hydrogen donor.

In aqueous solution, amino acids in the free state react with radicals formed by radiolysis of water, principally with OH· and e_{aq}^-, but structurally different amino acids exhibit a widely varying reactivity. A comparison of the interaction of amino acids with these radicals is shown in Table 3–4. Amino acid residues in peptide chains of proteins show a somewhat different reactivity in aqueous solutions of proteins; the most labile residues are cysteine and histidine, although the reaction rate constants for OH· and e_{aq}^- vary considerably with respect to different proteins.

Enzymes, such as lysozyme and ribonuclease, have been studied in relation to the effect of the gaseous atmosphere. Oxygen, when dissolved in aqueous solutions of enzymes, scavenges e_{aq}^- and H·, yielding the products HO_2 and O_2^-. Therefore, the

$$RH \rightsquigarrow R·^* \qquad \text{(Eq. 31)}$$

$$R· + O_2 \longrightarrow ROO· \text{ inactive enzyme molecule} \qquad \text{(Eq. 32)}$$

$$R· + H· \longrightarrow RH \text{ active enzyme molecule} \qquad \text{(Eq. 33)}$$

*Arrows interrupted by a zig-zag configuration indicate that exposure to ionizing radiations is involved. A straight arrow indicates, as usual, the direction in which a reaction proceeds.

OH radical is largely responsible for radiation injury, and O_2 has a quasi-protective effect which, however, is less pronounced during irradiation with densely ionizing radiations as compared with X-irradiation. Irradiation in an atmosphere of nitrogen involves the action of all three primary radical species resulting from radiolysis of water; the additional yield of H derived from the reaction of hydrated electrons with H^+ plays a significant role under these circumstances. The radiation sensitivity of lysozyme is 10 times greater on X-irradiation than on irradiation with densely ionizing types of radiation. The latter phenomenon probably reflects the action of the reducing radicals produced by delta-rays of high energy outside the core of the ionizing track. When enzymes are irradiated in an atmosphere of N_2O, which converts e_{aq}^- to OH^- (viz: $N_2O \rightarrow N_2 + OH + OH^-$), radiation damage is mainly due to the action of OH and H. The preceding discussion demonstrates that irradiation of aqueous solutions yields information which can be interpreted on the basis of the events associated with the radiolysis of water.

A variety of agents are capable of exerting protective effects which reduce the extent of radiation damage, if not abolish it completely. The protective action of cysteine is noteworthy in that it can react with all three radicals derived from water, as well as with one of the molecular products, hydrogen peroxide. The presence of cysteine, for example, in the solution will reduce the inactivation of lysozyme by radiation. The concentration of this or other protective agents under these conditions must be 1.5 to 2.0 times higher for a comparable degree of protection when densely ionizing radiations are used than when X-rays or other sparsely ionizing radiations are the agents.

The chemical processes which lead to inactivation of enzyme proteins in solution can be described reasonably well, but those responsible for inactivation of enzymes in the solid state are not nearly as well known. Existing observations are summarized as follows. Some of these same phenomena also occur in the irradiation of aqueous solutions of proteins.

a) Thermolabile fractions of solid, irradiated enzymes have been isolated in several instances.

b) Serological changes in the behavior of irradiated solid proteins have been reported.

c) Aggregate formation of enzyme proteins is known to occur.

d) ^3H_2S exchanges H at radical sites in irradiated proteins. The extent of this exchange varies with different amino acids residues. For example, lysyl residues exchange eight times more H for ^3H than glycl residues.

e) Mechanical properties change, particularly in fibrous proteins; this change can be correlated with physico-chemical changes.

f) Breakage of disulfide is often associated with radiation damage.

Factors such as temperature, the LET of the radiation used, the nature of solutes other than the enzyme protein present in solution, and the gaseous environment influence the extent of radiation damage to proteins in solution.

3.9 NUCLEIC ACIDS

The nucleic acids are in the form of another type of macromolecule which is damaged by ionizing radiation as well as by ultraviolet radiation. The results of radiation damage to these nucleic acids is death to the organism, when the damage is severe or so localized as to prevent replication, or mutation, when damage to the nucleic acid is such as to alter the coding in the replication processes. Inducement of mutation by X-irradiation of fruit flies is the classic example of mutation by ionizing radiation; and concern about the lethal and mutagenic effects of fallout from nuclear bomb tests, or from nuclear war is a modern example of these effects. The chemical damage which occurs as a result of ultraviolet irradiation is better understood than that which is the result of ionizing radiation irradiation. Some of the effects observed in irradiation of nucleic acids are summarized as follows:

a) Strand scission, either single or double strand scission.

b) Denaturation associated with changes in viscosity, changes in birefringence, and so forth.

c) Cross-linking of DNA molecules or fragments thereof.

d) Destruction of the nitrogenous bases, liberation of ammonia.

e) Destruction of the deoxyribose-phosphate moiety.

f) Conformational changes.

g) Impairment of priming ability, for DNA and RNA synthesis.

When the reactivity of DNA with respect to ionizing radiations is expressed on a "per nucleotide" basis, the resultant value is lower than that of its summed constitutive nucleotides. This can be accounted for by noting that the susceptible nucleotides are less accessible than the relatively less reactive deoxyribose moieties and the phosphate groups. All free nucleotides are reactive toward OH· and hydrated electrons but are only moderately reactive toward H·. Nucleic acids are damaged most extensively by the OH· radical. Sparsely ionizing radiations are most likely to cause single strand scission, whereas the probability of double strand scission is greatest with densely ionizing radiations. Radiation-induced strand separation, without strand scission, of the two strands of the double helix also occurs.

3.10 THE DIRECT AND INDIRECT EFFECTS OF RADIATION

A. Direct Action of Ionizing Radiations

Direct action of radiation entails in its simplest conceptualization the localized deposition of energy by high-energy charged particles or electrons within a discrete volume representing all or a portion of a given molecular structure. To the latter volume the term "target" is affixed, and the interaction of radiation with the target represents a "hit." One molecule may have more than one target site; thus, multiple hits may be scored on one molecule. The hits scored on the target produce chemical changes and may or may not alter the biologic activity of the irradiated molecule. Occasionally more than a single hit is necessary in order to alter the biologic activity of the irradiated molecule.

The stochastic nature of biologic responses to ionizing radiations implies that the relationship between radiation dose and biologic effect is reflected in an exponential curve, as demonstrated by four different models. These models are all adaptations of the simple first-order decay process in which alteration of the molecule is a function only of the concentration of the molecules and dose: $-(dN/dt) = KN$.

The Single-Hit, Single-Target Model. Equation 34 expresses this model, where N = number of individuals surviving after having received radiation dose D; N_0 = number of individuals present before irradiation; and v = volume of target (cm^3). The target may also be introduced as a sensitive area α. The dose required for $N = 0.37 N_0$, the D_{37} dose which 37 per cent of the irradiated individuals survive, is derived from the surviving fraction N/N_0 (see Equation 35). The dose D_{37} also represents the average dose which will generate one hit.

The Single-Hit, Multi-Target Model. The mathematical statement for this model, written in terms of the surviving fraction, is shown in Equation 36 (n = number of targets). When D is large, the equation reduces to that of Equation 37.

$$N = N_0 e^{-vD} \qquad \text{(Eq. 34)}$$

$$N/N_0 = e^{-1} = 0.37 = e^{-vD_{37}} \qquad \text{(Eq. 35)}$$

$$N/N_0 = 1 - (1 - e^{-vD})^n \qquad \text{(Eq. 36)}$$

$$N/N_0 = n e^{-vD} \qquad \text{(Eq. 37)}$$

The survival curve for this model has a sigmoidal shape; log N varies linearly with the radiation dose at high dose levels. This model is applied frequently when dealing with sigmoidal curves (for survival), primarily because of the simplicity of its application. By extrapolating the linear portion of the survival curve to the log N/N_0 coordinate, a value for n (extrapolation number) is found at the intercept with the log N/N_0 coordinate. Furthermore, the slope of the linear portion of the survival curve yields a value for $1/D_0$ which is equivalent to the target size α. The relationship between n and D_q is shown in Equation 38. $D_q = D_0 \ln n$, i.e., the "quasi-threshold dose." This mode of expressing the radiation dose is useful when dealing with dose fractionation and other special circumstances. The relationship between D_0, D_q, and D_{37} is given in Equation 39. Here D_0 is the dose obtained from the survival curve by drawing a line through N_0 and parallel to the linear portion of the survival curve. The value for D_0 is then obtained from this line by letting it intersect a line drawn horizontally to the 37 per cent survivors point on the log N/N_0 coordinate.

The Multi-Hit, Single-Target Model. This model requires that the inactivating dose be greater than m (hit number) and that the distribution of m follow the Poisson distribution curve. Log N does not vary linearly with dose, but the survival curve has a sigmoidal shape. Equation 40 expresses this model.

For the special case of m = 1, Equation 40 reduces to Equation 34, seen in the single-hit, single-target model. In Equation 40, m = one hit and i = a non-negative integer.

The Multi-Hit, Multi-Target Model. This model provides that at least m hits must be scored on each target in order to produce an inactivating event. The mathematical formulation is that shown in Equation 41. Equation 42 gives the value of B, where m = number of hits, n = number of targets, and α = size of target.

The relationship between dose and biologic effect for the mechanism of direct action of ionizing radiations is expressed by Equation 43, where N = number of undamaged molecules after irradiation; N_0 = number of molecules present prior to irradiation; and k = a constant (or $1/D_{37}$).

Since $1/D_{37}$ is equatable with the target size, the magnitude of a target size can be computed for a dose which is survived by 37 per cent of the irradiated population. For a D_{37} dose in rads, for the target size in Dalton units (1 Dalton = 1 molecular weight unit), and by assuming that the energy for each interaction between radiation and

---

(Eq. 38)
$$N/N_0 = 1 = ne^{-vD_q}$$

(Eq. 39)
$$D_{37} = D_0 - D_q$$

(Eq. 40)
$$N/N_0 = e^{-vD} \sum_{i=0}^{m-1} \frac{(vD)^i}{i!}$$

(Eq. 41)
$$N/N_0 = nB - n(n-1)/2!B^2 + n(n-1)(n-2)3!B^3$$

(Eq. 42)
$$B = \sum_{i=0}^{1=m-1} \frac{(\alpha D)^i}{i!} e^{-\alpha D}$$

(Eq. 43)
$$N = N_0 e^{-kD}$$

Target size in grams $= 1/[(D_{37} \text{ rad} \times 6.2 \times 10^{13} \text{ eV per rad}) (1/75 \text{ eV per interaction})]$ **(Eq. 44)**

Target size in Daltons $=$ (target size in grams) $(6.02 \times 10^{23}$ molecules per mole$) =$
$$(0.72 \times 10^{22})/D_{37}$$ **(Eq. 45)**

target is 75 eV, the size of the radiation target can be computed from the target size in grams which is obtained as in Equation 44 or 45.

B. Indirect Action of Ionizing Radiations

In concentrated solutions of organic or biologic molecules, such as are found in cells or other organized biologic systems, an appreciable fraction of the incident radiation is absorbed by the biologic or organic molecule, and the effects of the irradiation are the result of the radiation chemistry — i.e., ionization, fragmentation, radical formation, electron capture, and so forth — of the molecule in which the energy is deposited. This is called direct action. The direct action of ionizing radiation must be studied in non-biologic conditions where the target molecule can be isolated from other interfering molecules. Representative studies are those on radiation effects on amino acids, peptides, carbohydrates, the purines and pyrimidines of the nucleic acids, structural proteins, enzymes in solution, and so on. Extrapolation of the results of these isolated studies to a biologic system where many types of such molecules are not only in close proximity but often bound to each other is still very uncertain.

When the concentration of solute is low, as in many body fluids, the incident radiation is absorbed almost entirely by the water, and the primary products of the irradiation are the products of water radiolysis, which have been discussed at length above. Damage to the biologic molecules in the solution is then caused almost entirely by their reaction with $H^{\cdot}$, $OH^{\cdot}$, $HO_2^{\cdot}$, e_{aq}^-, and so forth; these reactions have already been discussed. Alteration in the solute molecules, then, is the result of H-abstraction, radical additions, electron additions, and such.

Transfer of electronic energy — excitation or ionization transfer — between water and solute molecules is probably a very minor contributor to the radiation damage processes, and of course such energy transfer between solute molecules cannot take place. The nature of the chemical alterations in many biologic molecules as the result of their interaction with the radicals, oxidizing, and reducing species formed in the radiolysis of water is still very imperfectly known or understood.

When the concentration of solute is such that the mechanisms of radiation damage are entirely those of indirect action, alteration of the solute $[G(-M)]$ and the G-values for formation of products (including the G-values for inactivation or alteration of any biologic function) are independent of the concentration of the solute and depend only upon the radiation dose.

References

1. Adelstein, S. J.: Radiation-induced changes in biologically active macromolecules. Radiol. Clin. N. Amer., 3:181, 1965.
2. Allen, A. O.: *The Radiation Chemistry of Water and Aqueous Solutions.* Princeton, N.J., D. Van Nostrand, 1961.
3. Augenstine, L. G., Mason, R., and Rosenberg, B. (eds.): *Physical Processes in Radiation Biology.* New York, Academic Press, 1964.
4. Augenstine, L. G., Mason, R., and Quastler, H. (eds.): *Advances in Radiation Biology*, Vol. I. New York, Academic Press, 1964.
5. Augenstine, L. G.: The effects of ionizing radiation on enzymes. *In* Nord, F. F. (ed.): *Advances in Enzymology*, Vol. 24. New York, John Wiley, 1962.
6. Ausloos, P. (ed.): *Fundamental Processes in Radiation Chemistry.* New York, John Wiley, 1968.
7. Mozumder, A.: Charged particle tracks and their structure. *In* Burton, M., and Magee, J. L. (eds.): *Advances in Radiation Chemistry*, Vol. 1. New York, John Wiley, 1969.
8. Okada, S.: Cells. *In* Altman, K. I., Gerber, G. B., and Okada, S.: *Radiation Biochemistry*, Vol. 1. New York, Academic Press, 1970.
9. Phillips, G. O. (ed.): *Energetics and Mechanisms in Radiation Biology.* New York, Academic Press, 1968.
10. Spinks, J. W. T., and Woods, R. J. (eds.): *An Introduction to Radiation Chemistry.* New York, John Wiley, 1964.

4 MOLECULAR BIOLOGY

Glenn V. Dalrymple, M.D., and Max L. Baker, Ph.D.

4.0 INTRODUCTION

The earlier chapters have traced the processes involved in the absorption of radiation and the transfer of energy to target molecules. Although living cells contain molecules of many types, the results of many studies performed during the past three decades indicate DNA (deoxyribonucleic acid) as a radiation-sensitive "target" of great importance. Since the DNA carries the genetic code, one should not be surprised that relatively subtle damage causes profound effects. This section will first review the biochemistry of three important macromolecules—DNA, RNA (ribonucleic acid), and protein. Later portions will deal with the alterations caused by radiation and how they are important in radiation biology.

4.1 THE BIOCHEMISTRY OF THE NUCLEIC ACIDS AND PROTEINS

A. The Structure of DNA

The compounds DNA and RNA are classified as nucleic acids. Fundamental building blocks of both types of nucleic acids are known as *bases*. There are two types of bases—the *purines* and the *pyrimidines* (Figure 4–1). The purines are *adenine* and *guanine;* the pyrimidines are *thymine, cytosine,* and *uracil.* As Figure 4–1 shows, the only difference between adenine and guanine lies in the peripheral groups; the heterocyclic rings are the same. The same principle holds for the pyrimidines.

The second set of building blocks are the five-carbon sugars, *ribose* and *deoxyribose.*

The only difference between these sugars is an –OH group at the 2' position (deoxyribose does *not* have an oxygen at the 2' position).

The next step in the ascending scale of complexity concerns compounds made up of a combination of a base and a sugar (Figure 4–2). These are known as *nucleosides.* If, in addition, a phosphate is present on the sugar, the compound becomes known as a *nucleotide.* In the literature, the nucleosides and nucleotides are frequently abbreviated. The sugars are R (ribose) and dR (deoxyribose). For the nucleosides the first letter of the name of the base is used. For example,

UR   Uridine (uracil + ribose)
CdR   Deoxycytidine (cytosine + deoxyribose)

This type of nomenclature is used very frequently to indicate compounds labeled with radioactive elements:

[3]HTdR   Tritiated thymidine
[3]HCdR   Tritiated deoxycytidine

Figure 4–3 carries the development a step further, showing the primary structure of DNA. The nucleotides are linked together by phosphate groups. This linkage provides the *phosphodiester backbone* of the DNA molecule. The point of attachment of the bases to the deoxyribose moieties* is also

---
*The term "moiety" means a chemical group which is a portion of a larger group. In this instance, the deoxyribose is a portion of the DNA molecule.

BASES

Purines

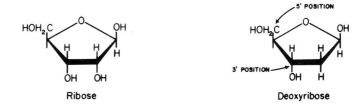

Adenine   Guanine

Pyrimidines

FIGURE 4–1 Chemical structures of the bases and sugars that make up the nucleic acids.

Thymine   Uracil   Cytosine

Sugars

Ribose   Deoxyribose

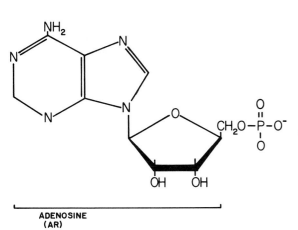

ADENOSINE
(AR)

ADENOSINE   MONOPHOSPHATE
(AMP)

FIGURE 4–2 Chemical structure of the nucleosides and nucleotides.

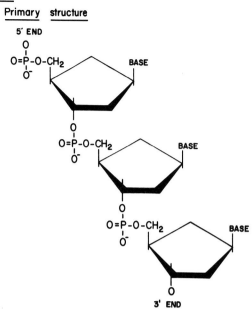

DNA

Primary structure

FIGURE 4-3 Primary structure of a section of the DNA molecule, showing the phosphodiester backbone in some detail. The positions of attachment of the bases to the sugar moieties are indicated.

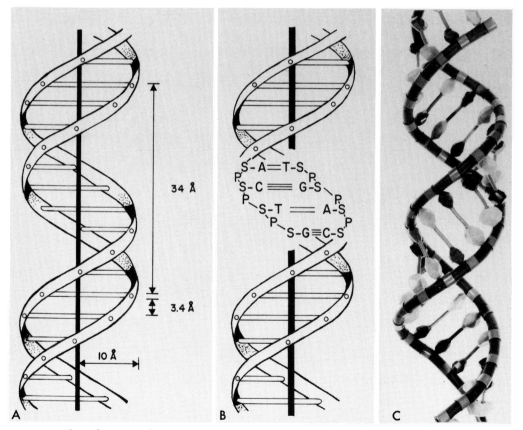

FIGURE 4-4 Three-dimensional structure of DNA. *A*, General form and dimensions of the doubly stranded helical structure of DNA. *B*, Schematic representation of DNA; S, P, A, T, G, and C represent sugar, phosphorus, adenine, thymine, guanine, and cytosine, respectively. *C*, Photograph of a model showing location of the bases in the double helix.

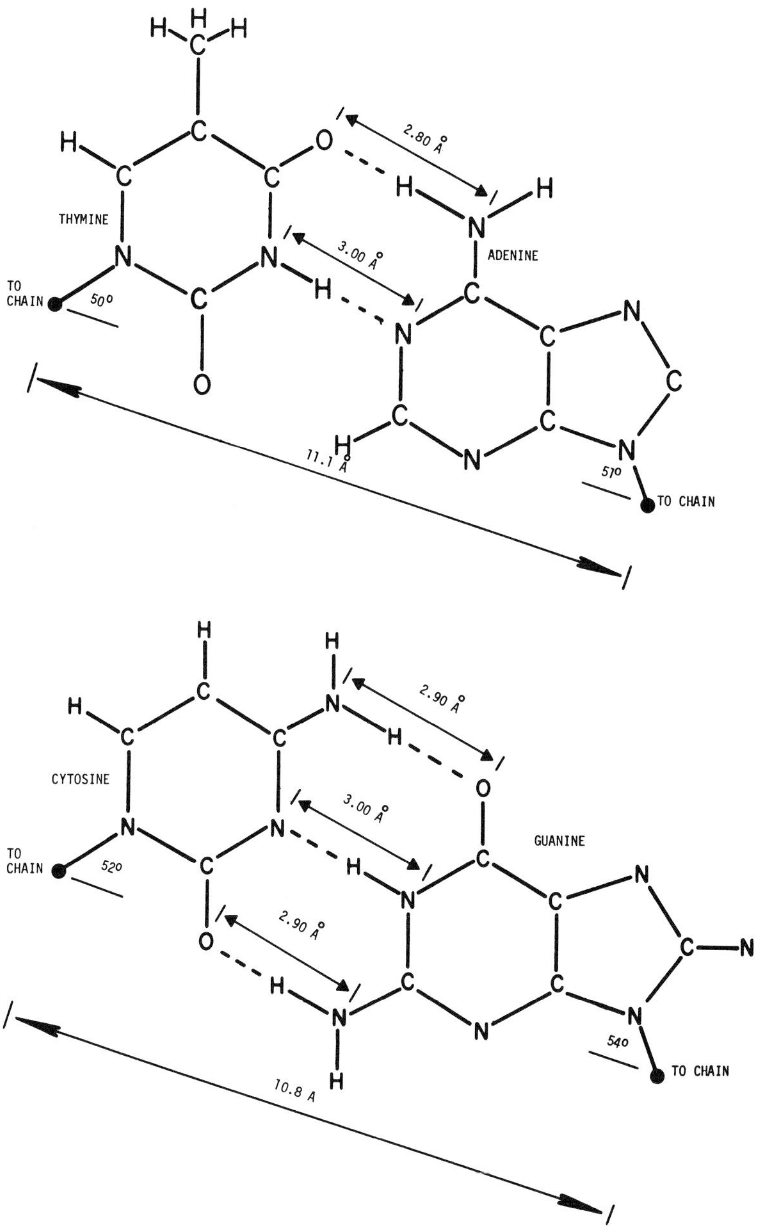

FIGURE 4–5 Hydrogen bonding between base pairs of DNA. The upper portion shows the A-T bonding, while the lower portion shows G-C bonding. These forces are important in holding the strands of the DNA double helix together.

indicated. The information carried by the DNA molecule is a result of the sequence of the bases.

The description of the *secondary* (three dimensional) structure by Watson and Crick (in 1953) gave tremendous impetus to the developing field of molecular biology. According to this model (and its later modifications) the DNA molecule is comprised of two strands arranged in the form of a double

helix (Figure 4–4). The radius of the double helix is about 10 Å; a distance of 3.4 Å separates the base pairs. A complete turn requires 34 Å.

The phosphodiester backbones of the strands are oriented to the "outside" while the bases are projected "inside." The sequence of the bases in the two strands is *complementary* in nature; that is, an adenine (A) moiety in one strand opposes a thymine

(T) moiety in the other. In a similar manner a guanine moiety opposes a cytosine moiety. Although, by definition, the number of adenine moieties must be equal to the number of thymine moieties (A = T), and the number of guanine moieties must equal the number of cytosine moieties (G = C), the relative amounts (ratios) of A + T and G + C varies greatly in DNA from different sources. In fact, an increased amount of G + C has been related to an increased radiosensitivity.

On the two strands, A is located opposite T and C is located opposite G as a consequence of the structure of these bases. As Figure 4–5 shows, thymine and adenine fit together in such a manner that hydrogen bonding between them can occur. Similarly, guanine and cytosine fit together. The differences in structure prevent adenine and thymine from forming hydrogen bonds with guanine or cytosine. The hydrogen bond, while a weak bond, helps maintain the paired strands of the DNA molecule in close proximity to each other.

The DNA molecule is the largest known biologic molecule. The molecular weight of the DNA of bacteria and bacterial viruses (also known as bacteriophages) generally falls between 2×10^6 and 10^{12} Daltons.* The molecular weight of mammalian DNA, however, may be a great deal larger (estimates of 10^{10} and 10^{12} Daltons have been proposed). These very high molecular weights, in fact, suggest that the DNA molecule is on the order of several *millimeters* to *centimeters* in length.

B. The Replication of DNA

The process of replication of the DNA is of great importance in the process of replication of cells. Without the ability to duplicate exact copies of the DNA molecule, the production of viable daughter cells would be very unlikely.

The enzymatic synthesis of DNA is accomplished, under the proper conditions, by the enzyme *DNA polymerase.** Under *in vitro* conditions, DNA synthesis can occur if the reaction mixture contains template DNA,† inorganic ions (such as magnesium), and the four deoxyribonucleotides (as triphosphates — dATP, dCTP, dTTP, and dGTP) in equal amounts. In the most basic terms the reaction is shown at the bottom of the page. In other words, in the presence of the template DNA, the new DNA is synthesized from the nucleotide triphosphates. The energy required to drive the reaction is provided by the high-energy phosphate bonds of the triphosphate. Pyrophosphate is a by-product of the reaction.

Recall that ATP (adenosine triphosphate) is very important in the transfer of energy in biologic systems. ATP (also written ARPPP) can be split such that

$$ARPPP \longrightarrow ARP + P \sim P$$

The compounds ARP (more familiarly, AMP, or adenosine monophosphate) and pyrophosphate ($P \sim P$) are produced.

The biosynthesis of DNA has been of great interest for a number of years. Very interesting experiments by Meselson and Stahl indicate that DNA is replicated by a

---

*The Dalton unit is used to express molecular weights. One Dalton is equal to the molecular weight of a hydrogen atom. The Dalton is synonymous with the atomic mass unit (AMU).

*This term is used simply to designate that enzyme which synthesizes DNA. The current literature suggests that cells possess multiple enzyme activities collectively termed DNA polymerase. Some of these synthesize DNA in repair processes, others function to duplicate DNA at the DNA synthetic period, or they may possess both functions.

†In the literature a distinction is made between *primer* and *template* DNA. For our purposes we will simply consider the DNA to be the template necessary for the synthesis of new DNA. Therefore, we will use the term "template DNA."

$$\text{Template DNA} + \begin{bmatrix} n \text{ dATP} \\ n \text{ dCTP} \\ n \text{ dTTP} \\ n \text{ dGTP} \end{bmatrix} \xrightarrow[\text{Mg}^{++}]{\text{DNA polymerase}} \text{Template} +$$

Newly synthesized DNA + $n\, P \sim P$ (Pyrophosphate).

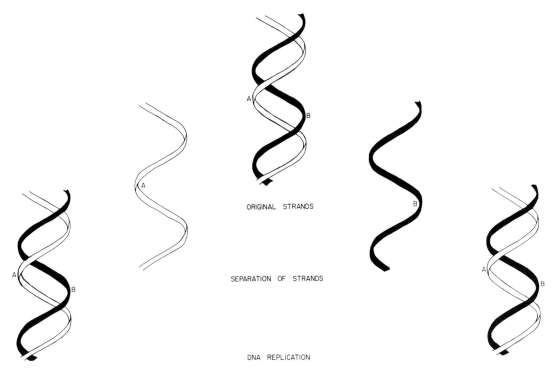

ORIGINAL STRANDS

SEPARATION OF STRANDS

DNA REPLICATION

FIGURE 4–6 Diagrammatic representation of semi-conservative DNA replication. The upper portion shows the original strands, A and B. Following separation of the strands, DNA replicative processes produce new DNA strands complementary to the original ones. The result is two identical DNA molecules.

semi-conservative mechanism. For this, the strands of the DNA molecule unwind and separate (the strands, however, do not break), with synthesis proceeding with the unwinding. Each strand, then, acts as a template to direct the synthesis of a complementary strand. The original molecule is comprised of two strands, *A* and *B*, which are complementary to each other. As the strands separate, the *A* strand directs the synthesis of a complementary strand which, therefore, is identical to the initial *B* strand. In the same way, the initial *B* strand directs the synthesis of a complementary strand. This strand, then, must have the same sequence as the original *A* strand. The final result is two identical molecules, each with *A* and *B* strands.

Thus the sequence of the bases of each complementary strand is exactly opposite that of the original strand (recall that when the original strand contains T the complementary strand will contain A; G in the original strand is opposed by C in the complementary strand, and so forth). The result, then, of the semi-conservative mechanism of DNA replication is two

double helical DNA molecules which are identical (Fig. 4–6).

Later we will be concerned with the *non-conservative* replication of DNA which is induced by radiation.

Recent studies have suggested that DNA synthesis may be "quantal" in nature. Higher organisms do not synthesize DNA from one end to the other as a continuous process. Instead, small portions are synthesized at varying positions along the length of the DNA molecule. These segments are connected so that a single new strand is formed.

C. The Structure, Replication, and Function of RNA; Protein Synthesis

Where DNA represents a polymer of deoxyribonucleotides, RNA is a polymer of ribonucleotides. RNA contains the bases uracil, adenine, guanine, and cytosine; thymine is not a natural constituent of RNA. The ribonucleotides are joined by a phosphodiester backbone in a manner similar to that in DNA. RNA, however, does not exist as a double helical structure. Instead, the RNA molecule seems to be a single polynucleotide strand which contains "hairpin" areas of bending of the molecule upon itself (Figure 4–7). This arrangement allows local hydrogen bonding.

RNA synthesis is similar in many respects to DNA synthesis. RNA synthesis requires equal amounts of the ribonucleotide triphosphates (ATP, UTP, CTP, and GTP), template DNA, and the enzyme RNA polymerase. The base composition of the RNA synthesized upon the DNA template is

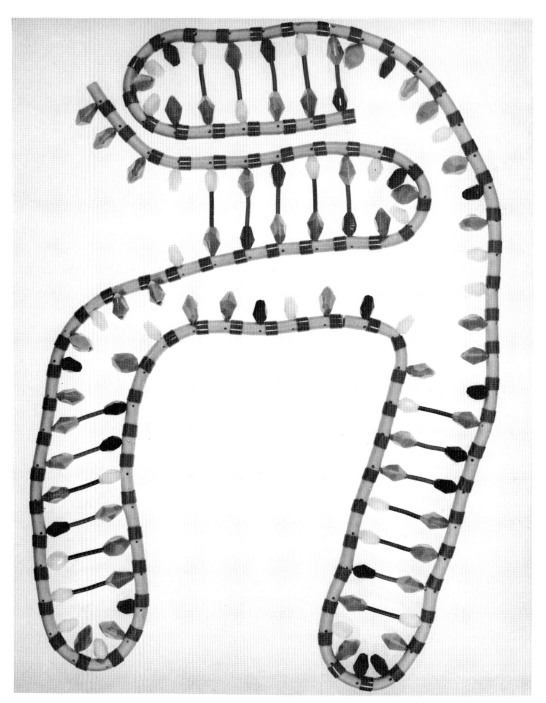

FIGURE 4–7   Model of the structure of RNA. This photograph shows that although the molecule is single-stranded, it does have regions which are double-stranded.

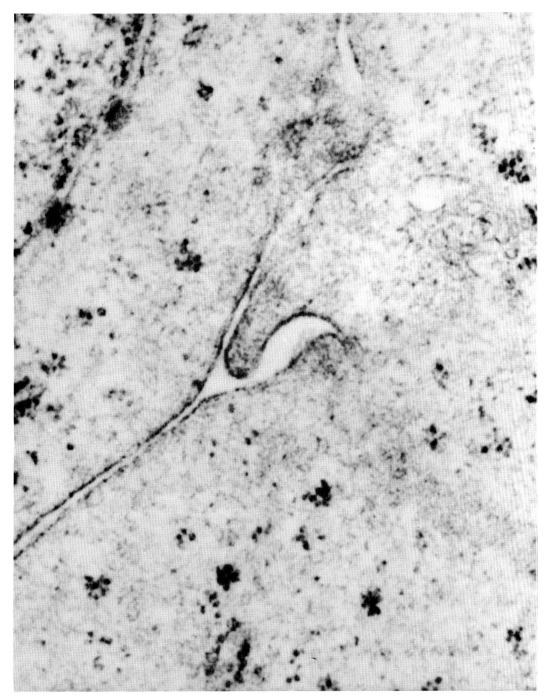

FIGURE 4–8 Electron photomicrograph of the lens of the eye from a chick embryo. The ribosomes appear as black grains ($\times$ 43000).

complementary. The pairings of the bases are the same as for DNA replication, except that the complementary RNA strand contains a uracil rather than a thymine moiety.

An important question concerns how the DNA double helix "opens up" to allow the bases to be read. If this did not occur, the sequence of bases could not be reached by RNA polymerase. The best available evidence indicates that the DNA strands separate and unwind for a distance and that this allows RNA polymerase to have access to the DNA and thereby to make RNA.

RNA has been shown to be very important in the transfer of information from the DNA molecule to protein. The first step concerns the synthesis of RNA on the nuclear DNA. The nucleus contains RNA polymerase and the nucleotide triphosphates. Because the RNA molecule is much smaller than the DNA molecule, only a portion of the information contained in the entire DNA molecule (genome) can be copied by the synthesis of a single RNA molecule. The process of copying the DNA is known as *transcription*. Transcription, then, produces a molecule of RNA—*messenger RNA*, or mRNA—which contains a specific portion of the information carried by the DNA molecule. The messenger RNA then passes through the nuclear membrane into the cytoplasm where it joins RNA–protein known as *ribosomes*. The RNA portion of the ribosomes is known as rRNA. A group of ribosomes linked by a messenger RNA molecule comprises a structure known as the *polysome*. (Polysomes and ribosomes can be seen with the electron microscope; see Figure 4–8.)

A third type of RNA, *transfer RNA* (tRNA or sRNA), is also important because it carries a specific amino acid to the polysome. Transfer RNA contains a sequence of three nucleotides at the *anticodon* end. The *codon* is the sequence of sets of three nucleotides on the messenger RNA. As a result, the proper tRNA molecule is directed to the proper position on the messenger RNA.

This step is most important. A separate species of tRNA molecules (with a unique sequence of nucleotides on the anticodon end) exists for each amino acid. Since the tRNA molecule actually carries the amino acid to the ribosome, the proper alignment of the codon (mRNA) and the anticodon (tRNA) ensures that the correct amino acid will be inserted into the correct position of the newly synthesized polypeptide. This step, called *translation*, is the process in

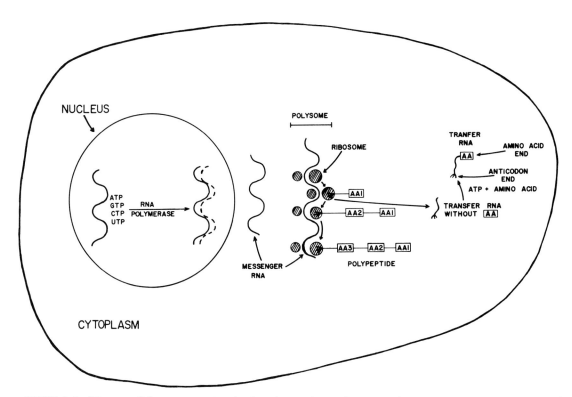

FIGURE 4–9 Diagram of the processes involved in the synthesis of protein. The messenger RNA is synthesized by RNA polymerase, using the nuclear DNA as a template. The messenger RNA then passes to the ribosome. By means of the code carried by the messenger RNA, a polypeptide is synthesized. The amino acids are represented by AA1, AA2, and so on. The transfer RNA, which brings the proper amino acid to the polysome, is regenerated by the tRNA regenerating system.

which the code which was transcribed from the DNA to the RNA has been translated into a protein.

After the tRNA has given up its amino acid, the *amino acid activating system* (including enzymes and ATP) catalyzes the attachment of another amino acid to tRNA. This provides a sufficient supply of "charged" tRNA molecules (bearing amino acids) to maintain protein synthesis. Figure 4–9 summarizes the steps involved in protein synthesis.

The *genetic code* is based upon sets of three nucleotides. A great deal of effort has been devoted to learning which codes specify which amino acids. An example is the sequence on messenger RNA of U U U codes: when U U U appears in the messenger RNA, it will direct the placement of a molecule of the amino acid phenylalanine in the newly synthesized polypeptide. In this case, protein synthesis proceeds as follows: the DNA has a sequence of nucleotides—for example, A A A; this results in the formation of mRNA which contains a U U U code; and this code, in turn, directs the placement of a phenylalanine molecule. (See also Table 5–2.)

How important is the exact sequence of amino acids? The change of a single amino acid means the difference between normal hemoglobin and the hemoglobin of a patient with sickle cell disease. How universal is the genetic code? A very interesting experiment has shown that if transfer RNA from *E. coli* is mixed with rabbit polysomes, rabbit hemoglobin is synthesized. This indicates that the amino acids (carried by the transfer RNA) from bacteria can be used to make mammalian protein, which shows that the code is similar between bacteria and mammals.

Throughout this discussion, the point that has become known as the "central dogma" of molecular biology has been stressed. This idea, that DNA codes for RNA which in turn codes for protein, may not always be the case. There is now evidence in certain viral systems of a reverse transcription. In these systems, a virus which contains only RNA directs the synthesis of DNA within a host. Thus the RNA is actually coding for the DNA. Reverse transcription seems to occur only in a few limited systems, however, and for the most part the "central dogma" still applies.

4.2 RADIATION EFFECTS ON MACROMOLECULES

Next we will consider the effect of ionizing radiation upon the macromolecules DNA, RNA, and protein. During the past three decades, many experiments have pointed to DNA as the radiosensitive "target" responsible for loss of viability. As examples:

a. Studies with microbeams of radiation showed the nucleus to be more radiosensitive than the cytoplasm.

b. "Suicide" experiments were performed in which different compounds were heavily labeled with tritium-containing compounds (³HTdR for labeling DNA; ³HUR for labeling RNA, and ³H amino acids for labeling protein). The greatest killing efficiency, by far, occurred when the DNA was labeled with ³HTdR. Labeling the RNA and protein produced much less cell killing.

c. Experiments with the compound bromodeoxyuridine (BUdR) provide a third bit of evidence. As Figure 4–10 shows, the structure of thymine and bromouracil are very similar. Consequently, BUdR is incorporated into DNA in the same manner as TdR. If as little as one per cent of the T molecules in the DNA molecule of bacteria or mammalian cells are replaced with BU moieties, the cells are greatly sensitized to the effects of both UV and ionizing radiation. This degree of replacement, however, does not cause any other observable alteration of the cell's function.

Therefore, a mass of evidence points to DNA as the "target" of greatest radiobiologic importance.

A. DNA Breaks

As a starting point in the study of the effects of radiation, we will consider the simplest natural DNA-containing particles —the bacterial viruses. Many of these viruses are made up of a double-strand DNA molecule covered with a thin protein coat. If these viruses are infective, they are able to penetrate the host bacteria and replicate. For this, the phage provides the DNA but uses the RNA and protein synthetic capabilities of the bacterium.

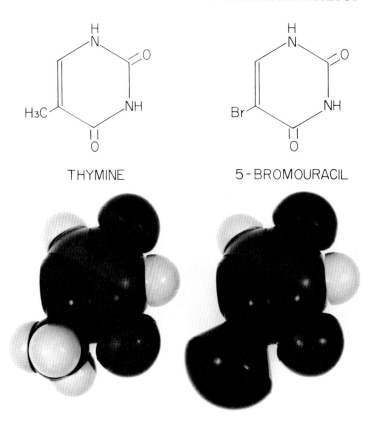

THYMINE   5 - BROMOURACIL

FIGURE 4–10 A comparison of the structure of thymine and 5-BU. Since the radius of the Br atom is almost the same as the radius of —CH$_3$, BU can serve as a thymine analog. The photographs of the models show the relative sizes of the —Br and —CH$_3$ moieties.

Many experiments have indicated that radiation can cause breakage of one or both DNA strands. If the bacteriophage DNA contains a single-strand break, the phage is infective; it can replicate within the bacteria. The host bacterium contains enzymes which rejoin single-strand DNA breaks. After the broken strands are rejoined they are normal in all respects; they can function as templates for the synthesis of more strands. Consequently, the single-strand break would represent nonlethal injury. Double-strand DNA breaks, on the other hand, are associated with loss of infectivity. This is also not surprising because a double-strand break would mean that *both* strands were broken and an intact strand would not be available to serve as a template to direct enzymes necessary to rejoin the breaks.

Experiments with bacteria have shown that radiation indeed produces large numbers of single- and double-strand DNA breaks. The available evidence suggests that at least two factors may be responsible for the production of the breaks. First, the ionization *per se* is responsible for many of the breaks. Second, the radiation may cause damage which results in actual breaks by the actions of enzymes (nucleases) present within the cell.

As would be supposed from the bacteriophage studies, the single-strand DNA breaks are rapidly repaired while the double-strand breaks are not. In addition, more recent studies with mammalian cells grown in culture have shown single-strand DNA breaks to be rapidly rejoined after irradiation.

The results found in experiments such as these have led to the development of models to describe the mechanisms involved. The single-strand break could represent reparable injury if an enzyme were available which rejoined DNA breaks. The presence of an opposite and intact strand seems necessary to provide both the coding to direct the rejoining as well as to maintain continuity. With an intact complementary strand and a certain enzyme, then, the result is DNA which is entirely normal.

One enzyme that rejoins single-strand DNA breaks has been described. This enzyme, DNA ligase (also known as DNA sealase, DNA rejoining enzyme, and polynucleotide joining enzyme), rejoins a specific type of single-strand break (the break must have $5'PO_4$; $3'OH$ termini). Other types of DNA change have been postulated which are thought to involve breaks in the deoxyribose ring, damage to the bases, and so forth. It is very likely that many types of DNA breaks are produced by radiation.

The double-strand DNA breaks seem to represent irreparable injury because a scission through the molecule at any level should be associated with a considerable separation of the fragments and consequent loss of structural integrity. Rejoining, if it occurred, would likely result in sufficient alteration of the genetic code that lethality would follow.

There are also other points to be considered here. The rate of rejoining of single-strand breaks by mammalian cells is very rapid. In fact, DNA rejoining occurs some three to five times faster than the repair of sublethal injury, as measured by cell survival experiments (see Chapter 6). Also, prevention of DNA rejoining does *not* necessarily cause loss of the ability of cells to repair sublethal injury. Therefore, the true biologic significance of post-irradiation DNA breaks is not known. Because of the great biologic importance of DNA, however, any post-irradiation changes in the DNA molecule deserve careful attention.

B. Other Responses of DNA to Irradiation

In addition to breaks, radiation also causes other effects on DNA. Large doses of radiation cause *unscheduled DNA synthesis*, i.e., DNA synthesis occurring at a time when it normally does not occur (for example, DNA synthesis in the G_1 and G_2 phases of the cell cycle*). A similar and possibly related phenomenon is known as *repair replication* or repair synthesis. By definition, this is *non-conservative* DNA replication. DNA precursors, such as ³HTdR, are taken up into DNA strands which have already been synthesized. Recall that semi-conservative DNA synthesis requires that the *new* DNA strand be synthesized upon a pre-existing strand. In repair replication, ³HTdR would be taken

up into the already existing strand. At present, the importance of unscheduled DNA synthesis and repair replication in the repair of radiation injury by mammalian cells is not known.

Another potential form of damage to the DNA molecule is base damage. For this, the radiation is assumed to cause alterations in the structure of the bases such that the genetic code is changed, DNA synthesis is inhibited, or both occur. Ultraviolet radiation produces several types of alterations of DNA structure. One type of damage is the formation of pyrimidine dimers (see Section 4.6). Although synthesis can progress normally in the normal portion of the DNA molecule, the presence of dimers severely restricts the synthesis of DNA past that point. The biologic significance of base damage after irradiation with ionizing radiation, however, is not known. X- and γ-rays, for example, do not produce pyrimidine dimers.

Experiments with bacteria have demonstrated that large doses of radiation cause massive degradation of DNA during the immediate post-irradiation period. The bacterium, apparently, attempts to rid itself of DNA damage by degrading a large portion of the molecule and then resynthesizing the degraded portion. As we have seen before, one strand could be completely degraded and the opposite strand could direct resynthesis of the degraded strand. Current evidence indicates, however, that mammalian cells do not extensively degrade DNA after irradiation. Results such as these suggest that mammalian cells repair radiation injury by processes somewhat different than those used by microorganisms.

C. Effects of Radiation on DNA and RNA Synthesis

A very important question concerns the effect of radiation upon the synthesis of DNA and RNA. In the broadest sense at least four questions must be considered: (a) Are the observed changes due to alterations of enzyme systems responsible for DNA synthesis or RNA synthesis? (b) Are the observed changes a consequence of alteration of the previously existing DNA (the template)? (c) Are the changes due to alterations in pools of precursors needed

---

*See Chapter 6 for details of the cell cycle.

to make DNA or RNA? (d) Are combinations of these factors operating?

For mammalian cells the problem is compounded because DNA synthesis occurs in a discrete portion of the cell cycle, the S period. Many experiments have indicated that radiation decreases the uptake of labeled precursors (such as thymidine) into DNA. These results, however, are subject to some question because of the possible alteration of pool sizes of the natural DNA precursors. For example, if radiation caused a local increase in TdR concentration, we would anticipate decreased uptake of ^{3}HTdR into DNA because of the "mass action" phenomenon. This would be in spite of a normal DNA synthesis. Also, the choice of precursors can alter the results. A given dose of radiation may depress the uptake of TdR into DNA, but the incorporation of ^{32}PO$_4$ may remain normal.

The available evidence suggests that once the enzymes necessary for DNA synthesis are present, very large doses of radiation are necessary to stop the enzymatic synthesis. If, however, the enzymes are not present, but are in the process of being induced, radiation can prevent the appearance of enzymes necessary for DNA synthesis and thereby prevent that synthesis. This circumstance can be shown experimentally by using the regenerating liver. Partial hepatectomy of a rat is followed by a quiescent period of some 18–20 hours, after which many of the remaining cells enter mitosis. During the period before the onset of mitosis, many of the enzymes necessary for DNA synthesis are synthesized. As would be expected, irradiation during this period causes a profound depression of DNA synthesis. Irradiation at a later time, after synthesis of the enzymes has been completed, however, does not depress DNA synthesis.

There are still more problems. One of the important effects of radiation is to cause a transitory (in some cases, permanent) mitotic arrest. This leads to a decreased number of cells passing through mitosis and, therefore, a decreased number of cells entering the S period. As a result, the relative incorporation of DNA precursors into a given tissue (or cell culture) is depressed because fewer cells are in the S period. Although the amount of DNA synthesized

per cell in the S period is normal, the *total* amount of DNA synthesized is depressed.

Certain evidence indicates that radiation produces sufficient damage to the DNA molecule that it cannot serve effectively as a template for both DNA and RNA synthesis. This damage could have a profound impact upon the cell because both DNA duplication and the synthesis of messenger RNA would be altered by radiation. *In vitro* experiments support this notion. However, *in vivo* studies in which the incorporation of precursors into RNA is measured after irradiation have not produced results which are identical to the *in vitro* experiments. In some cell systems, radiation causes an increased incorporation of RNA precursors, such as ^{3}H uridine. In others, radiation causes a depression. If DNA extracted from irradiated cells is used as a template for RNA synthesis, an interesting result follows. The DNA seems to offer many "sites" for the attachment of RNA polymerase. The amount of RNA synthesized, however, is lower than in the case of non-irradiated DNA. The best available evidence, then, suggests that radiation may cause some alterations of RNA synthesis (and thereby transcription) as a consequence of alteration of the DNA template.

The enzymatic reactions required to synthesize RNA are not sufficiently radiosensitive to be an important factor in limiting or altering transcription. In addition, radiation probably does not cause significant changes in the synthesis and function of tRNA and ribosomal RNA except after very large doses.

Experimental results also suggest that sufficient precursors are available to prevent a depletion of some key compound from inhibiting DNA, RNA, or protein synthesis. Earlier work suggested that, since radiation causes uncoupling of oxidative phosphorylation in some radiosensitive tissues (and thereby depresses intracellular ATP levels), alterations in energy metabolism were possibly of great importance. Later studies, however, showed that extreme depression of energy metabolism (such as by treating with dinitrophenol) does not inhibit the ability of cultured mammalian cells to repair sublethal radiation injury. Therefore, the fact that radiation does cause changes in energy metabolism in some tissues does not seem to have important consequences.

The end product of the DNA-transcription-translation sequence is protein; alterations at any point in the sequence could have extreme results. As indicated before, the change in one DNA codon for a single amino acid can yield a non-functional protein or, worse, a protein which causes a disease. The available technology is just reaching the point where detailed sequences of proteins can be analyzed to allow the study of the final result of radiation damage to DNA and RNA.

D. Effects of Radiation on Proteins

Large doses of radiation are usually required to destroy the function of proteins such as enzymes. This occurs, not because proteins are radioresistant *per se*, but rather, as a consequence of the relatively small size of the protein molecule (as compared with DNA) and the relatively large number of protein molecules within the cell. Also, large doses of radiation are necessary to depress the incorporation of protein precursors into newly synthesized protein. Therefore, where damage to DNA or RNA from relatively low doses may yield an abnormal protein, the *synthesis* of protein *per se* is radioresistant.

Present evidence suggests that certain proteins, such as *histones* and *protamines*, may be important for the regulation of gene activity. These proteins (as well as other classes of proteins) combine with DNA to make up a DNA-protein complex known as *nucleoprotein*. Nuclear chromatin is primarily composed of nucleoprotein. Histones and protamines are basic proteins—they contain amino acids which have large numbers of amino groups (e.g., arginine). They complex with DNA, via electrostatic bonds, in such a manner that RNA synthesis is diminished or completely stopped. By this means these proteins serve as repressors because their presence prevents the synthesis of messenger RNA. As a result, transcription is stopped and protein synthesis is altered. Radiation has been found to cause damage which is manifested by disturbances in certain physicochemical properties of the DNA-protein complex. Such a "lesion" could cause improper gene expression which, in turn, could change the cell's metabolic machinery.

SUMMARY

This section reviews those aspects of molecular biology relative to the effects of radiation at the molecular level. The structure, synthesis, and function of DNA, RNA, and protein are described. The importance of DNA as a target and the types of damage covered by ionizing radiation are considered. The influence of radiation upon macromolecular synthesis and the importance of these effects are described. The mechanisms of repair of radiation damage to DNA are reviewed. The chapter concludes with a consideration of the potential importance of radiation upon the DNA-RNA-protein axis.

References

1. Casarett, A. P.: *Radiation Biology.* Englewood Cliffs, N.J., Prentice-Hall, 1968.
2. DuPraw, E. J.: *Cell and Molecular Biology.* New York, Academic Press, 1968. See Chaps. 12–15.
3. Ingram, V. M.: *The Biosynthesis of Macromolecules.* New York, W. A. Benjamin, 1965.
4. Kanzir, D. T.: Radiation-induced alterations in the structure of deoxyribonucleic acid, and their biological consequences. *In* Davidson, J. N., and Cohn, W. E. (eds.): *Progress in Nucleic Acid Research and Molecular Biology*, Vol. 9. New York, Academic Press, 1969.
5. Kaplan, H. S.: Biochemical basis of reproductive death in irradiated cells. Amer. J. Roentgen., 90:907–916, 1963.
6. Pizzarello, D. J., and Witcofski, R. L.: *Basic Radiation Biology.* Philadelphia, Lea and Febiger, 1967. See Chaps. 12–18.
7. Smith, K. C., and Hanawalt, P. C.: *Molecular Photobiology; Inactivation and Recovery,* New York, Academic Press, 1969.
8. Steiner, R. F.: *The Chemical Foundations of Molecular Biology.* Princeton, N.J., D. Van Nostrand, 1965.
9. Watson, J. D.: *The Molecular Biology of the Gene.* New York, W. A. Benjamin, 1965.

Ultraviolet Effects

John Jagger, Ph.D.

4.3 THE NATURE OF ULTRAVIOLET RADIATION

Electromagnetic radiations are usually characterized by their wavelength. In the range of ultraviolet and visible radiation, it is common to measure the wavelength in units of *nanometers* (1 nm = 10^{-9} meters = 1μ = 10 Å). Visible light lies in the range of 380 to 780 nm. Wavelengths shorter than visible lie in the ultraviolet range (see Figure 4–13), which we divide into two regions; the *near ultraviolet* or "near UV" (300 to 380 nm), which is present in sunlight; and the *far ultraviolet*, "far UV" or "UV" (below 300 nm), which is not present in sunlight but is strongly absorbed by biologic material.

Unlike X-radiation, far ultraviolet (UV) does not ionize atoms and molecules; it loses energy to matter solely in the form of electronic excitation. Such excitation in the UV region can occur only in certain molecular structures, chiefly conjugated systems (alternating single and double bonds in a carbon chain) such as the benzene ring; it usually does not occur in single atoms or in highly saturated molecules such as carbohydrates and lipids. Therefore, absorption of UV in biologic material is *non-random* and occurs primarily in nucleic acids, proteins, and coenzymes, which usually possess conjugated structures. The efficiency for absorption of UV by these systems is very high. In addition, once a UV photon has been absorbed, it disappears and does not give rise to further radiation, as occurs with X-rays. Therefore, UV does not penetrate very far into biologic material, and most of it is absorbed within the first 10 microns.

We see, then, that UV differs from X-radiation in three important respects: (a) it does not ionize; (b) its interaction with biologic material is non-random; and (c) its ability to penetrate biologic material is very low.

For biologic systems under normal conditions (vegetative state, at room temperature or at 37°C), there is very little similarity in the damages produced by ionizing and ultraviolet radiation. The most obvious evidence for this lies in the observations that the oxygen effect (which influences about two-thirds of X-ray damage) does not occur with UV, and photoreactivation (which influences about two-thirds of UV damage) does not occur with X-rays.

4.4 WHY ULTRAVIOLET EFFECTS ARE RELEVANT TO RADIOLOGY

In view of these important differences between ionizing radiation action and UV action, one may wonder why a study of UV effects is relevant to radiology. There are several reasons:

The primary target is the same. The genes of a living cell are unique, irreplaceable, and usually essential components made of DNA. In addition, nucleic acids are effective absorbers of both ionizing and UV radiation. These facts mean that DNA is far and above the most important target for both X-rays and UV.

Some of the damages may be similar. Damages produced in the DNA of cells in the solid state (frozen cells or spores) may to some extent be similar for the two types of radiation. In addition, some of the short-lived intermediates (for example, free radicals) involved in base damage to DNA may be similar for the two radiations.

Some of the repair mechanisms may be similar. This is much more likely than that the damages would be similar. Extensive repair of UV damage to the DNA of biologic systems is carried out by enzymes normally present in the cell. These repair systems are capable of acting to some extent on damages induced by chemical agents such as nitrogen mustard. Some of them appear to be effective against X-ray damage. For example, certain bacterial mutants (*rec*⁻ mutants) are more sensitive to UV (indicating a loss of UV reparability) and are also more sensitive to X-rays. These mutants lack repair systems apparently related to the systems used in genetic recombination; the latter is such a fundamental capability of cells that one is not surprised that a repair system based upon genetic recombination may operate on a wide variety of damages.

The same experimental approaches may be useful. This is probably the most important reason why someone interested in X-ray damage should study what is known about UV damage. The techniques that have been developed in UV research, involving (a) isolation of mutants of varying radiation sensitivity, (b) isolation and characterization of specific photoproducts produced in DNA, and (c) use of *extremely* low dose rates, will undoubtedly prove fruitful in X-ray studies and have, in some instances, already been so applied.

4.5 THE NATURE OF ULTRAVIOLET DAMAGE TO CELLS

Some of the action of far-UV radiation on large cells may be due to absorption in proteins or in coenzymes. However, in bacteria, which far UV above 220 nm can easily penetrate, as well as in many cells of higher organisms, nucleic acid is overwhelmingly the most important target molecule for the biologic effects commonly studied, such as mutation and killing (compare Figures 4–11 and 4–13). This is because, every base being aromatic, nucleic acid is a better absorber of UV (above 220 nm) per unit weight than almost any other biologic molecule (Figure 4–11), and be-

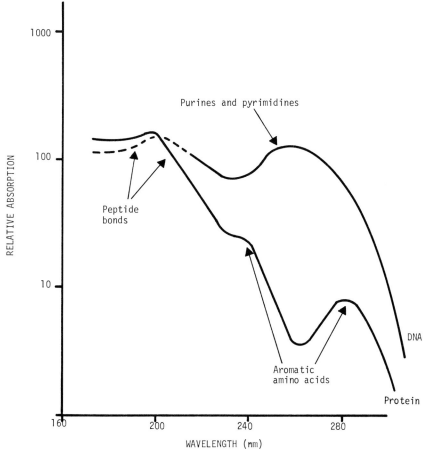

FIGURE 4–11 Ultraviolet absorption spectra of 1 per cent solutions of a typical protein (bovine serum albumin) and of DNA at pH 7. (After Smith, K. C., and Hanawalt, P. C.: *Molecular Photobiology: Inactivation and Recovery.* New York, Academic Press, 1969.)

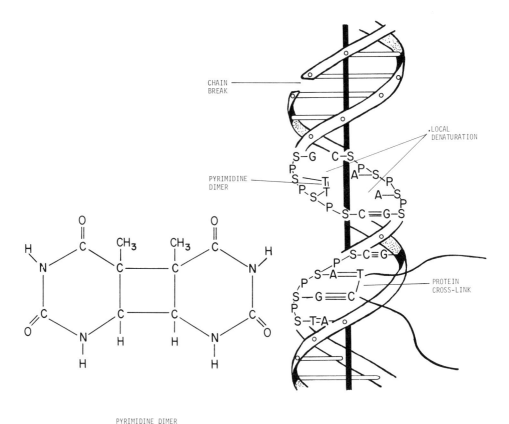

CHAIN BREAK

.LOCAL DENATURATION

PYRIMIDINE DIMER

PROTEIN CROSS-LINK

PYRIMIDINE DIMER

FIGURE 4–12 Schematic illustration of alterations found in DNA extracted from cells that have been irradiated with ultraviolet light. (After Smith, K. C., and Hanawalt, P. C.: *Molecular Photobiology: Inactivation and Recovery.* New York, Academic Press, 1969.)

cause the genetic material of cells is unique and, therefore, crucially important to the cell. The latter fact suggests that DNA would be a much more important cellular target than RNA, and this view is supported by many experimental data. In the rest of this section, we shall, therefore, consider only ultraviolet damages to DNA.

Being essentially saturated compounds, the phosphate and sugar moieties of DNA do not absorb radiation above 220 nm; they are therefore of little importance in UV effects. This leaves the purine and pyrimidine bases, both of which absorb far UV strongly. Studies with individual bases and with polynucleotides, however, indicate that the pyrimidines are about 10 times more susceptible to UV damage than the purines, and energy absorbed in purines is generally either dissipated or transferred to pyrimidines. Consequently, *the far-UV photo-*

biology of small cells is concerned primarily with effects on the pyrimidines of DNA.

Figure 4–12 illustrates the types of damages that UV may produce in DNA. It is now clear that the most important UV photoproduct under normal biologic conditions is the *pyrimidine dimer*. It occurs in a reaction in which two adjacent pyrimidines in the same DNA strand form covalent bonds at their 5,6 positions, thus producing a cyclobutane ring (Figure 4–12). These dimers are quite stable. Their formation involves loss of the 5,6 double bond, with consequent loss of the aromaticity of the pyrimidine ring and the characteristic 260 nm absorption peak of the pyrimidine (Figure 4–11).

DNA molecules may become cross-linked to other DNA chains upon UV irradiation, as evidenced by *in vitro* experiments as well as by observations on inactivation of bacteria in different humidities or physical states. There is also evidence in bacteria and in mammalian cells for UV-induced linkage of DNA to protein, with some indication that this might involve pyrimidine-cystine bonds. The DNA-protein binding is not photoreactivable but may account for a major portion of non-photoreactivable damage.

We can now estimate the relative importance of various lesions in the DNA of cells under normal conditions. Pyrimidine dimers are overwhelmingly the most important lesion, representing about 60 to 90 per cent of the total damage. DNA-protein cross-links are probably the second most important damage, although little is known about them. Various base damages other than pyrimidine dimerization (not discussed here) probably rank third in importance. Single-strand chain breaks are quite rare and represent less than one per cent of the total damage, while double-strand breaks do not occur at all.

4.6 REPAIR OF ULTRAVIOLET DAMAGE TO DNA

A. Photoreactivation

We now have an elementary understanding of this effect, in which damage induced in biologic systems by far-UV radiation may be partly eliminated by subsequent irradiation with near-UV, violet, or blue light (300 to 500 nm). The effective wavelengths often differ in different systems (Fig. 4–13). Extracts of photoreactivable cells (yeast, *Escherichia coli*) can mediate *in vitro* photoreactivation of the biologic

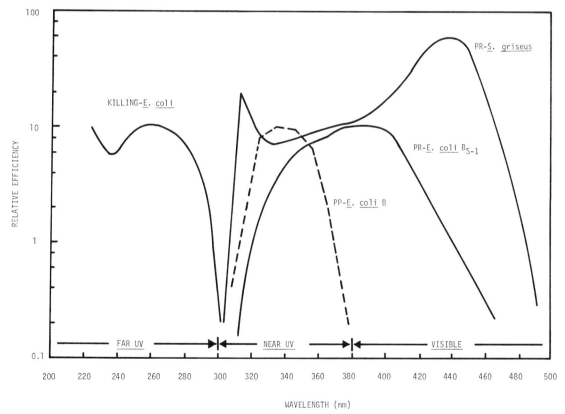

FIGURE 4–13 Action spectra for killing in *Escherichia coli,* photoreactivation (PR) in *E. coli* and *Streptomyces griseus,* and photoprotection (PP), or indirect photoreactivation, in *E. coli* (broken line). Curves have been normalized to similar efficiencies for display purposes; actually UV is much more efficient in killing than in photoreactivation. (Data from Smith, K. C., and Hanawalt, P. C.: *Molecular Photobiology: Inactivation and Recovery.* New York, Academic Press, 1969, and Jagger, J., Takebe, H., and Snow, J. M. Photochem. Photobiol., *12*:185, 1970.)

activity of transforming DNA (a DNA whose biologic activity can be assayed). The active factor is an enzyme, and the process takes the following course: (a) the enzyme forms a complex (E-DNA) with far-UV-damaged DNA (it is specific for this damage and will not combine with DNA damaged in other ways); (b) the complex absorbs photoreactivating light; and (c) the complex dissociates into enzyme and repaired DNA:

$$E + DNA \rightleftharpoons E\text{-}DNA \xrightarrow{\text{light}} E + DNA$$

It is now known that the DNA photoreactivating enzyme functions by splitting pyrimidine dimers. This appears to be its only function. Details of the reaction are not understood and the chromophore (light-absorbing molecular structure) remains unidentified.

Photoreactivation may be of two different types, either or both of which may occur in one biologic system. The predominant type is *direct photoenzymatic reactivation*, which utilizes the photoreactivating enzyme, shows a strong dependence upon temperature during photoreactivation, and shows saturation effects at high dose rates of the photoreactivating light. A second type is called *indirect photoreactivation*. This is mediated by a narrower band of wavelengths (300 to 380 nm, with a peak at 340 nm) and is similar in mechanism to photoprotection, showing little or no dependence upon temperature and no dose-rate-saturation effects.

B. Excision-Resynthesis Repair

There is now much evidence that cells repair, in the absence of photoreactivating light, most of the genetic (DNA) damage inflicted upon them by UV. It has been

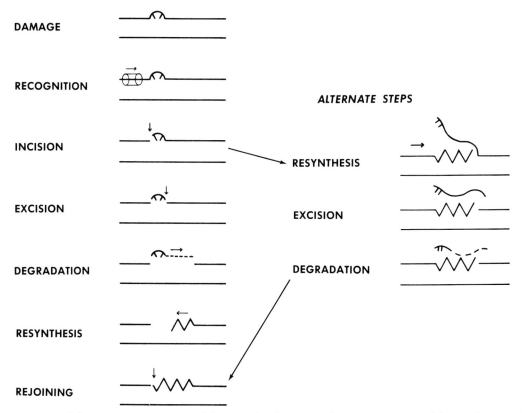

FIGURE 4–14 Schematic representation of the postulated steps in the excision repair of damaged DNA. The steps in the left-hand column illustrate the "cut and patch" sequence. An initial incision in the damaged strand is followed by local degradation before the resynthesis of the region has begun. In the alternative "patch and cut" model, the resynthesis step begins immediately after the incision step and the excision of the damaged region occurs when resynthesis is complete. In both models the final step involves a rejoining of the repaired section to the contiguous DNA of the original parental strand. (After Smith, K. C., and Hanawalt, P. C.: *Molecular Photobiology: Inactivation and Recovery*. New York, Academic Press, 1969.)

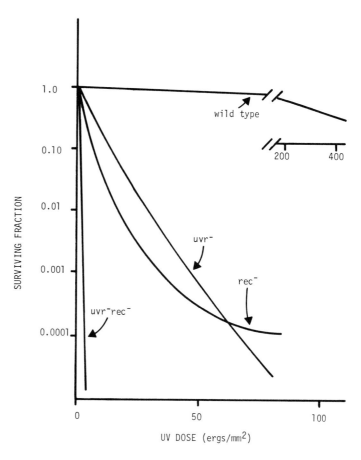

FIGURE 4–15 The sensitivity of colony-forming ability to ultraviolet light in several UV-sensitive bacterial mutants. The mutant strain uvr^- is unable to excise thymine dimers. The rec^- mutant is defective in genetic recombination. The double mutant $uvr^-\ rec^-$ is deficient in both excision and recombination and it is more sensitive than either single mutant. (After Smith, K. C., and Hanawalt, P. C.: *Molecular Photobiology: Inactivation and Recovery.* New York, Academic Press, 1969.)

shown that pyrimidine dimers are removed from the DNA of UV-resistant strains, but not from the DNA of very sensitive strains. The process (Figure 4–14) is considered to require production of a single-strand break, or "incision," near the dimer; removal of an oligonucleotide containing the dimer ("excision"); resynthesis of the removed segment along the intact complementary strand, which it uses as a template; and rejoining of the ends of the original and the resynthesized strand to form a continuous and "native" double-stranded DNA. The first step of "excision-resynthesis" repair (namely, incision) has been demonstrated in the test tube, using bacterial extracts (which contain the incision enzyme) and phage DNA. Bacterial mutants which *lack* the incision enzyme are nevertheless capable of repairing X-ray damage, since X-rays produce the incision (single-strand break).

One consequence of the induction of pyrimidine dimers in DNA is that the two pyrimidines involved lose their hydrogen

bonding to the complementary strand. This results in a local denaturation of the double-stranded DNA (see Figure 4–12) which may serve as a recognition site for repair-enzyme systems (Figure 4–14).

The excision-resynthesis system appears to be able to repair as much as 98 per cent of a far-UV damage in bacteria. Thus, a mutant bacterium lacking this system $(uvr^-)^*$ is some 50 times more sensitive to UV killing (compare 37 per cent survival for "uvr^-" and "wild type" in Figure 4–15).

C. Recombination Repair

Bacteria able to excise pyrimidine dimers but deficient in the ability to undergo genetic recombination $(rec^-)^*$ are also

---

*In genetic terminology, the "wild type" is the normal, unmutated strain. Mutants are referred to by a three-letter code. Thus, a "rec^-" mutant is a strain that has mutated to a state where it can no longer engage in genetic recombination (sex at the molecular level). "uvr^-" means lacking UV repair of the excision-resynthesis type.

some 50 times more sensitive to UV killing than the wild type (compare curves for "*rec⁻*" and "wild type" in Figure 4–15). Therefore, the recombination-repair system (about which little is known) appears to be fundamentally different from the excision-resynthesis system and presumably is closely related to the process of genetic recombination. A cell deficient both in excision-resynthesis repair and in the ability to recombine (*uvr⁻rec⁻*) becomes extremely sensitive to UV, showing a 37 per cent survival dose of only about 0.2 erg/mm²,† which corresponds to about one pyrimidine dimer per cell. This is presumably, therefore, the most UV-sensitive cell that could exist. It is approximately 2000 times as sensitive as the wild-type strain, which implies that bacteria are capable of repairing in the dark some 99.95 per cent of their far-UV damage. In addition, photoreactivation can repair two-thirds of the remaining damage, making a total of 99.98 per cent of the cellular damage that can be repaired.

D. Repair Treatments

The three repair systems just discussed —namely, direct photoenzymatic reactivation, excision-resynthesis repair, and recombination repair—are repair *mechanisms* that are controlled by specific genes. A variety of repair *treatments* are known that will encourage various of these mechanisms.

Photoprotection is a decreased far-UV sensitivity (three-fold decrease in slope of survival curve) induced by near-UV irradiation *before* the far-UV irradiation. It is similar in mechanism to *indirect photoreactivation*, the initial action being apparently a purely photochemical effect outside of DNA (which does not absorb near UV). It does not operate by splitting pyrimidine dimers, but is believed to involve inactivation of isoprenoid quinones of the electron transport system (in mitochondria or in bacterial cell walls). The illumination (effective wavelengths 300 to 380 nm, with a peak at 340 nm; see Figure 4–13) induces growth delays and division delays which presumably permit more time

for "dark-repair processes" (repair processes other than photoreactivation) to operate. It is, therefore, easy to see why the illumination may occur either before (photoprotection) or after (indirect photoreactivation) the far-UV irradiation. *Escherichia coli* B_{s-1}, which has very little dark-repair ability, shows only direct photoenzymatic reactivation, and *E. coli* B *phr⁻*, which can conduct dark repair, but lacks active photoreactivating (phr) enzyme, shows only indirect photoreactivation. Many strains, like *E. coli* B, show both direct and indirect photoreactivation.

Liquid-holding recovery is a higher survival (three-fold decrease in slope of survival curve) of bacteria after holding them in a liquid for a few hours. This treatment appears to enhance excision-resynthesis repair. Also, it appears to involve repair of essentially the same damage as does photoprotection.

E. Some Other Aspects of Repair

The questions of the extent to which mutational damage may be similar to lethal damage and the extent to which it may consist of pyrimidine dimers are still under debate. Mutational damage can generally be photoreactivated, which strongly suggests that much of it is induced by pyrimidine dimers. Some mutational damage, however, may be induced by different photoproducts.

All earlier studies on UV killing indicated that dose rate is not important (provided that a constant total dose is applied), from which it was correctly concluded that the initial action of a far-UV photon is purely photochemical (not requiring enzymes). Recent studies, however, have shown that UV-resistant bacteria, which presumably have good dark-repair systems, show a much higher survival when the *dose rate* is extremely low (for example, if the dose is administered continuously over a 24-hour period). This does not reflect a difference in the initial action of the photons, but rather an inefficiency in the dark-repair process under the usual irradiation conditions (namely, high UV doses and normal dose rates) which permit lesions to accumulate before they are repaired.

---

†"Erg/mm²" is a measure of energy per unit area, and is the common way of expressing UV doses.

4.7 OCCURRENCE OF THE BACTERIAL PHENOMENA IN HIGHER ORGANISMS

Thymine dimers induced by far-UV radiation have been found in all types of living cells that have been tested. Photoreactivating enzyme has been found in all types of living cells with the notable exception of cells of placental mammals, and it is present at only low concentration in the non-placental mammals (marsupials). However, indirect photoreactivation may well occur in mammalian cells.

"Repair replication" is a term describing an unusual DNA replication often observed after radiation treatment and believed to reflect resynthesis of excised regions of DNA (Figure 4–14). In few cases, however, has such observed unusual replication been clearly shown to involve a repair process. "Repair replication" occurs in mammalian cells, and has recently been correlated with enhanced survival. In cells of higher organisms, "unscheduled DNA synthesis" means synthesis outside the normal synthesis (S) period; it may occur after radiation treat-ment, but has not yet been shown to involve true repair resynthesis.

Although it is clear that pyrimidine dimers are produced in mammalian systems, in only a few cases have workers been able to observe excision of these dimers. It has recently been shown that normal diploid human skin fibroblasts can excise up to 70 per cent of their dimers, but that fibroblasts derived from individuals suffering from the human skin disorder xeroderma pigmentosum excise less than 20 per cent of their dimers. Xeroderma pigmentosum is a disease characterized by increased sensitivity to the small amounts of far UV present in sunlight leading to skin malignancies of various types. The increased sensitivity may be explained as an inability to excise pyrimidine dimers. This is the first time that pyrimidine dimers *per se* have been experimentally implicated in the process of carcinogenesis.

Reference

1. Smith, K. C., and Hanawalt, P. C.: *Molecular Photobiology; Inactivation and Recovery.* New York, Academic Press, 1969.

5 GENETIC EFFECTS OF RADIATION[*]

Mary Esther Gaulden, Ph.D.

5.0 INTRODUCTION

Genetics is the study of the inheritance of observable characters, which include molecular as well as morphological and behavioral traits. In 1927, H. J. Muller discovered that X-rays could induce permanent changes called mutations in the hereditary units (genes). He was awarded the Nobel Prize in 1946 for this work which was done with the fruit fly *Drosophila* and which has made an enormous impact on our knowledge of all biologic systems, including man. Mutations can occur spontaneously (cause unknown) or can be induced by a variety of physical and chemical agents, radiation being one of the most efficient mutagens known. Mutations can occur in somatic cells, with consequences only to the individual who is exposed, and in germ cells, with consequences to future generations. Perspective on the possible consequences of mutation can be gained by remembering that the growth, organization, function, reproduction, adaptability to environment, and survival of an organism are all under genetic control.

As described in the previous chapter, the hereditary material is DNA and is located in the chromosomes. Radiation-induced changes in or destruction of molecules and structures that occur in great numbers in a cell (e.g., enzymes and mitochondria) have little or no effect on the cell unless a large proportion is damaged. Because DNA is a unique molecule in the cell, it is a primary target for radiation action. This means that the very small doses of radiation, such as those encountered in diagnostic radiology, may produce genetic effects of far-reaching consequences. Many of the radiation effects on the cell discussed in subsequent chapters may, in the final analysis, be explained by initial lesions in the DNA, especially at low to moderate doses.

Because mutations can be induced by very low doses of radiation, geneticists have long cautioned that the gonads should be shielded whenever possible during medical radiation exposure. Most radiation-induced mutations are recessive in expression and cannot, therefore, be detected for a number of generations, if ever, in man. This fact explains why geneticists are not surprised that no gene mutations have been observed in the first generation offspring of atomic bomb survivors or of individuals known to have received large amounts of radiation. Radiation-induced recessive genes may, however, have some deleterious effect, even in the heterozygous condition (undetectable without breeding or pedigree studies). The recessive nature of most induced mutations is responsible for the dilemma geneticists face when trying to convince others of the genetic hazards of low doses of X-rays. The physician uses diagnostic radiation to alleviate an *immediate* health problem of a particular patient, whereas the geneticist is concerned with X-ray-induced heritable changes that may be harmful to *future* generations. In this connection it is of interest to recall the

[*]Manuscript prepared under support of U.S. Public Health Service Training Grant 5-T01-CA-05136.

TABLE 5–1   SOME MAXIMUM PERMISSIBLE WHOLE-BODY (CRITICAL ORGANS) DOSES*

The values are in addition to medical and background exposure. The units of dose are those in use at the indicated dates. The *R* (Roentgen) is equivalent to absorption of 83 ergs per gram of air. The *rem* (Roentgen equivalent man) is the amount of radiation which causes in man the same biological damage as 1 R of X- or gamma-radiation. The *rad* (radiation absorbed dose) represents an energy absorption of 100 ergs per gram of any material; in the human it is nearly equivalent to the Roentgen. Currently the R is used as the unit for exposure and the rad for absorbed dose.

For the Individual Occupational Worker:

Year	*Exposure or Dose*
1925	0.1 of an erythema dose/year**
1934	0.1 R/day or 0.5 R/week
1949	0.3 rem/week or 15 rem/year
1956 to present	0.1 rem/week or 5.0 rem/year

For Individuals in the Population:

Year	*Exposure or Dose*
1952	0.03 rem/week
1958	5 rem/30 years
Present	0.170 rem/year

*As established by the International Commission on Radiological Protection and the United States Council on Radiation Protection and Measurements. See Morgan, K. Z., and Turner, E. J. (eds.): *Principles of Radiation Protection.* New York, John Wiley, 1967. See also *Basic Radiation Protection Criteria.* Report No. 39, National Council on Radiation Protection and Measurements, January 15, 1971 (P.O. Box 4867, Washington, D.C. 20008).

**Estimated to be approximately equivalent to 25 and 50 R/year from X-rays produced by 100-kv and 200-kv potentials, respectively.

reluctance of early radiation workers to acknowledge the harmful effects of X-rays. In spite of the facts that 55 deaths attributable to X-ray injuries were reported within one year after Roentgen's discovery of the radiation, and that definitive evidence for X-ray-induced fetal death in guinea pigs (without skin burns) was published in 1901, the dangers of X-rays were ignored or explained away in favor of the enormous diagnostic gains they offered. International and national efforts to establish guidelines for limiting the exposure of radiation workers were not begun until the 1920's. Limitations on exposure of the population-at-large were proposed in 1952; they do not include medical-dental radiation exposure. Table 5–1 shows the decreases in maximum permissible doses over a 47-year period. The radical reduction after 1949 reflects, in large part, recognition of genetic effects of radiation on both somatic and germ cells.

Acceptance of the probability that diagnostic radiation induces mutations in man requires somewhat the same attitude as acknowledgement, for example, of the fact that water is made up of two atoms of hydrogen and one of oxygen. Established principles of chemistry and physics lead us to accept the molecular constitution of water and its behavior under varying conditions without ever demonstrating to ourselves in the laboratory that they are indeed true. The principles of radiation genetics are well established on the basis of innumerable experiments with all types of organisms, both plant and animal. Limited experimental evidence, as well as the unity of nature, indicate that man's genetic behavior is essentially like that of all other organisms. Appreciation of the genetic hazards of low doses of radiation requires some understanding of the principles of genetics. Knowledgeable patients are becoming more concerned about genetic effects of radiation, which is not surprising in view of the fact that high school students are learning molecular and human genetics at an increasingly sophisticated level. The lay press has given much attention to the number of human conditions which are associated with specific chromosome mutations and has, thereby, further increased public interest. The concern about mutations is beginning to surface in litigation against members of the medical profession. In this chapter, therefore, the basic principles of genetics and radiation-induced mutation will be discussed, and experimental data will be related to genetic hazards of radiation in man.*

5.1 GENES AND GENE ACTION

A *gene* is a segment of DNA with a finite number of nucleotides. The information (genetic code) contained in the gene resides in its linear sequence of bases. This sequence in DNA determines the linear sequence of nucleotides in messenger RNA, which in turn determines the linear sequence of amino acids in a specific protein. The "information" in the genes is coded for protein synthesis only, which is sufficient for cell and organism function because all enzymes (limiting factors in the synthesis of any compound) are proteins.

Current estimates suggest that an average gene consists of about 1500 linearly arranged base pairs. Our knowledge of the molecular aspects of the gene is derived mainly from studies on viruses and bacteria, but all the evidence from experimental organisms, including human cells grown *in vitro*, reveals that there is one basic genetic code for polypeptide synthesis in all organisms. In other words, a gene that codes for a given enzyme will be found in all organisms that synthesize that enzyme, be they amoebae or men. Thus, we are justified in extrapolating to a certain extent from data obtained on gene action and mutation in experimental organisms to these phenomena in man.

A. Gene Action

In man the study of gene action must be carried out mainly by *Mendelian genetic analysis*. This classic method involves description of the end product, the *phenotype*, which is an observable character that results from the expression of one or more

genes. In molecular terms the phenotype can ultimately be reduced to one or more specific proteins. The term *genotype* is used in different contexts to denote a single pair of genes for a specific character or a number of the genes in a cell or an organism. Analysis of genotype is accomplished by breeding experiments or, in man, by pedigree study. *Genome* refers to the entire genetic constitution of a cell or organism.

Genes occur along chromosomes in linear order like beads on a string, and the position of a gene in a chromosome is referred to as its *locus*. Each normal human cell has 46 chromosomes: 23 are derived from the mother and 23 from the father. One pair of the chromosomes determines sex (XX in female and XY in male); the other 22 pairs are referred to as *autosomes*.

Each of a pair of chromosomes normally has the same genes for given characters in identical linear sequence; the two chromosomes are said to be *homologous*. Alternative forms of a gene at a given locus on a chromosome are called *alleles*. For example, production of the β polypeptide chains of normal hemoglobin is controlled by a gene (designated Hb^A) and those of the abnormal sickle-cell hemoglobin by an allele (Hb^S) of that same gene. Several dozen abnormal alleles of the normal hemoglobin gene have been identified in the human population, but only two of them will occur in a single individual. Different alleles of a gene arise by mutation.

When the members of a pair of genes are alike, they are said to be *homozygous* ($Hb^A Hb^A$ or $Hb^S Hb^S$); when they are different they are said to be *heterozygous* ($Hb^A Hb^S$). When one gene has been deleted from a chromosome, the gene at that locus on the other chromosome is said to be *hemizygous* (Hb^A).

The expression of a gene can be classified as *dominant* or *recessive*. A dominant gene by definition expresses itself in the presence of a recessive allele, the expression of which is either ineffective or suppressed. For example, an individual who inherits from one parent the dominant gene for brachydactyly and from the other parent the recessive normal gene will be brachydactylous (heterozygous). For a completely recessive gene to be expressed, an individual must possess only the recessive genes (i.e., must be homozygous recessive).

---

*A complete list of references covering the material in this chapter can be obtained from the author upon request.

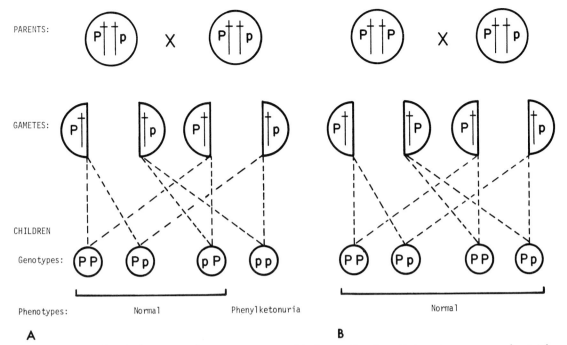

FIGURE 5–1 Mode of inheritance of a recessive gene, with the one for phenylketonuria as an example. *A*, The genotypes and phenotypes resulting from the various possible combinations of gametes when both parents are heterozygous (one chromosome has the normal dominant gene, designated P, and one has the recessive abnormal gene, p. Note that the gametes have only one chromosome of a pair. See Section 5.4). *B*, One parent is homozygous dominant and the other is heterozygous.

The disease phenylketonuria is caused by a recessive gene that leads to a body deficiency of the enzyme phenylalanine hydroxylase with accompanying mental retardation and the presence of phenylpyruvic acid in the urine. Figure 5–1 shows the mode of inheritance that yields one-fourth phenylketonuric offspring from normal parents heterozygous (both Pp) for this recessive gene. If only one parent is heterozygous for the gene, half of the offspring will carry the recessive gene, but none will be affected.

It should be pointed out that not all genes are completely dominant; some permit expression of the recessive allele, the extent of expression varying with different genes. For example, the recessive gene responsible for the skin disease xeroderma pigmentosum can express itself in heterozygotes; the skin of such individuals shows a greater than normal amount of freckling. The skin of homozygotes for the dominant gene shows a "normal" reaction to sunlight, whereas the skin of homozygotes for the recessive gene develops degenerative areas that become cancerous and lethal.

The Y sex chromosome in the human has genes that determine maleness but has very few other known genes. The X chromosome, on the other hand, has many genes which, because they have no sister alleles on the Y chromosome, are hemizygous in the male. For this reason many recessive sex-linked genes have been identified in man, such as hemophilia, Hunter's disease, and Duchenne-type muscular dystrophy.

In addition to classifying genes as dominant or recessive, we can also classify them as nonlethal, sublethal, or lethal. A *sublethal* gene is one that causes death in childhood or before reproductive age is reached. Epiloia is caused by a dominant sublethal gene in man, and Tay-Sachs disease is caused by a recessive sublethal. A *lethal* gene does not permit survival of the embryo or the infant. Anencephaly in the human is a homozygous recessive lethal condition that is detectable as early as the third week of embryonic development. Much sterility and abortion in the human are probably caused by genetic change.

The preceding discussion might lead one to think that each character of an organism is determined by a single pair of genes. The opposite appears to be true in that many characters are undoubtedly the result of expression of several to many genes (*polygenic*) (e.g., height, weight, intelligence, and so on). Uncovering a mutation in a polygenic situation is difficult if not impossible in the absence of selective breeding. In man, therefore, mutations in the many polygenically determined characters will escape detection. The inheritance of more than 800 individual genes has been definitely worked out in man, and that of another 1000 genes tentatively defined. These figures, however, are small in view of the total number of gene pairs in a human cell, which is estimated to be many thousands.

5.2 GENE MUTATION

Mutation can be defined as an unusual permanent change in the primary structure of DNA or in the nuclear content of DNA. In general, a gene mutation involves a change in the primary structure and a chromosome mutation a change in the amount of DNA. Because the methods for detecting and analyzing the two types of mutation differ, they will be discussed separately.

In Mendelian terminology, a gene mutation is called a point mutation, a change in the hereditary material which is not microscopically detectable, but which results in an altered phenotype. Elucidation of the primary structure of DNA and of molecular details of gene expression has revealed some of the small changes in a DNA molecule that can cause gene mutation.

Data on the mutagenic effects in various organisms of nonionizing ultraviolet radiation and of chemicals demonstrate that small changes in DNA base composition or sequence, or both, are responsible for gene mutation. Definitive data on the effects of ionizing radiation at the level of the DNA molecule have only recently begun to appear. X-rays have been shown to produce breaks in one or both of the strands (backbone) of DNA (see Chapter 4), but the biologic significance of such breaks is not understood. It seems likely that effects on the bases are more important and are directly involved in the production of gene mutations.

The substitution, gain, or loss of one or more bases in a DNA molecule can cause gene mutation. Substitution can arise from mispairing of bases, that is, when a base does not pair with its usual base partner at replication. Mistakes in base pairing can be caused by ionization of bases (Figure 5-2A) and by tautomeric shifts* in the position of atoms (Figure 5-2B). The four common bases of DNA can all exist in tautomeric forms that represent single proton shifts. The usual or preponderant tautomer of A pairs with T, but an unusual tautomer of A can pair (mispair) with C. This unusual tautomer would, during replication of the DNA, cause the substitution of a C where a T should be in the newly synthesized DNA chain. During transcription of the resulting "mutant" triplet, RNA would be formed with G substituted for U. This could result in a *missense* codon (i.e., one that codes for a different amino acid) or a *nonsense* codon that codes for no amino acid. Either instance would be a mutation. If the codon that results is a *sense* codon (i.e., one that codes the same as before the change), there would be no evident mutation. The production of either a missense or a nonsense codon may cause a gene mutation. Examples are given in Table 5-2.

A striking example of a mutation that results from the substitution of only one base is the sickle-cell anemia gene. Sickle-cell hemoglobin differs from normal hemoglobin by a single amino acid substitution: glutamic acid is replaced by valine at the sixth residue position in the beta chain (there are 146 amino acids in each of the alpha and beta chains of hemoglobin). The mRNA base triplet GAA codes for glutamic acid and GUA codes for valine; thus, substitution of only one base in a DNA molecule (adenine substituted for thymine) can produce this mutation, which has severe effects.

Substitution can also be caused by base analogues, such as the halogenated pyrimi-

*Tautomerism is a form of stereoisomerism in which the compounds are interconvertible. It occurs under normal conditions and results in an equilibrium mixture of the compounds. The more frequent tautomers of thymine (T) and guanine (G) are the keto forms and of adenine (A) and cytosine (C), the amino forms. The enol and imine forms are rare.

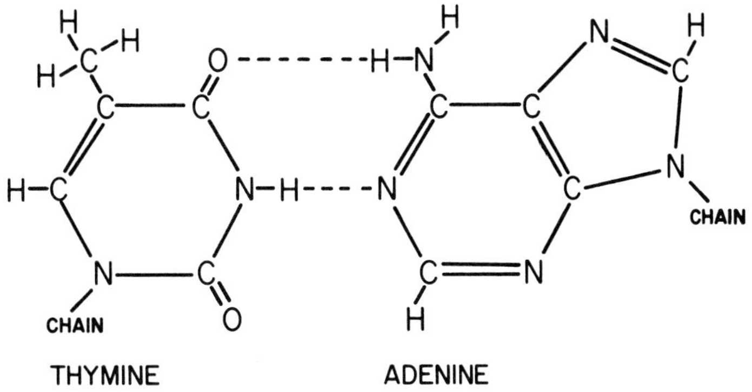

FIGURE 5–2A Ionization of a base in DNA can cause mispairing of the bases of DNA. Thymine normally pairs with adenine (*top*). If a proton is lost (−) from the 1-position of thymine, a keto tautomer is formed which will mispair with guanine. The dotted lines represent hydrogen bonds.

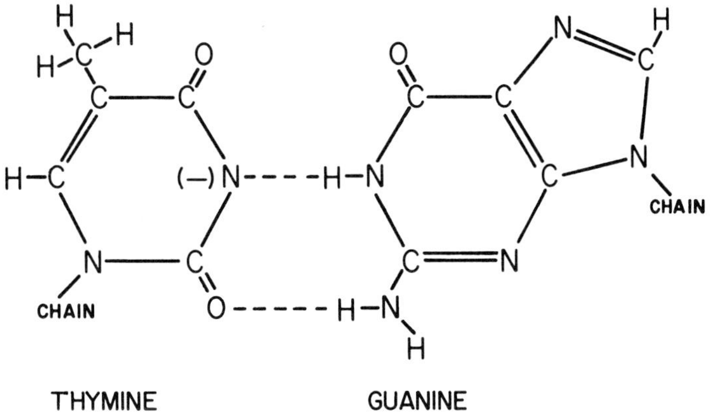

THYMINE   ADENINE

THYMINE   GUANINE

ADENINE

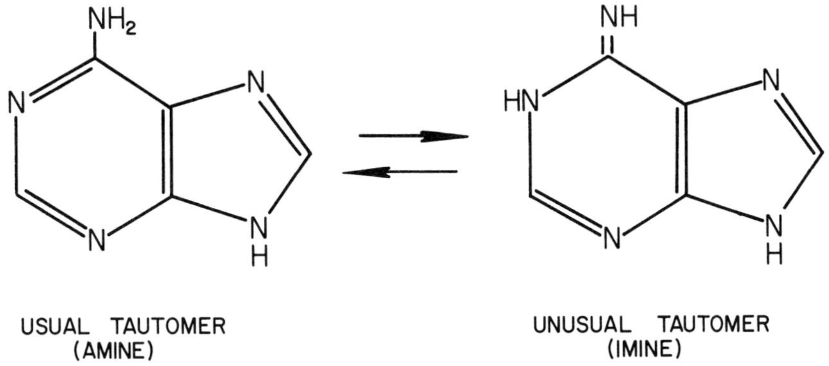

USUAL TAUTOMER
(AMINE)

UNUSUAL TAUTOMER
(IMINE)

FIGURE 5–2B Amine-imine tautomerism as exemplified by the two forms of adenine.

TABLE 5–2 EXAMPLE OF THE CONSEQUENCES OF THE SUBSTITUTION OF ONE OR OF TWO BASES IN THE DNA TRIPLET AAA

Code (Sequence of Bases) in DNA	Condon (Sequence of Bases) in Messenger RNA	Amino Acid	Type of Codon
AAA	UUU	phenylalanine	sense (normal)
AAC	UUG	phenylalanine	sense
ACA	UGU	cystine	missense
ATC	UAG	none	nonsense

dines which are incorporated into DNA. Such substitution, with its consequences for DNA replication and transcription, probably accounts, in part at least, for the increased sensitivity of analogue-containing cells to the lethal effects of radiation (see Chapter 4).

Rotational substitutions of bases occur if the bonds that connect a base pair to their sugars are broken and the pair rotates 180° with re-formation of bonds. This would lead to an incorrect base sequence in one triplet in each of the two strands of the DNA molecule affected.

X-radiation may cause the gain or loss of one or a few nucleotides, resulting in what is known as a *frameshift mutation*, in which the linear sequence of nucleotides is changed not only for the triplet containing the insertion or deletion but also for the successive triplets. The "frame" of reading is shifted (Figure 5–3) so that the triplets are different and may code for missense or nonsense codons. Thus, even though only one base may be involved initially, a frameshift mutation is more drastic than one resulting from a base substitution.

The mechanism for the acquisition or loss of nucleotides is not known, but a plausible hypothesis, which fits some of the data on identified frameshift mutations in microorganisms, has been proposed that invokes "misrepair." It states that during repair of a single-strand break, mispairing errors occur that lead to gain or loss of bases in the repaired strand, as diagramed in Figure 5–4.

READING FRAME SHIFTS

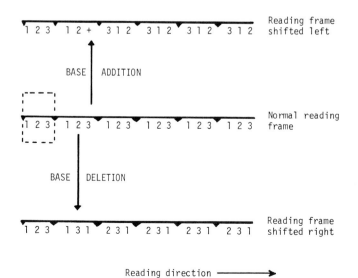

FIGURE 5–3 Frameshift mutation. The genetic code or information is the linear sequence of bases in the DNA. The DNA serves as the template that determines the linear sequence of bases in messenger RNA, which moves from the chromosome to the cytoplasm to direct protein synthesis. The "message" in messenger RNA consists of the sequential arrangement of units of three bases (codons), each of which "codes" for a specific amino acid. The linear sequence of codons in messenger RNA, therefore, determines the linear sequence of amino acids in the protein being synthesized. Successive triplets of bases are "read" through a "frame" (dotted). A frameshift mutation can occur if a single base is inserted or deleted in a DNA molecule. This causes the linear sequence of bases to be changed not only for the triplet directly affected but also for all successive triplets, as illustrated in the top and bottom lines of this figure. (Modified from Drake, J. W.: The Molecular Basis of Mutation. San Francisco, Holden-Day, 1970.)

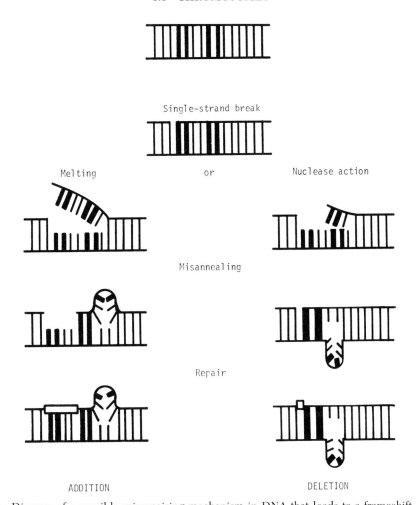

FIGURE 5–4 Diagram of a possible misrepairing mechanism in DNA that leads to a frameshift mutation. The horizontal lines represent the backbones of the molecule, the vertical lines the base pairs, the heavy bars identical (homologous) base pair sequences, and the horizontal open bars in the bottom line newly synthesized DNA.

A single-strand break in a DNA molecule causes localized breakage (melting) of the hydrogen bonds that hold the two strands together or in digestion (removal) of a short piece of the broken strand by an enzyme. If the homologous bases then mispair (misanneal, or form new hydrogen bonds) and the break is repaired by synthesis of new DNA, the repaired strand will now either have four additional bases or will have lost four bases. Either situation results in a frameshift mutation. (Modified from Drake, 1970.)

5.3 CHROMOSOMES

Unlike microorganisms, which have only one chromosome consisting of a single, circular DNA molecule, higher organisms have a number of chromosomes, each of which contains DNA, protein, and some RNA. The molecular organization of the chromosomes of higher organisms has not been worked out, but the genes are known to occur in a linear order along the length of each chromosome.

Major advances in human cytogenetics were made possible in 1960 with the devel-

opment of a technique for analyzing the metaphase chromosomes of the lymphocytes in peripheral blood. A few drops of blood are placed in appropriate culture medium containing phytohemagglutinin, which stimulates the lymphocytes to undergo cell division. When a large number of the lymphocytes begin to divide (about 60 to 70 hours after the beginning of culture), an alkaloid, colchicine, is added to the culture for several hours to disorganize the spindles in the cells at metaphase. Without a spindle the chromosomes cannot divide, and cell division is prevented. The

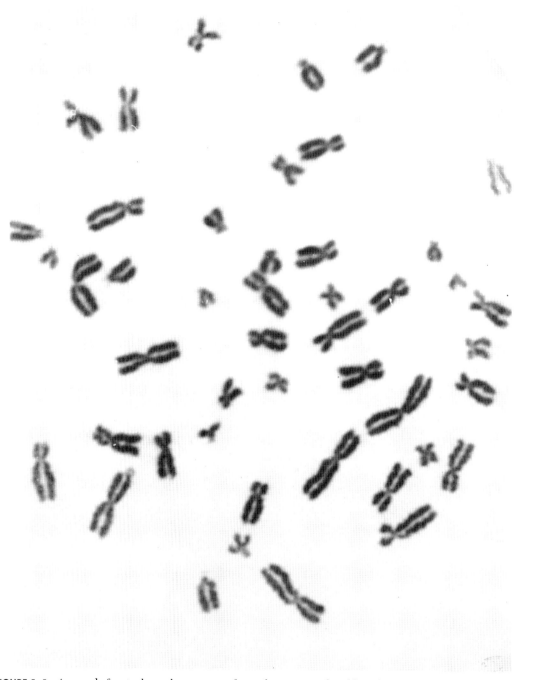

FIGURE 5–5 A spread of metaphase chromosomes from a human peripheral lymphocyte. The fixed cell is dropped onto an iced slide and dried immediately. This procedure causes the cell to break open, so that the chromosomes spread out and each one can be easily observed.

cells are then fixed and put on slides so that the individual chromosomes are spread out, as shown in Figure 5–5.

The morphology of a chromosome is shown in Figure 5–6. The terms in this figure are useful for distinguishing specific chromosomes. To prepare a *karyotype*, the chromosomes are cut out of a photograph and arranged in order of decreasing size, as shown in Figure 5–7. By international

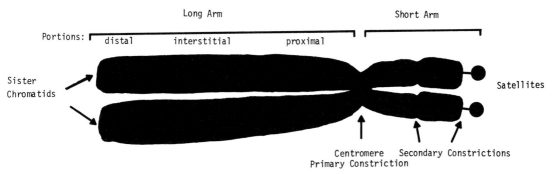

FIGURE 5-6 Morphology of a metaphase chromosome.

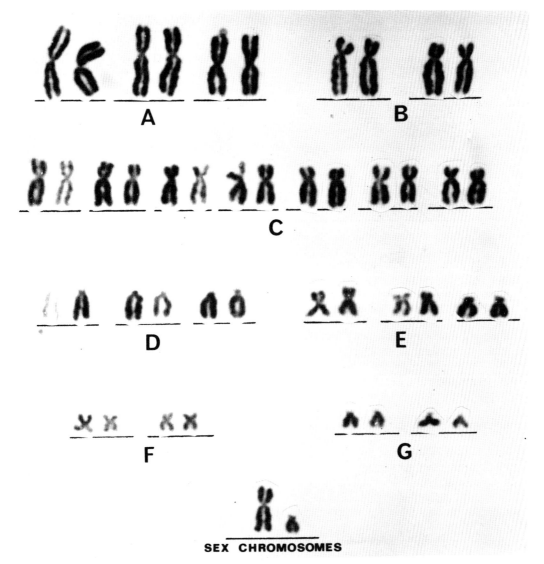

FIGURE 5-7 A karyotype prepared with the chromosomes shown in Figure 5–5. There are no chromosomal abnormalities. The 22 pairs of autosomal chromosomes can be referred to by number, the longest being number 1 and the smallest pairs 21 and 22. Of the sex chromosomes, the larger is the X and the smaller the Y. (The small sphere at the top of one of the third pair of chromosomes is debris.)

agreement, cytogeneticists arrange the human autosomes in seven general groups, designated A to G.

Identity of the chromosome pairs within some groups (e.g., the B and D groups) can be established arbitarily by their pattern of uptake of tritiated thymidine into DNA late in the S phase. The S (synthesis) phase is that part of the cell cycle in which the chromosomes are duplicating or replicating themselves (see Chapter 6). When the chromosomes are spread out on a slide, stained and covered with a photographic emulsion, the beta rays from each incorporated tritium atom will "expose" the emulsion directly above the chromosome. After development the changed individual grains in the very fine emulsion will be visible above each chromosome that contains radioactive thymidine. This type of preparation is called an *autoradiogram.* Because human chromosomal DNA is replicated in segments (replicons) at varying positions along the length of the chromosome (not in zipper fashion continuously from one end to the other) and because the order in which specific segments replicate is always the same, it is possible to identify the segments that are labeled near the end of the S phase. For example, chromosome five is labeled late in the S phase in its short arm, whereas chromosome four is labeled during the same period in the proximal portion of the long arm.

Recently, staining procedures have been developed that reveal "banding" patterns (light and dark staining regions) characteristic for each human chromosome. This is the most promising method yet devised for distinguishing the chromosomes within each group, for identifying mutant chromosomes, and for grossly locating known human genes.

5.4 MITOSIS AND MEIOSIS

The equal distribution of the genes at cell division to the two new daughter cells, which is vital for genetic continuity, is accomplished by the process of *mitosis.* In most mammalian cells mitosis occupies approximately 5 per cent of the total cell cycle (see Chapter 6). Four consecutive stages of mitosis can be defined on the basis of chromosome morphology and movement. *Prophase* begins when the chromosomes can first be recognized as slender double threads that gradually coil and thereby become condensed (Figure 5–8). At the beginning of *metaphase* the nuclear membrane disappears, and the chromosomes (at minimum size) move to the equator of a spindle to lie in one plane, called the metaphase "plate." Each chromosome is attached to the spindle at a specific locus, the centromere or spindle fiber attachment point. The spindle consists of many fibers, and those attached to chromosomes direct their movement. The cell enters *anaphase* when each centromere of the two chromosome halves (chromatids) begins to move to a pole of the spindle, pulling the rest of the chromatid with it. In this manner chromosome halves are distributed to opposite poles. At *telophase* the cleavage furrow forms in the plane of the spindle equator, dividing the cell in half (*cytokinesis*). The chromosomes decondense, and each daughter cell enters the intermitotic (*interphase*) period, during which the chromosomes replicate.

Meiosis (Figure 5–8) is the process by which the chromosome number is reduced by one-half in the production of germ cells. It requires two cell divisions and occurs only in the gonads. It ensures that the chromosome (gene) number of a species remains constant, each parent contributing half of the genetic material.

At the beginning of *prophase I* of meiosis the two homologues of each pair of chromosomes come together in close contact to form a *bivalent,* the genes on one chromosome pairing specifically by some unknown mechanism with their alleles on the homologous chromosome. Each chromosome has two chromatids, so a bivalent has four chromatids. At several points in a bivalent, one chromatid in each homologue breaks and the ends are exchanged, the result being genetic crossing-over and recombination between the two chromatids. For example, prior to pairing the sequence of genes in a segment of one homologue might be A B C D E and in the other homologue a b c d e. After crossing-over between the second and third genes, the sequence in the first homologue would be A B c d e and in the other a b C D E. This is the mechanism for gene interchange between homologues

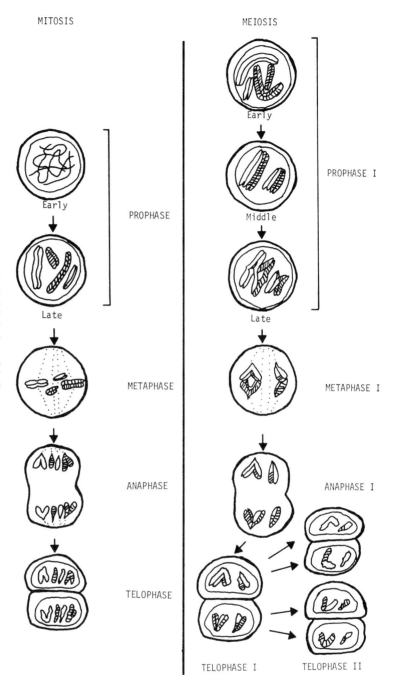

FIGURE 5-8 Diagram of chromosomal changes and distributions in mitosis and meiosis. For simplicity, only two pairs of chromosomes are shown. The cross-hatched chromosomes are from one parent and the open chromosomes from the other. For the second division of meiosis, the prophase, metaphase, and anaphase stages are omitted from the diagram.

that results in the great variety of genotypes in a population.

Subsequent to pairing and crossing-over, the homologues repel each other and are held together only where the chromatids are intertwined as a result of crossing-over. The chromosomes coil and contract until they are quite short by *metaphase I*, when they orient on the equator of the spindle.

At *anaphase I* the chromosomes (each with its two chromatids) of a bivalent go to opposite poles of the spindle; thus, the homologues of each chromosome pair are separated, and the two daughter cells have half the number of chromosomes of the mother cell. A short, incomplete interphase (no synthesis of DNA) is followed by the second division which is strictly mitotic in that the chromatids of each chromosome at *anaphase II* go to opposite poles. Thus, for example in man, meiosis provides for the distribution of the four chromatids of each of the 23 bivalents to four cells, each of which has one set of 23 chromosomes.

In summary, chromosome duplication in mitosis is followed by one cell division and in meiosis by two. Only in meiosis do the homologues pair and segregate into the two daughter cells, causing a reduction in chromosome number.

5.5 RADIATION-INDUCED GENE MUTATION IN MICE

Prior to the late 1940's most of our knowledge about the efficacy of radiation in producing mutations in higher organisms was limited to the fruit fly, *Drosophila.* After World War II, experiments were initiated at the Oak Ridge National Laboratory by Drs. W. L. and L. B. Russell to determine the mutagenic effects of ionizing radiation on the germ cells of mice. Thousands of animals were used, and the data obtained remain the best from which to extrapolate to man.

To detect radiation-induced mutations in the mouse a specific locus method was used. Seven specific dominant genes (loci) were selected that control recognizable phenotypic characters, such as coat color and patterns, and ear and tail defects. Mutations in these characters could be easily detected among the offspring. In addition, spontaneous mutation rates of these seven genes were known in the male mouse. Animals bred to be homozygous dominant for all seven genes were irradiated and mated at varying times after irradiation with unirradiated animals which were homozygous recessive for these genes (Figure 5–9). Those offspring that arose from a germ cell containing no radiation-induced mutation would show the dominant phenotype, whereas those arising from a germ cell carrying a mutation in one or several of the specific genes would show the recessive phenotype (most radiation-induced mutations are recessive).

Two of the genes studied, namely, short ear and dilute coat color, are very closely linked; that is, they are quite close together on the chromosome and crossing-over (see Section 5.4) between them does not occur. Thus, mutation in one of these and not in the other in an offspring is good evidence that gene, and not chromosome, mutations are being studied.

Because germ cells are produced from stem cells[*] at different times in the life cycle of the male and female mammal, and because the frequency of gene mutations varies with the cell type irradiated, radiation-induced mutations in the two sexes will be discussed separately.

---

[*]A stem cell is a progenitor cell that divides to produce one cell like itself and another cell that differentiates with or without further division.

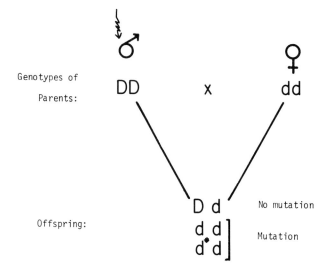

FIGURE 5–9 The specific locus method used for detecting radiation-induced recessive mutations in the first generation after irradiation. Illustrated is the situation when the male homozygous for the dominant gene (DD) for a given character is irradiated and mated with a female homozygous for the recessive gene (dd). Offspring with no mutation will have the dominant phenotype; those with a mutation will have the recessive phenotype.

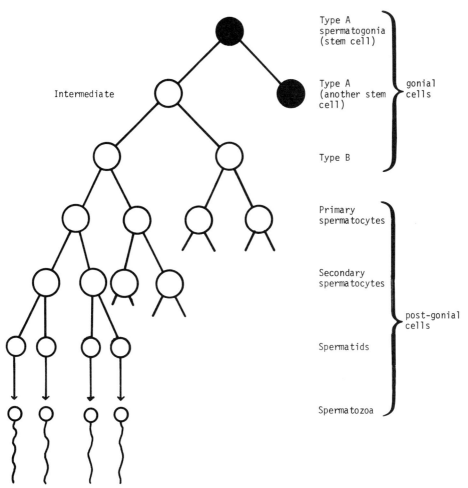

FIGURE 5–10   Cell types produced between division of a stem cell (solid) and production of mature sperm. In the mouse the time from the gonial division to mature sperm is about 6 weeks, in man about 10 weeks.

A. Germ Cell Production in the Male Mammal

The spermatozoa arise from the germinal epithelium in the seminiferous tubules of the testes, and their production in the mammal is continuous from puberty until death. Figure 5–10 shows the sequential cell types that occur in the mouse and human testes. The time required from the division of a gonial (stem) cell to the production of a mature sperm in the mouse is about six weeks and in the human about ten weeks.

Some of the gonial cells are quite sensitive to the lethal effects of radiation. The type A spermatogonia evidently comprise at least two populations of cells. One consists of the stem cells, which are relatively resistant to the lethal effects of radiation and can withstand exposures of 100 to 1000 R. The other population, which is the pro-

liferating and differentiating group, is quite sensitive, as are the intermediate and Type B spermatogonia. The LD_{50}* of these sensitive cells is in the range of 20 to 25 R; the lethal effects of 3 R can be readily detected. Thus some progenitor cells of sperm are killed by a very low dose of X-rays.

The effects of radiation on fertility are not immediately apparent because the post-gonial cells are relatively resistant to the lethal effects of radiation. After exposure to moderate or even high doses, there is an initial fertile period followed by decreased fertility or temporary sterility, the length of this latter period depending on dose and on the proportion of the stem cell (gonial) population that is killed. Temporary aspermia in the mouse is produced by exposures

---

*LD_{50} is the dose lethal to 50 per cent of the cells.

of about 300 R, and permanent sterility occurs only after doses of over 1000 R.

Much the same response to radiation is observed in the human testis. A group of human volunteers (prisoners) received 8 R to 600 R to the testes and were later vasectomized. Weekly sperm counts and biopsies were made for one year before and up to three years after irradiation. Data on these individuals plus observations on radiotherapy patients and radiation accident victims can be summarized as follows: Low doses (8 to 50 R) kill some type A and B spermatogonia and cause a reduction in sperm count. For example, 25 rads (acute) cause about a 30 per cent reduction in sperm count, first detectable six weeks after exposure; recovery occurs at about 40 weeks. A dose of 50 rads may result in a short period of temporary sterility. Medium doses (100 to 300 rads) kill not only some type A and B gonial cells but also some spermatocytes. Recovery from aspermia is slow. High doses (400 to 600 rads) cause a quick decline in sperm count with prolonged aspermia and retarded recovery over periods of months. Obvious damage to some gonia and spermatocytes can be observed as early as four hours after irradiation. Temporary aspermia at nine to ten months after exposure has been reported in radiation accident victims who received about 200 R to the groin; complete recovery was effected at about 20 months. A dose of about 250 rads may cause temporary sterility for one to two years; an acute dose of about 600 rads or fractioned doses totaling about 1500 rads over 10 days will induce permanent sterility in many males. Contrary to popular belief, sterility in the human male does not produce significant changes in hormone balance, libido or physical capability. In general, there is a slower initial rate of the decrease in the number of human gonia, but cellular degeneration persists longer and recovery of sperm counts is much later than in the mouse. The human data, therefore, parallel the mouse data except for the time scale.

B. Gene Mutation Induction in the Male Mammal

The data on the male mouse can be summarized as follows:

A. The number of mutations induced by a given dose of radiation varies with the cell stage at the time of exposure. Mutation frequency induced in the post-gonial cells (Figure 5–10) is twice that in the gonial cells. This was determined by varying the time between irradiation and mating; for example, the offspring of irradiated males mated six weeks after irradiation would arise from sperm that were Type A spermatogonia at the time of irradiation.

Post-gonial cells are short-lived, so the gonial cells are the more important ones from the standpoint of human fertility and genetic hazards. Because the highest mutation frequency occurs in the post-gonial cells, males should be advised to refrain from procreation during the first few months after radiation exposure. This will reduce, but *not* eliminate, the number of mutations transmitted to the offspring.

B. The average mutation frequency in the mouse is 15 times higher than had been reported in *Drosophila,* so extrapolation from mouse to man indicates greater human radiation genetic hazards than had been expected on the basis of extrapolation from the fruit fly to man.

C. There is no evidence that spermatogonia containing an induced gene mutation are less viable than those that do not contain a mutation. It was observed that in offspring derived from irradiated gonia, there is no change in mutation frequency with increasing time between irradiation and mating up to two years (normal mouse lifespan). Thus, mutations induced in a stem cell will be propagated throughout the remainder of a male mammal's life.

D. There is a differential mutation rate (calculated as the number of mutations per locus per gamete) for different loci; that is, some genes are either more susceptible to mutation or are able to undergo less recovery from radiation damage than are other genes. The mutation rate varied by a factor of 30 between the locus with the highest rate and the one with the lowest rate. It was also observed that the *relative* mutation rates for two loci may vary with sex and cell type at the time of irradiation, but do not vary with exposure rate between 1000 R per min and 0.001 R per min.

It should be noted that the spontaneous mutation rates for the different specific loci do not vary in the same manner as radiation-induced rates. In fact, data on 7 million mice show a reverse rank order for four of the loci (i.e., the gene with the highest radiation-induced rate has the lowest spontaneous rate). In other words, knowing the mutation rate of a gene under one condition does not enable us to predict the rate under another condition.

E. Breeding of offspring derived from irradiated males showed that radiation-induced mutations have predominately severe effects: three-fourths of the mutations are lethal in the homozygous condition and most of them are deleterious in the heterozygous condition. Therefore, a radiation-induced recessive mutation may have an undesirable effect in the first-generation offspring of irradiated parents.

F. At a given dose the mutation frequency is lower at low exposure rates than at high ones. Five exposure rates were used: 90, 9, 0.8, 0.009, and 0.001 R per min. At rates of 0.8 R per min or lower the mutation frequency was one-fourth to one-third that observed after the higher exposure rates. This is a highly significant difference. The decreased number of radiation-induced mutations at the lower exposure rates is observed only when the offspring arise from cells irradiated as spermatocytes or gonial cells; there is no exposure-rate effect when spermatozoa are irradiated.

These effects can be interpreted to mean that at low exposure rates there is some repair of radiation damage to DNA, but there appears to be a certain level or a certain type of injury that is not reparable, because even at the lowest exposure rate

(0.001 R per min) some mutations are observed.*

The exposure rate experiments with male mice were done with relatively high total doses (300 rads or more). It is possible, therefore, that at low doses some repair of mutations might occur even with high exposure rates. This idea has been tested and the number of mutations has been found to remain strictly proportional to dose down to 37 R, the lowest dose used.

C. Germ Cell Production in the Female Mammal

In the female mammal the production of mature germ cells follows a different time course than in the male. The cell types and the production of a mature ovum are shown in Figure 5-11. All cells in the oogonial stages progress to the oocyte stage in the embryo. By three days after birth all of the oocytes of the mouse and the human are in a resting stage, so there is no cell division. In the adult, therefore, there are no stem (oogonial) cells, but there are three types of follicles: mature, nearly mature, and immature. The three polar bodies produced with the ovum degenerate and are of no biologic significance.

A dose of about 50 rads causes permanent sterility in the female mouse. This results from lethal effects on cells in the immature

---

*The exposure rate used in diagnostic radiology differs with the procedure; for example, the average exposure rate for fluoroscopy is low, 4 R/min (to skin), but for radiography is high, 240 R/min.

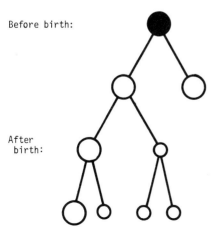

Before birth: — Oogonial cell

Primary oocyte - resting (Immature follicle)
(Nearly mature follicle--oocyte has begun meiosis)

Secondary oocyte and polar body (Mature follicle) Sec. oocyte completes division on fertilization (In human, this division starts at ovulation)

After birth:

Ovum and 3 polar bodies (In human, this division is completed in the tube)

FIGURE 5-11 Oogenesis in the mouse.

follicle stage. In the human female a single dose of 50 rads to the ovaries will cause temporary sterility in some individuals. An acute dose of about 400 rads or a fractionated dose of about 1500 rads (over 10 days) will induce permanent sterility in most women. Radiation-induced sterilization of women induces pronounced hormonal changes comparable to those occurring at natural menopause.

D. Gene Mutation Induction in the Female Mammal

The data obtained with mouse oocytes revealed that their mutational response to radiation differs from that of spermatogonia in three respects:

(1) The decrease in frequency of mutations with increasing time between irradiation and mating approaches the near zero level. The first and second litters (early mating period) after irradiation were derived from ova exposed in the mature and nearly mature follicle stages, respectively. The mutation frequency was very high. All subsequent litters (late mating period) were derived from ova exposed in the immature follicle stage. In these the mutation frequency was extremely low; in fact, it was probably not significantly higher than the spontaneous mutation frequency in the male (spontaneous frequency in the female has not been precisely determined for all seven specific loci).

(2) Oocytes in mature or nearly mature follicles showed a reduced mutation frequency with reduction in exposure rate, from 90 to 0.8 R per min, that was comparable to that found with spermatogonia. But, unlike spermatogonia, oocytes exhibited a further lowering of mutation frequency when the exposure rate was reduced to 0.009 R per min.

(3) The frequency of mutations detected in the early mating period is less after small doses (50 rads) of high exposure rate radiation than after moderate to high doses. In other words, in contrast to the male, there appears to be some repair of mutations in the female at low doses, which may be comparable to mutational repair mechanisms described in microorganisms.

In summary, the data on the mouse indicate that offspring conceived soon after irradiation of either the male or female parent have more mutations than later conceptuses. If extrapolation from mouse to man is justifiable, men and women should be advised to avoid procreating during the first few months after exposure of the gonads to diagnostic radiation. After this initial post-irradiation period fewer radiation-induced mutations are passed on to offspring by the female than by the male. The most likely explanation for this at present is that the oocytes of the female are either more efficient in repairing damage or are less sensitive to the induction of damage than are the male germ cells. Men and women whose gonads are exposed to high doses during radiotherapy would be well-advised to avoid procreation at any time in the future.

It should be pointed out that the mouse data were obtained from mature animals. The oogonia and oocytes of the female fetus are comparable to the germ cell stages found in the mature male. The radiation-induced mutation frequency in the female fetus, therefore, may be quite different from that in the mature female. Because the frequency may be relatively high, as is the case in the mature male, irradiation of the human fetus should be avoided whenever possible for this reason, as well as for others.

5.6 CHROMOSOME MUTATION

A change in the number of whole chromosomes, which alters the amount of DNA, and the production of one or more breaks in a chromosome, which alters the amount of DNA, the linear sequence of genes, or both, are called *chromosome mutations*. Strictly speaking, small alterations in the number or sequence of nucleotides in a short segment of DNA are chromosome mutations, but the use of the term will be limited to those gross changes that can be analyzed with the light microscope.

A. Changes in the Number of Whole Chromosomes

Euploidy or polyploidy. This condition results from an increase in the number of whole sets of chromosomes, a set being equal to the number found in a gamete (*haploid*), which is 23 in man. A zygote contains two homologous sets of chromosomes, or the *diploid* number. A change in the number of chromosome sets can result from destruction of the spindle or prevention of cleavage furrow formation so that cell division does not follow mitosis. It can also result from *endoreplication,* a duplication of the chromosomes that is not followed by mitosis and cell division. Radiation-induced polyploidy is probably for the most part a secondary effect resulting from those chromosome aberrations (e.g., dicentrics) that make impossible the separation of chromosomes at anaphase.

The more common types of polyploidy are triploidy (three sets) and tetraploidy (four sets). Euploidy in every cell of the body is not a viable human condition. A small per cent of spontaneous abortuses are triploid and probably arise from union of one haploid and one diploid gamete. Rarely, a triploid full-term infant is born; it does not live long. An occasional individual has been reported to be mosaic for diploid and either triploid or tetraploid cells. Euploidy is most commonly observed in tumors, and it ranges from triploidy to many multiples of 23. Single cells in carcinoma of the colon have been reported to have as many as 2000 chromosomes.

Aneuploidy. Aneuploidy is a change in the number of one or more specific chromosomes of a set.

Hypodiploid cells have less than the diploid number of chromosomes. A *nullisomic* cell is one in which both members of a pair of chromosomes are absent. In a *monosomic* cell or organism one member of a pair of chromosomes is missing. The majority of patients with Turner's syndrome (phenotypic females with streak gonads) are monosomic for the sex chromosome (i.e., they are XO instead of XX).

A *hyperdiploid* cell or organism has one or more additional chromosomes, the most common type being trisomy, or one extra chromosome. Individuals with Down's syndrome or mongolism are *trisomic* for chromosome 21 — they have three members of chromosome 21 instead of the usual two. Some mongoloids have two normal chromosomes 21 and the additional genes of chromosome 21 are represented in a translocation, which is discussed later, to another chromosome. There is evidence that some males with an extra Y chromosome (XYY)

tend to be antisocial. In several court cases, lawyers have contended that such individuals, on trial for murder, were not mentally fit to be tried because of their extra Y chromosome. A *tetrasomic* cell or organism contains an extra pair of chromosomes, for example, the XXYY individuals with Klinefelter's syndrome.

Aneuploidy arises from *nondisjunction* of chromosomes at anaphase, which causes both sister chromatids to go to the same cell rather than one to each daughter cell. Nondisjunction during somatic cell division results in one trisomic cell and one monosomic cell for the chromosome affected. Nondisjunction at meiosis results in varying degrees of aneuploidy in the gametes, the exact change depending on whether one or both of the meiotic divisions are involved. An individual derived from such a gamete will be uniformly aneuploid. Nondisjunction during embryogenesis gives rise to a *mosaic* individual, some cells or tissues being normal and some aneuploid. The severity of the clinical manifestations is generally related to the types of tissues and the number of cells that are aneuploid. A number of individuals have been reported to be mosaic for varying numbers of sex chromosomes. Aneuploidy is found in 20 to 50 per cent of spontaneous abortuses, with XO monosomy and trisomy of chromosome 16 being among the more common abnormalities. Mosaics constitute about 20 per cent of abortuses that are visibly abnormal.

Nondisjunction is induced by radiation in experimental animals, but only after exposures of about 100 R or more. Preconceptual exposure of humans to diagnostic radiation has been implicated, but certainly not proved, as a cause of aneuploidy in offspring.

B. Chromosome Breaks

Chromosome mutations that involve gross structural changes (also called aberrations, anomalies or lesions) arise when radiation breaks a chromosome at one or more points along its length. A break can result in a change in the number of genes (and consequently, the amount of DNA) in the cell, or in the linear sequence of genes, or both. This type of break at present cannot be equated with the DNA strand breakage discussed in Chapter 4.

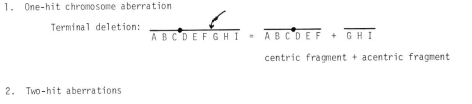

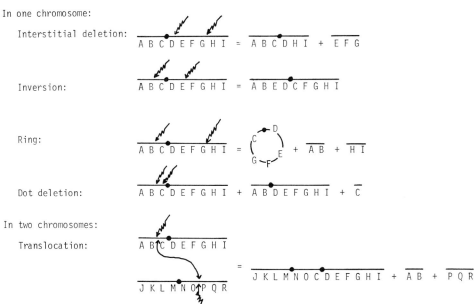

FIGURE 5–12 Some typical chromosome mutations. The dot (●) represents the centromere, the letters individual genes, and the jagged arrows the points of radiation-induced breaks in the chromosomes.

The broken ends of a chromosome may rejoin (restitute) so that no lesion results, or they may heal without rejoining, or they may join with broken ends of other chromosomes. A broken end can only join with another broken end and *not* with a normal unbroken end. It is estimated that approximately 90 per cent of individual chromosome breaks restitute so that recovery is complete and no lesion is formed.

A *chromosome break* occurs when both chromatids (see Figure 5–12) are broken at the same locus (also called isochromatid break); they may be induced by breakage before or after chromosome replication. *Chromatid breaks* involve only one chromatid and occur when the cell is irradiated after replication.

A chromosome that differs from the normal chromosomes as a result of gross structural changes and that is found in many cells is referred to as a *marker* chromosome. A number of neoplasms have been reported with distinctive marker chromosomes,

which suggests that each tumor arose from a single cell. Some of the more common types of chromosome mutations are described in the following paragraphs. They are classified on the basis of the number of breaks in one or two chromosomes (Figure 5–12).

Single-Break or One-Hit Aberrations. A *terminal deletion* occurs when the two ends of a break heal separately, a centric and an acentric fragment being produced. Because the *centric fragment* contains a centromere, it will move to a pole of the spindle during cell division along with the other unbroken chromosomes and, therefore, will be included in a daughter nucleus. The *acentric fragment* usually remains in the cytoplasm and is eventually resorbed. Thus, a block of genes is deleted, leading to a deficiency or loss in the amount of DNA in one nucleus, in the case of a chromatid, and in both nuclei, in the case of a chromosome deletion. If vital genes are contained in an acentric fragment, produced by terminal deletion or by other types of chromosome change described in this and the next section, the mutation will probably be lethal only if the cell divides and the genes are lost to a nucleus. This is the basis of the Law of Bergonie and Tribondeau, set forth in 1906, which states that dividing cells are more radiosensitive than nondividing cells. It accounts in part for the fact that the embryo and fetus are more susceptible than adults to radiation, which may also be the case for some tissues in young children. It should be noted that there are exceptions to the "Law," one of which is the small lymphocyte that is radiosensitive but does not usually divide. The production and loss at mitosis of acentric fragments are evidently involved in the killing of some tumor cells by therapeutic doses of radiation. Some investigators have reported that in squamous cell carcinoma of the uterine cervix, reliable prediction of tumor response to radiation can be made by determining the chromosome mutation frequency in a biopsy taken after an initial exposure to 500 R. Presence or absence of mutations indicates that tumors will be sensitive or resistant, respectively, to the therapy.

Almost 90 per cent of patients with chronic myelogenous leukemia (CML) have an identifiable terminal deletion of half of the long arm of one G chromosome in cells of blood and bone marrow, but not in other tissues. This mutation, the "Philadelphia" (Ph[1]) chromosome, named for the place of its discovery, is used for diagnosing CML, the only human neoplasm now known to be associated with a *consistent* chromosome mutation. The genes responsible for maintaining control of leukopoiesis are thought to be located in the deleted portion. A small proportion of CML patients lack the chromosome mutation, but their disorder represents a different clinical entity — for example, their median survival time is much shorter and their white blood cell and platelet counts are lower than in patients with the chromosome mutation; their response to chemical therapy is poor. Such patients possibly have gene mutations in both chromosomes in the segment that is missing in the one Ph[1] chromosome and perhaps in other chromosomes as well.

Two-Break or Two-Hit Aberrations In One Chromosome. *Interstitial deletion* results when there is loss of the chromosome seg-ment between two breaks. The end result of this type of two-hit aberration cannot be unequivocally distinguished from a terminal deletion resulting from one break unless analysis for the missing genes or missing stained chromosome bands (see Section 5.3) can be made.

An *inversion* occurs when the chromosome segment between two breaks is turned end for end and rejoining occurs to give a rearrangement of genes. An inversion may have no detrimental effect on a somatic cell if the changes in base sequences are not vital. During meiosis, however, an inversion will result in abnormal pairing of the chromosomes which may lead to genetically unbalanced gametes. This type of mutation can be identified in man if distinctly staining chromosome bands are involved.

An inversion that includes the centromere is called pericentric; one that does not include the centromere is paracentric.

Ring chromosomes are formed when the two broken ends of a chromosome join with each other. If the ring does not contain a centromere, it is lost as any other acentric fragment. A centric ring is usually an *unstable* aberration; its formation always results in the loss of those genes in the two acentric fragments; interlocking of replicated rings, making their separation impossible and leading to their loss, may occur. Rings can, however, be stable aberrations; a few individuals have been reported with a ring chromosome, usually chromosome 13. The mental deficiency evident in such individuals probably reflects the loss of those genes in the acentric fragments.

A *dot deletion* is produced when two breaks are quite close together so that only a minute portion of the chromosome is deleted. It can be a one-hit phenomenon when a photon passes through a sharp turn in a chromosome. Unequivocal identification of a dot deletion is impossible in man. The cell will be hemizygous for the undeleted genes in the other chromosome of the pair; if they are recessive, they will be expressed.

An unstained segment between two aligned portions of a chromosome, as seen with the light microscope, is called a *gap*. That a portion of the chromosome has not been deleted can be inferred from the fact that gaps are not accompanied by acentric fragments. Electron microscopy has revealed that a thread of material connects the two chromatid segments on either side of the gap. Thus, a gap might be viewed as an exaggerated secondary constriction. The nature of this type of abnormality is not known, but its frequency has been shown in experimental organisms to increase linearly with dose of radiation, which suggests that it is a one-hit phenomenon. The presence of gaps at specific loci in some chromosomes is heritable; whether they are originally induced by radiation cannot be determined. Members of seven generations of one family have been described with a large gap in the long arm of chromosome 16, which is inherited in a Mendelian dominant manner.

Two-Break or Two-Hit Aberrations In Two Chromosomes.   Two breaks, one in each of two chromosomes, that are followed by joining of the different broken ends result in a *translocation* (interchange) of genes from one chromosome to another. In the case of a reciprocal translocation between two nonhomologous chromosomes, no genes are lost from the cell; only the linear order of some genes is changed. When no detectable effects of such a translocation are observed, it is said to be *balanced.* This type of chromosome mutation will cause no difficulties during ordinary cell division, but can lead to abnormal pairing patterns during meiosis and thereby to defective germ cells that may not be viable. There are individuals who have been described with identifiable balanced translocations who are unable to conceive.

When a centric fragment is translocated to another centric fragment, a single *dicentric* chromosome and two acentric fragments are formed. If the two centromeres of the dicentric go to opposite poles at anaphase, they will be connected at the point of union, forming a *bridge.* At cytokinesis the bridge is usually broken at some point (not necessarily at the point of union), causing a genic imbalance in addition to that caused by loss of the acentric fragments. If both centromeres of a dicentric move to the same pole at cell division, the mutation will be stable until the centromeres of the dicentric move to opposite poles at some subsequent division. When a dicentric moves into one daughter cell,

there will also be genic imbalance in both daughter cells, extra genes in one and deficiency for those genes in the other cell.

In addition to the chromosome breakage discussed above, radiation can also induce the phenomenon of *chromosome stickiness* when cells are irradiated just before or during metaphase with doses of about 100 rads or more. The nature of this so-called "physiological" effect is not understood, but it appears to be a surface effect that causes individual chromosomes to stick together and form clumps, the degree of stickiness being roughly proportional to dose. At anaphase numerous bridges are formed which lead to simultaneous breakage of many chromosomes and unequal distribution of genes in the daughter nuclei.

For convenience, gene and chromosome mutations have been discussed as separate entities, but both types of mutation can occur in the same cell at the same time. The frequency of viable gene mutations is greater than the frequency of viable chromosome mutations in *Drosophila*, the only higher organism in which their relative frequencies have been tested. This is to be expected because a chromosome mutation usually involves a number of genes. In this connection, it is of interest that approximately half of spontaneous abortuses contain chromosome mutations, whereas only about 2 per cent of induced abortuses have them. The agent responsible for these mutations is not known, but it is possible that medical radiation induces some of them.

5.7   RELATION OF MUTATION FREQUENCY TO RADIATION DOSE

In all higher organisms that have been studied, the number of detectable gene mutations increases linearly with increasing dose, with the possible exception noted in female mice. There is no evidence for a threshold dose; even very low doses—in the one rad range—can induce mutations, although the number will be quite small. Thus, we are justified in assuming that the doses of radiation used for diagnosis can induce mutations. It is estimated that in man one R of X-radiation induces an average of one gene mutation in every 500 gametes, which is about 1/70 of the *total* detectable spontaneous mutation rate. This rate cannot be ignored.

The dose-effect relation of chromosome mutations differs for one- and two-hit breaks (each break apparently being produced by one photon) (Figure 5–13A, B). At low exposures only one-hit breaks are observed and their frequency bears a linear relation to dose. There is no threshold dose for the induction of single breaks by X-rays, the lowest dose used with human lymphocytes being five rads and with experimental organisms one rad. In human lymphocytes one rad doubles the frequency of chromosome mutations that occur spontaneously. Exposure rate does not affect single-break frequency.

Two-hit aberrations are the result of two single hits which must occur close together in space and time. One would expect, therefore, to find more two-hit aberrations after a high dose than after a low dose and to ob-

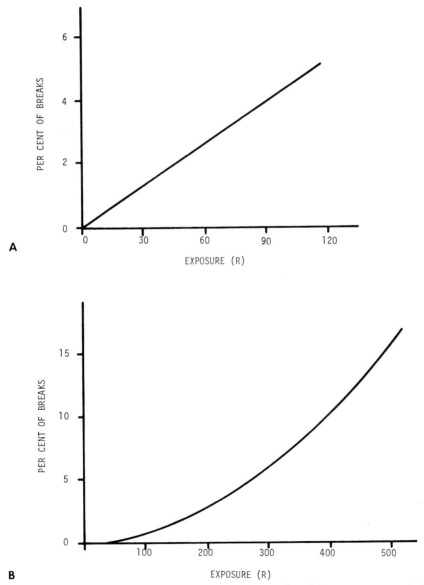

FIGURE 5–13 Dose-effect relations of chromosome mutations induced by X-rays. *A*, Single-hit chromosome break frequency in grasshopper neuroblasts. *B*, Two-hit chromosome break frequency in *Tradescantia* microspores. (Modified from Casarett, A. P.: Radiation Biology. Englewood Cliffs, N.J., Prentice-Hall, 1968.)

serve a threshold dose for the production of two-hit chromosome mutations. This is generally true, and the frequency of two-hit breaks increases more rapidly than a single power of the dose (about 1.7 power) (Figure 5–13B). Exceptions would include dot deletions, discussed earlier. Also, recent data obtained with *Drosophila* indicate that low exposures of X-rays (10 R) to sperm induce about one and one-half times more chromosomal rearrangements (two-hit breaks) than occur spontaneously, and the frequency of translocations in human lymphocytes exposed to a few rads of X-rays suggests that one-hit kinetics may be involved in the production of these two-break aberrations.

5.8 CHROMOSOME MUTATION IN MAN

It is impossible to determine the frequency of gene mutations induced in the germ cells of man by diagnostic radiation. The frequency of chromosome mutations, however, can be obtained with the peripheral blood technique described on page 59. This provides some idea of the magnitude of radiation effects on the genetic system in the human. The available data are not extensive, but they indicate that real and significant cytogenetic effects of low doses of radiation, such as are encountered in diagnostic radiology, can be demonstrated in man. It should be noted that viruses and some medications can temporarily increase the frequency of chromosome mutations in peripheral lymphocytes, so data on radiation-induced mutations must be obtained in the absence of such factors. All of the data discussed in the following section were obtained with peripheral lymphocytes.

A. Patients Receiving Diagnostic X-rays

Blood samples taken immediately after, and at varying intervals up to several months after, exposure of patients to several types of diagnostic X-rays have been examined for chromosome mutations. When skin exposures were 20 mR to 3R (chest films and intravenous pyelograms) no mutations were observed. After 4 to 12 R (cardiac catheterization) fragments and gaps were observed; after 12 to 35 R (upper GI series

and barium enema) chromosome fragments, dicentrics, and ring chromosomes were observed.

B. Radioactive Isotopes

Isotopes may be potentially quite hazardous because of their localization in cells. Radioactive iodine (^{131}I) is widely used to treat thyrotoxicosis. A patient who has a 30-g gland with 60 per cent uptake and who is treated with 5 mCi of ^{131}I by mouth will receive the following average tissue doses: five rads whole body, 9000 to 10,000 rads thyroid gland, 2 to 5 rads hemopoietic tissue, and about 1 rad to the testes or 2 rads to the ovary. None of these doses is genetically insignificant to the patient, and that to the germ cells may be of consequence to future generations.

It has been shown that in patients receiving 5 mCi of ^{131}I by mouth, about 6 per cent of the peripheral lymphocytes two hours later had chromosome aberrations and about 5 per cent one year later; in the control subjects there were aberrations in only 0.7 per cent of the lymphocytes.

Therapeutic doses of ^{131}I used to treat thyroid carcinoma are capable of inducing sterility in the human female. The effects of intraperitoneal injection of ^{131}I (0.2 to 0.7 μCi) on offspring have been studied in mice. It was found that when such males were mated to untreated females, the number of dead embryos was significantly increased over that from matings with untreated males. These data indicate that ^{131}I induced lethal gene or chromosome mutations in the male germ cells or their stem cells. Even though intraperitoneal injection is not used medically, the dose levels in these experiments were much less than those used by the oral or intravenous routes for diagnostic medical purposes.

Administration of the isotope to pregnant women should be avoided. ^{131}I has been found to be concentrated in an 18 week old fetus and in its immature Graafian follicles, making possible genetic effects in the oogonia and oocytes.

C. Radiology Personnel

Chromosome mutation frequency has been found to be significantly increased in radiotherapy nurses who received a total dose of 63 to 116 rads over a period of ten years. Several studies have been made on radiologists and most of them reveal significant increases in chromosome mutation frequency. It is usually impossible to estimate, much less determine, the amount of radiation these professional individuals have received; film badge records are in-adequate because badges are not always worn routinely. The author has found that, in general, the number of cells with chromosome mutations is increased in those individuals with a number of years of occupational exposure to radiation. Figure 5–14 is a karyotype of a cell from one radiologist whose lymphocytes had a number of chromosome mutations.

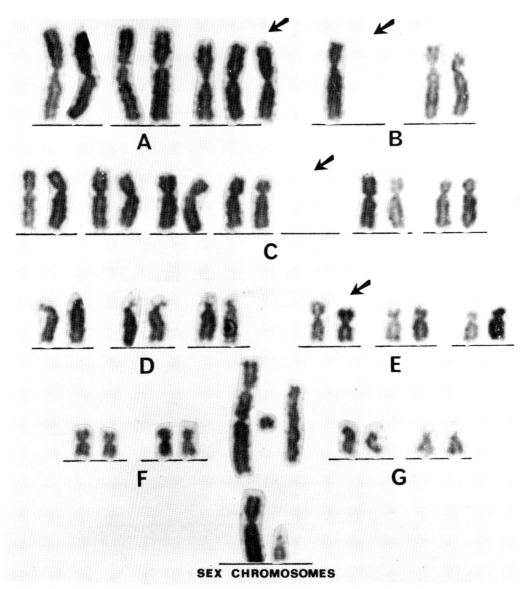

SEX CHROMOSOMES

FIGURE 5–14 Karyotype of a lymphocyte from a diagnostic radiologist who has been practicing for a number of years. Note that chromosome 3 is trisomic, 4 is monosomic, 10 is nullisomic and 16 is "mismatched" (probably normal). Between the F and G groups are a dicentric chromosome and two acentric chromosome fragments. Seven per cent of this individual's peripheral lymphocytes had one or more chromosome mutations; 2 per cent of the cells from the matched control subject (not occupationally exposed to radiation) had mutations, most of which were of a less drastic nature than those in the radiologist (e.g., no dicentric chromosomes). The dot and circle over the far right D chromosome are debris.

D. Nuclear Installation Workers

That very low levels of exposure over a long period of time can significantly increase the number of chromosome mutations has been shown by studies on radiation workers at a nuclear installation. Rigid observance of safety precautions and the routine use of personal monitoring devices by these workers provided reliable exposure records; it was estimated from these records that they received an average dose of about 1.4 R per year over a 15-year period. The number of chromosome aberrations observed was significantly greater than in a group of individuals who had not worked with radiation.

5.9　IMPLICATIONS FOR MAN

A. Significance of Mutations in Lymphocytes

Analysis of chromosome mutations in peripheral lymphocytes is the easiest method yet devised to examine the effects of low doses of radiation on man *in vivo* and *in vitro*. Their main significance lies in the fact that they serve as an *index* to the frequency of gene and chromosome mutations (equal numbers produced by low doses) that one might expect to occur in other cells in the body. Approximately 95 to 99 per cent of the skin dose received in diagnostic X-radiation is absorbed by the body. Therefore, if the frequency of chromosome mutations observed in lymphocytes is much above the normal level (1 to 3 per cent), it might be expected that some mutations would also be present in the stem cells in the bone marrow.

What relation does the frequency of chromosome mutations found in lymphocytes bear to an individual's future health? The answer to this question must await further research on the correlation of mutation frequency and the incidence of specific biologic effects of radiation—for example, neoplasia, as determined in defined human populations by epidemiological methods. In the meantime, several relevant points should be kept in mind. Evidence is accumulating that radiation workers, including radiologists, have higher than normal frequencies of chromosome mutations. There is little doubt that the cause of

neoplasia is directly related to malfunctioning DNA, one aspect of which is mutation (another is the derepression of those genes controlling cell growth). In mice the lowest dose tested (10 R) has been shown to increase the incidence of leukemia. A cause-effect relation has been strongly invoked for a terminal chromosome deletion and chronic myelogenous leukemia in man, a type of mutation that could be induced by as little as one R of X-rays. Among the Japanese survivors of the atomic bomb explosions there still exists, over 25 years later, an increased risk of leukemia as compared to their unirradiated controls. This is true even for those individuals exposed to less than 50 rads, which suggests that there may be no threshold dose. These data are complicated by a neutron component in the radiation, but they give us pause in view of the fact that despite increased radiation safety practices, radiologists, dermatologists, and urologists suffer a disproportionately large number of leukemia deaths as compared with other medical specialists, and especially as compared with the general population.

In mice a direct correlation between frequency of chromosome mutations in liver cells and aging has been noted, and a dose-dependent decrease in life span has been shown for doses down to ten rads (the lowest examined). Several studies have shown that until recent years radiologists had shorter life spans and possibly more congenital malformations among their offspring than was true for other medical specialists. The studies concerned with congenital malformations involved only male radiologists, so if a real effect exists, it could only be explained on the basis of mutation.

Chromosome mutation frequency in lymphocytes has been used as a rough dosimeter in radiation accidents. Further research is needed on the kinetics of lymphocyte growth and on radiation response *in vitro* and *in vivo* before the method can be "calibrated." Another difficulty is that large numbers of cells must be analyzed when very low doses are involved. Some aspects of karyotype construction, a necessary part of analysis and a most laborious task at present, have been automated. It is expected that when the whole process is automated, within the next few years, significant advances will be made in our knowledge of the effects of low doses and also in the use of the lymphocyte as a dosimeter. When this is accomplished, film badge records will probably be supplemented with routine karyotype analyses in many cases, which will probably give more reliable and accurate indices of exposure. Also, if a patient wants to know how much radiation he has received, a few drops of blood from a finger puncture will yield enough lymphocytes for chromosome analysis. Automation of karyotyping may increase the amount of litigation dealing with genetic hazards of medical-dental radiation.

B. Genetically Significant Dose of Medical Radiation

Medical-dental radiation is the largest source of man-made radiation to the human population. The following figures, taken from a survey made in the United States in 1964, give some idea of the scope of exposure: 66 million persons were given medical radiographic examinations, 46 million received dental radiographic exams, 7.8 million were given fluoroscopic exams, and 600,000 persons received radiation therapy. It is estimated that these numbers will double by about 1977.

The radiographic examinations are the

TABLE 5–3 ESTIMATED AVERAGE GONAD DOSE PER SELECTED EXAMINATION (U.S. 1964)*

Examination	Dose in Millirads		Average No. of Films per Examination
	Testicular	Ovarian	
Skull	<1	4	3.7
Cervical spine	8	2	3.1
Upper extremity (excluding shoulder)	2	1	2.3
Lower extremity (excluding hip)	96	<1	2.4
Chest			
Radiography	5	8	1.4
Photofluorography	<1	8	
Fluoroscopy	1	71	
Thoracic spine	196	9	2.1
Shoulder	<1	<1	1.8
Upper gastrointestinal series			
Total†	137	558	
Radiography	130	360	4.4
Fluoroscopy	7	198	
Barium enema			
Total†	1585	805	
Radiography	1535	439	3.5
Fluoroscopy	50	366	
Cholecystography	2	193	3.7
Intravenous or retrograde pyelography	2091	407	5.0
Abdomen	254	289	1.7
Lumbar spine	2268	275	2.5
Pelvis	717	41	1.5
Hip	1064	309	2.3

*From Penfil, R. L., and M. L. Brown: Genetically significant dose to the United States population from diagnostic medical roentgenology, 1964. Radiology, 90:209–216, 1968.

†Totals were derived by addition of radiography and fluoroscopy since most of these examinations include both fluoroscopy and one or more radiographic films.

most important for calculating the magnitude of genetic effects in the population. Table 5–3 presents the estimated *average* gonadal doses per selected medical examination in the United States. Even though they are not whole-body exposures, some of these values make the average natural background dose to the population of 100 millirads per person per year look small.

In order to estimate the genetic hazards of medical radiation exposure to the population as a whole, the average gonadal dose actually received by individuals who are potential parents is projected statistically to give an estimated dose that theoretically is received by every potential parent. This estimated gonadal dose to the whole population has been called the *"genetically significant dose"* (GSD), but a more accurate designation would be "mutagenic equivalent dose." The validity of the concept of the GSD is predicated mainly on the following points derived from experimental animals: (1) Mutations produced in the precursor cells of ova and sperm are cumulative. Therefore, the number of new radiation-induced mutations that an individual will transmit to offspring depends on the amount of radiation his gonads have received from his own conception to the time each of his offspring is conceived. (2) Any dose of radiation, no matter how small, has a finite probability of producing a mutation, and the number of mutations produced bears a linear relation to dose. (3) The genetic significance of new mutations to a *population* is determined by the *total* number transmitted, regardless of how many mutations are transmitted by how many individuals. In other words, the potential population import of the number of mutations produced in 1000 people by 0.020 rad of X-rays to each is the same as that produced in one person by 20 rads.

Four variables are involved in the calculation of the GSD: (1) the number of potential parents in the population (fetuses, children, and adults); (2) the number of children these individuals can be expected to produce; (3) the number of X-ray examinations given to potential parents of all ages; and (4) the average gonad dose received in these examinations. It should be emphasized that the GSD is *not* a measure of biologic effect, but rather a means of

estimating the genetic impact of low levels of radiation on a population.

In 1964, the GSD for the United States population was 55 millirads. This was the second highest GSD among the six countries in which reliable doses could be calculated. *It has been estimated that the GSD of 55 millirads could easily be reduced to 19 millirads by simply limiting the beam size of all X-ray machines to film size.* As has been pointed out by the American College of Radiology,* this would constitute a significant reduction in the amount of medical radiation that the population receives without altering the benefits that patients derive from diagnostic X-ray procedures.

The GSD of 55 millirads is calculated from data on both males and females, but 82 per cent of the dose is derived from X-ray examinations of males. The testes usually receive more radiation than the ovaries, but more significant is the fact that the number of radiation-induced mutations transmitted by sperm is probably much greater than those transmitted through ova.

On the basis of the present rate of increase in the number of X-ray examinations and the continued high levels of gonad doses, it has been predicted that by 1990 the GSD from medical X-rays, which is now estimated to be about half that of background radiation, will be two to four times that of background.

C. Gene Mutation and Selection

Gene mutation is responsible for the different characters that distinguish one species from another and for the variety of phenotypes that occurs within a single species. Adaptive evolution does not, however, result from mutation alone, but from the interaction of mutation and selection. *Selection* is that process by which genetic constitution either prevents or favors the

---

*In *X-ray Examinations, A Guide to Good Practice,* prepared by the American College of Radiology Commission on Radiologic Units, Standards and Protection with the assistance of the Public Health Service Bureau of Radiological Health and with the cooperation of the American Medical Association. For sale as stock number 5505-0003 for 35 cents from the Superintendent of Documents, U.S. Government Printing Office, Washington, D.C. 20402.

survival and reproduction of an organism in a given environment. Mutation in man is not rare: it is estimated that 20 per cent of the population carries at least one mutation that was produced in one parent of each individual. The importance of radiation-induced germ cell mutations for man is determined by natural selection against the harmful ones. Because most mutations are deleterious, we tend to think that they are eliminated relatively quickly from the population by natural selection. This is true for the dominant ones with lethal or sublethal effects, but a recessive mutant gene can remain in the population for varying periods, the time depending on the severity of its action in the heterozygote and in the much less frequent homozygote. If a recessive gene, even a sublethal or lethal one, has very little expression in the heterozygote, its frequency in the population will gradually increase over a large number of generations to reach an equilibrium. As the number of heterozygous individuals increases, the chances increase that two of them will mate. From such a mating one-fourth of the offspring will be affected because they are homozygous for the recessive gene (the other one-fourth will be homozygous for the dominant normal gene and one-half will be heterozygous). If a recessive gene has some degree of expression in the heterozygote that is detrimental but not immediately lethal, it may persist in the population.

Most radiation-induced mutations are recessive, and even though they may exert some deleterious effects in the heterozygous condition, they cannot be identified without selective breeding. An additional complication is that many phenotypes (e.g., intellect) are probably determined by a number of genes acting in concert. In man, therefore, we cannot expect to detect the new mutations for many generations, if ever. The human population has been exposed to medical radiation only since 1895, when Roentgen discovered X-rays. If a generation is defined as 30 years, less than three full generations have been completed; thus, precise assessment of the harmful effects of the radiation-induced mutation "load" in the population cannot even be approached for a long time. It is estimated that only 4 to 7 per cent of radiation-induced gene mutations in man are eliminated in the first few generations, after which the rate drops to 1 to 2 per cent per generation. All evidence on mutation, taken together, indicates that we should not assume that the radiation-induced mutations in man will be quickly removed from the population by selection.

Let us examine a few factors that are known to influence the frequency of some undesirable human genes in the population. (1) *Spontaneous mutation* can keep a deleterious gene in the population. Achondroplastic dwarfism is a human condition characterized by short legs and arms and by stubby fingers; the head and trunk sizes are normal. The gene responsible for this condition is a dominant mutant which is lethal in the homozygous condition. Dwarfs are heterozygotes. They have a low reproductive rate; parturition frequently requires Cesarean section and the infants are subject to high mortality. In addition, there is cultural pressure against reproduction of dwarfs, because they are not what modern society considers attractive individuals. This gene does not disappear because the normal gene has a relatively *high spontaneous mutation rate*, approximately one in 24,000 gametes, so that the supply of the dominant gene is being constantly replenished in the population.

(2) Sickle cell anemia is caused by a recessive gene. The spontaneous mutation rate of the normal dominant gene to the recessive gene is very low—1 per 100,000 gametes—which makes the mutation rare. The frequency of this deleterious recessive gene has increased in some populations by a phenomenon known as *genetic polymorphism*. The sickle cell anemia gene is lethal to individuals homozygous for it (death usually occurs before adolescence). It bestows a distinct survival advantage to heterozygotes in that they have a decreased mortality from falciparum malaria as compared to individuals who are homozygous for the dominant normal gene. Therefore, malaria serves as a selection factor for keeping this gene in the population, and there are some areas of the world in which 40 per cent of the population have the sickle cell anemia gene.

(3) *Medical progress* can alter the frequency of a gene in the population. Dia-

betes mellitus is caused by a recessive gene with incomplete penetrance. (A gene is said to be incompletely penetrant when its presence does not always produce a given phenotype; this can apply to certain dominant and recessive genes in both the heterozygous and homozygous conditions.) An individual homozygous for the recessive gene may or may not develop the disease; environmental factors, such as diet, tend to increase penetrance (i.e., the ability of the genotype to express itself). The widespread use of insulin has enabled increased numbers of diabetics to reach reproductive age and has strengthened their reproductive ability, thereby leading to an increased frequency of this gene.

The porphyria gene is a dominant one that causes affected individuals to excrete excessive amounts of porphyrin (a breakdown product of hemoglobin); they have no discomfort unless exposed to sunlight which may cause their skin to develop blisters and abrasions. The gene is rare in most populations (its presence in one per cent of the Dutch Afrikaners can be traced to a single immigrant who came to South Africa in 1698). In the past this gene has been relatively harmless, but in the environment of modern medicine it can be detrimental, in fact, lethal: individuals with the gene are acutely sensitive to barbiturates and certain other drugs. Modern medicine can, therefore, select *against* this gene.

(4) *Disease* can be a powerful selection factor. Genes for resistance to a given disease can be linked with genes for other characters; this causes a simultaneous selection for the other characters. Thus, survivors of a disease can be genetically different from those who succumb to it. The susceptibility of man to diseases (e.g., pulmonary tuberculosis) has been demonstrated to be genetic in several population studies.

No mutant genes in the human population are definitely known to have been induced by either background or medical-dental radiation, but there is good reason to believe that some arise from these sources. A portion of so-called spontaneous mutations may in fact be induced by both types of radiation. In the absence of evidence to the contrary, we must assume that medical-dental radiation produces some gene mutations, which most probably are deleterious and some of which remain in the population with varying degrees of selective value.

D. Fetal Irradiation and Mutation

When an unsuspected conceptus has been exposed to diagnostic radiation, the first concern always seems to be with possible developmental effects. They cannot be ignored, but other, possibly more important effects of low doses of radiation should be weighed in helping a patient reach a decision on the advisability of therapeutic abortion. *In utero* irradiation may increase the chance of neoplasia sometime in childhood. More data are needed to determine unequivocally the dimensions of this problem; but the study with the largest sample — approximately 750,000 children (MacMahon, 1962) — indicates that the effects may be real.

The possible induction of gene and chromosome mutations should be given great weight in an abortion decision. From 20 to 50 per cent of spontaneous abortions have been found to have one or more chromosome mutations and those with such mutations tend to abort earlier than those without. Of the spontaneous abortions with no detectable mutations, a sizeable portion may contain a very small chromosome or gene mutation. A cause-effect relation of chromosome mutation to spontaneous abortion is implicated by the fact that only 2 per cent of induced abortions have recognizable mutations.

Fetal waste in the population is relatively high. About ten per cent of recognized pregnancies end in spontaneous abortion; the actual figure is probably higher because very early embryo losses are difficult if not impossible to detect. About 2.5 per cent of liveborn infants have physical anomalies detectable at birth, which prevent or make difficult a normal existence. Dr. I. M. Cushner, an obstetrician, has pointed out, "It seems reasonably clear that at least a segment of these anomalies are radiation-induced, either by direct somatic effect upon the current fetus or — and more terrifying — by previous genetic injury to its ancestors. If this be true, it becomes urgent that obstetricians and all other physicians caring for pregnant women be familiar with this aspect of preventive medicine."

TABLE 5-4 CHROMOSOME MUTATION IN IRRADIATED FETUSES*

Case	Estimated Dose or Exposure	Type X-ray Examination	Fetal Age at Exposure	Age at Chromosome Analysis	Tissue Studied	Chromosome Mutations	Reference
1	0.19 rad	abdominal, hysterosalpingograph	10, 11 wks.	12 wks.**	—	none	c
2	3.0 R	—	6 wks.	6 wks.**	skin, lung	translocations, monosomics, trisomics	d
3	3.9 rads	barium meal, enema	6 wks.	6 wks.**	chorionic fragments	deletions, dicentrics	c
4	—	"radiopelvimetry"	1 wk.	25 mos.	lymphocytes, fibroblasts	mosaic for 1–3 markers (extra)	b
5	—	radiation therapy	20–30 wks.	1, 2, 3, 4 years	lymphocytes	all types	a

*References: a) Kucerova, M.: Long-term cytogenetic and clinical control of a child following intrauterine irradiation. Acta Radiol. [Ther.] (Stockholm), 9:353–361, 1970.

b) Lejeune, L., et al.: Mosaïque chromosomique, probablement radio-induite in utero. C. R. Acad. Sci. [D.] (Paris), 259:485–488, 1964.

c) Sato, H.: Chromosomes of irradiated embryos. Lancet, 11:551, 1966.

d) Thiede, H. A., and Salm, S. B.: Chromosome studies of human spontaneous abortions. Amer. J. Obstet. Gynec., 90:205–215, 1964.

**Induced abortuses.

Chromosome mutations found when fetuses have been irradiated at known stages of development are shown in Table 5–4. Chromosome mutations of the type caused by two hits were observed after a dose as low as three rads. Note that three of the cases were exposed during the first six weeks of development, the period when a woman often does not know she is pregnant.

The child designated as case 4 (Table 5–4) was first examined at age 25 months because of retarded intellect and abnormal physical growth. Case 5 is particularly interesting. This child, who received radiation in the fifth and sixth months during therapy of the mother for cervical carcinoma, was delivered by Cesarean section at the eighth month with a birth weight of 1960 g and a length of 44 cm (normal range), and showed *no congenital malformations*. She sat at 9 months, stood at 12 months, walked at 21 months and began to talk at 36 months. At 12 months, she had "febrile convulsions later followed by epileptic seizures of the type major epilepsy." At 4½ years there was evidence of slight anemia and leukocytosis, as well as microcephaly with a mental development equivalent to that of a two year old. Chromosomes of peripheral lymphocytes were analyzed at ages one, two, three, and four years of the child, and at one and two years after treatment of the mother. As expected, the number of chromosome mutations in both subjects was significantly high, but, unexpectedly, the frequency of unstable types of mutations in the child did not change appreciably over the four years. This case demonstrates that absence of detectable developmental defects at birth gives no assurance that morphological and behavioral abnormalities will not show at a later age.

It is possible that the chromosome mutations observed in the irradiated fetuses and children (Table 5–4) were not induced by the radiation. The presence, however, of two-hit type chromosome mutations militates against this interpretation, because such mutations are extremely rare in the absence of radiation. Until more data can be obtained on induced abortuses after diagnostic irradiation, it would be prudent to give careful consideration to the data in Table 5–4. This view gains weight in light of court decisions on possible, not proved, radiation damage to fetuses.

E. Reduction of Genetic Hazards

Several simple steps practiced by all physicians using X-ray equipment would reduce the genetic hazards that accompany exposure of somatic and germ cells. As mentioned previously, collimation of the beam size of every X-ray machine to film size will reduce the gonadal dose to the reproducing population by approximately two-thirds of the present dose. Further reduction could be effected by the routine use of gonad shields in all examinations in which their use does not interfere with diagnosis.

Limitation of the radiation field to the area being diagnosed would also reduce somatic cell exposure. This practice is particularly important with babies and children and is aided by the use of commercial baby holders that prevent movement. The American Academy of Pediatrics, taking cognizance of the radiation sensitivity of growing tissues and the accumulation of mutations in germ cells, has urged its members to call upon their radiologic colleagues for expert use of fluoroscopy and radiography in an effort to reduce exposure of both somatic and germ cells in children.

Most radiography now is performed by radiologic technologists and not by radiologists, so patient exposure could also be reduced by limiting the operation of X-ray machines to skilled technologists, thereby reducing the number of examinations that must be repeated because of poor image quality.

Exposure of embryos and fetuses could be considerably reduced by employing the elective booking method for abdominal radiography and fluoroscopy of women of reproductive age. This method, which limits X-rays to the first ten days after the beginning of the last menses, prevents irradiation of most unsuspected conceptuses.

5.10 SUMMARY

Mutation is an unusual, permanent change in the amount of genetic material (DNA) or in its primary structure. Radiation is one of the most potent mutagens known. Radiation-induced gene and chromosome mutations occur in somatic cells, with consequences only to the individual exposed, and in germ cells, with consequences to future generations. There is no threshold dose for the induction of mutation, and the frequency of mutations bears a linear relation to dose.

In experimental organisms, most radiation-induced gene mutations are recessive in expression; thus, we would not expect to detect them in the first generation of offspring in the absence of controlled breeding, as in humans. Many of the recessive mutations are deleterious in the heterozygote and lethal when homozygous.

Mutations are accumulated by the stem cells of ova and sperm, so the number of new mutations transmitted by an individual will depend on the amount of radiation his gonads have received from his conception to the time his offspring are conceived. The genetic significance of new mutations to a population is determined by the total number transmitted, regardless of how many mutations are transmitted by how many individuals.

Extrapolation from data on mice to the situation in the human leads us to expect that the greatest number of radiation-induced mutations transmitted to offspring might occur when procreation takes place within the first few months after exposure of either the male or female. Further delay of procreation will reduce, but probably not eliminate, especially in males, the number of radiation-induced mutations transmitted.

Analysis of chromosomes in peripheral lymphocytes provides the best available index to radiation genetic effects in man. The available data indicate that certain diagnostic radiologic procedures cause a significant increase in the frequency of chromosome mutations in man.

Much more research is needed to define the extent of genetic effects of low doses of radiation in man, but in the absence of definitive data we have every reason to assume that man's genetic system responds to radiation in approximately the same manner as that of experimental mammals.

Diagnostic radiology is a valuable, indeed an integral and indispensable, part of modern medicine, and physicians must have some knowledge of the genetic effects of radiation in order to weigh more confidently the benefits of a given radiologic procedure against possible hazards, especially in the fetus and young child. The use of methods to keep radiation exposure of the population at a minimum commensurate with good medical care is an important aspect of preventive medicine. A physician's cognizance of the genetic hazards of medical radiation inspires the confidence of patients.

References

1. American Academy of Pediatrics Statement on the Use of Diagnostic X-Ray. Pediatrics 28:676–677, 1961.
2. Brecher, R., and Brecher, E.: *The Rays; A History of Radiology in the United States and Canada.* Baltimore, Williams & Wilkins, 1969.
3. Carter, C. O.: *An ABC of Medical Genetics.* Boston, Little, Brown, 1969.
4. Cushner, I. M.: Irradiation of the fetus. *In* Barnes, A. C. (ed.): *Intra-uterine Development.* Philadelphia, Lea and Febiger, 1968.
5. Green, E. L.: Genetic effects of radiation on mammalian populations. Ann. Rev. Genetics, 2:87–120, 1968.
6. Lewis, E. B.: Ionizing radiation and tumor production. *In* M. D. Anderson 23d Annual Symposium on Fundamental Cancer Research: *Genetic Concepts and Neoplasia.* Baltimore, Williams & Wilkins, 1970.
7. MacMahon, B.: Prenatal X-ray exposure and childhood cancer. J. Nat. Cancer Inst., 28:1173–1191, 1962.
8. McKusick, V. A.: Human genetics. Ann. Rev. Genetics, 4:1–46, 1970.
9. Report of the United Nations Scientific Committee on the Effects of Atomic Radiation. Supp. No. 13 (A/7613), 1969.
10. Russell, W. L.: Recent studies on the genetic effects of radiation in mice. Pediatrics (supp.), *41*:223–230, 1968.
11. Spar, I. L.: Genetic effects of radiation. Med. Clin. N. Amer., 53:965–976, 1969.
12. Wills, C.: Genetic load. Sci. Amer., *222*:98–107, 1970.

Radiology and the Human Embryo and Fetus

Roberts Rugh, Ph.D.

5.11 INTRODUCTION

In considering anomalies that might be induced in the human embryo or fetus by ionizing radiations, one must distinguish clearly between those anomalies that result from mutational effects inherited through the germ cells (sperm or ova or their predecessors) and those congenital effects induced in the embryo or fetus by diagnostic X-rays or radiation therapy. Mutational effects are permanent, heritable changes that can be studied best by breeding experiments or analyses. Congenital effects that are not inherited are structural or functional deviations from the normal that result from some traumatic situation imposed during development. In this discussion, we will not include the genetic effects of radiation, but rather will cover the direct effects on the embryo or fetus and the consequences, both immediate and delayed.

Some preliminary remarks are essential, since there has arisen considerable misunderstanding about the nature of human fetal effects. The literature contains many papers* reporting individual or isolated cases involving presumed effects on the newborn resulting from exposure of a gravid uterus to medical radiation. It is unscientific and totally unjustifiable to attribute an anomaly to ionizing radiation in an isolated instance, because major recognizable congenital anomalies occur in 5 to 6 per cent of the human population even without a history of radiation exposure. An isolated case can have no statistical significance or validity. It is probable that for some time there will be no clear-cut and incontrovertible evidence that associates a causal relation of radiation to an anomaly of the human fetus. This is partly because statistical and control data are simply not available. In light of the accumulating knowledge of the biologic effects of ionizing radiations the temptation does exist to blame them exclusively for the presentation of an abnormal child who had previously been exposed to diagnostic or therapeutic radiation of the mother. It is unlikely that two cases involving identical variables will ever occur. Thus, while the literature may suggest that irradiation of the gravid uterus resulted, in a particular case, in harelip, microcephaly, microphthalmia, leukemia, or perinatal death, there are so many possible contributing factors (including heredity) that a cause and effect relationship could not be proved. This is fortunate because some indiscreet members of the legal profession and avaricious citizens, in attempts to make a malpractice suit out of sincere and intelligent efforts on the part of radiologists to arrive at a proper diagnosis or treatment, bypass the possibility that heredity or a host of traumatic situations can cause birth anomalies. The radiologist must remember that he has a marvelous tool for diagnosis and therapy, but also a potent one for damaging cells and tissues. It is our contention, in this section, that this tool is indeed misused *when used unnecessarily*, particularly with respect to the germ cells, embryo, or fetus which are particularly radiosensitive.

*The author has compiled a list of over 250 references in the scientific literature on the effects of ionizing radiations on the human fetus. A copy of this list may be found appended to his seminar paper #007, February, 1970, obtainable from The Environmental Health Service, U.S. Department of Health, Education and Welfare, c/o Mr. Burt Kline, Radiation Health, 1901 Chapman Ave., Rockville, Maryland 20852.

How, then, are we to gain a baseline of reliable information about possible radiation effects on the human embryo or fetus, since we cannot experiment with the human? Other mammals, such as the rodents, reproduce in quantity and with relatively short gestation periods. Rodent embryonic development can be compared directly with that of the human even though the gestation periods are 20 and 266 days, respectively, and humans rarely have litters of more than one. We in experimental radiobiology and embryology firmly believe that extrapolations from mouse to human effects of fetal radiation are valid on a qualitative basis so that we can now state, with considerable probability, those times in the development of any mammal when radiation insult could cause certain specific congenital anomalies. The extrapolation cannot be quantitative until we (if ever) have quantitative data directly from the human; consequently, dose extrapolations should be viewed as estimates. For example, with respect to mutational effects the germ cells of the mouse appear to be 15 times as radiosensitive as the germ cells of the genetically valuable fruit fly *Drosophila*, so that direct extrapolations of dose from *Drosophila* to mouse give rough estimates with respect to tissue or organ radiosensitivities. If, however, the germ cells of the mouse are so much more radiosensitive than are those of *Drosophila*, what would we expect from exposure of human germ cells? No one can predict except to apply an intelligent guess that at least the reactions may be different, and that the human germ cells are at least as radiosensitive as are those of the mouse. Cleavage, implantation, placentation, organogenesis, and refined differentiation of the various organs all occur in mammals in the same basic sequence but on different time scales. Thus, if the human fetus is subjected to X-rays at a developmental stage comparable to that of the mouse at a time when it is known to react by becoming hydrocephalic, we can suggest the probability (or possibility) that the human would react by developing the same anomaly. Here the prolific breeding of the mouse is of statistical advantage over the one-offspring-a-year human. But it must be emphasized that the dose required to produce a given anomaly may differ for man and mouse. We need data on the human to determine dose levels that produce particular anomalies.

We have presented in Table 5–5 a schedule of mouse and human development showing that the sequence is the same but the time scale is different, not only in length but in rate at different stages. If we anticipate our thesis, it is the fact of *development with differentiation* that makes the fetus uniquely vulnerable to radiation, so that this table would also be useful in predicting which human organs might react by becoming anamolous if subjected to X-rays at any of the gestation stages.

Reliable data on effects of X-irradiation on the human fetus are rare and come mainly from atomic bomb survivors, accidental exposures, occupational exposures, and from both diagnostic and therapeutic radiation exposure of patients who happen to be pregnant. Obviously, reliable cause and effect data could eventually be obtained if the dosimetric and radiation records were more accurate and complete.

If one scans the literature on radiation-induced congenital effects in the human, it becomes immediately evident that the principle area of effect is the central nervous system (CNS). It is known that prior to differentiation, when the presumptive CNS is in the neurectoderm stage, it is moderately radiosensitive—about 400 rads will kill all its cells. After complete neuron formation about 10,000 rads are needed to destroy a brain tumor. However, the embryo after about 17 days, the fetus throughout gestation, and even the newborn for several weeks are all permeated with the transitional stage neuroblasts which are so radiosensitive that they can be destroyed by 25 rads. All of the 100 billion neurons of the adult must, at some time, have gone through

TABLE 5–5 COMPARABLE EARLY POST-CONCEPTIONAL STAGES OF MOUSE AND MAN

Mouse Age (Days)	Human Age (Days)	Developmental Activity, Probable Susceptible Tissue
0	1	Fertilization
1	2	Cleavage: 1- to 4-cell stage
2	3	Cleavage: 5- to 8-cell stage
3	4	Morula
4	5–6	Blastula
5	7–9	Gastrulation, early implantation
6	10–12	Continued implantation, primitive streak
7	13–16	Earliest neurogenesis
8°	17–20	Neurogenesis; head process; eye, thyroid, and heart primordia; allantois and first 4 somite pairs
9°	21–25	Anterior neuropore; primitive germ cells and hemopoiesis in yolk sac; heart, vitelline vessels, aortic arches; perforate oral membrane and jaw parts; otic invagination; gut, liver; rapid increase in number of somite pairs
10°	25–29	Active organogenesis throughout; all primary brain parts separating; myocardial pulsations and circulating blood; all sense organs and optic lens developing; lung primordia; posterior limb buds; mesonephric tubules
11°	30–34	Early pre-skeletal chrondrification; pharyngeal pouches and pancreas; spinal nerves and sympathetic system; semicircular canals; posterior limb buds; bronchia, migrating germ cells; corpus callosum
12°	35–39	Differentiation of appendages and sense organs; all brain parts distinct; cortical differentiation; reflex pathways forming
13°	40–43	Early fetus: basic organogeny completing; atrioventricular valve; primary lid folds
14	44–50	Chondrification of ribs; muscles of esophagus, epithelial cords of testis; enucleate erythrocytes; active hemopoiesis; neuromuscular associations.
15	51–65	Cartilage in humerus; nucleate RBC 25%; gonad differentiation
16	66–105	Nucleate RBC 1%; cerebellum fused at midline; corpus callosum forms; alveoli; gastric glands; ossification of centrum

°Period of maximum radiosensitivity in the mouse; probably same in the human.

TABLE 5-6 ANOMALIES REPORTED FOLLOWING HUMAN EMBRYONIC AND FETAL X-IRRADIATION*

1. Microcephaly (most frequent)	16. Nystagmus
2. Hydrocephalus	17. Stillbirth increase
3. Porencephaly	18. Live birth weight decrease
4. Mental deficiency	19. Neonatal and infant death increase
5. Mongolism	20. Ear abnormalities
6. Idiocy	21. Spina bifida
7. Head ossification defects	22. Cleft palate
8. Skull malformations	23. Deformed arms
9. Micromelia	24. Clubfeet
10. Microphthalmus	25. Hypophalangism
11. Microcornea	26. Syndactyly
12. Coloboma	27. Hypermetropia
13. Strabismus	28. Amelogenesis
14. Cataract	29. Odontogenesis imperfecta
15. Chorioretinitis	30. Genital deformities

*All of the above anomalies reportedly caused by human fetal X-irradiation have been experimentally produced in the mouse or rat when they could be recognized and analyzed. (Obvious exceptions: 4–6.)

this sensitive stage in their metamorphosis, and it is known that there is no regeneration of neural tissues, no "repair" or "recovery" after damage by ionizing radiations. It is, therefore, logical that the structural and functional congenital anomalies of the CNS are the most frequent sequelae of embryonic or fetal X-irradiation.

In Table 5–6 are listed those anomalies reported in the literature as resulting from human embryonic or fetal irradiation, and every one which could be identified in a rodent has been produced by such radiation. Experiments with mammals other than the human are, therefore, not only justified but should be urgently pursued, with the reminder that extrapolations are legitimate for qualitative effects only. Thus far the only quantitative data from large human populations that appear to be statistically significant are those for neoplasia incidence.

5.12 EXTRAPOLATION FROM EXPERIMENTAL DATA TO MAN

We can now proceed to make some generalizations about radiosensitivity of the mammalian embryo and fetus, which are based on animal experimentation, and which are sometimes corroborated with human data. They are at least highly suggestive for the human.

First, there is evidence that the embryos and fetuses of pure lines (homozygous for most genes) of animals are more radio-

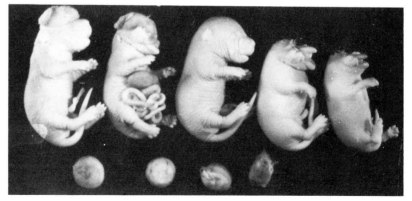

FIGURE 5–15 Entire litter of mice at birth showing variety of congenital anomalies from X-radiation. The members of this litter were exposed to the same field of X-rays, but each reacted differently with respect to the induced congenital anomalies: exencephaly (brain hernia) in mouse at far left; exencephaly with everted viscera; stunted; and two anencephalics. Below are the remains of four implantations that were killed. The variations in response may be due to genetic variations in radiosensitivity.

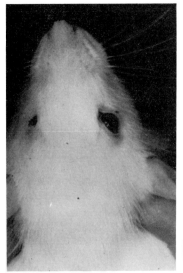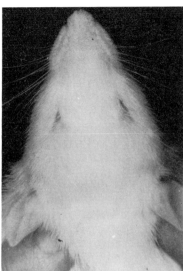

FIGURE 5-16 Two rats of the same litter exposed while *in utero* to X-rays, illustrating the fact that variations in response occur not only within a litter but, as here, within an individual. Rat on left shows one rather normal eye and a degree of microphthalmia in the other eye. Almost complete anophthalmia occurs in both eyes of rat to the right.

sensitive than are heterozygous lines. This is not surprising because heterozygosity tends to mask debilitating recessive genes, thereby increasing general vigor and resistance to all traumatic situations. The human individual is most certainly heterozygous, more so in certain cultures and regions than others, so the circumstances of human society ensure some built-in genetic radioresistance in man. No two individuals subjected to the same field of whole-body penetrating radiation would react in exactly the same manner, and the $LD_{50/30}$* whole-body dose is 400 rads, killing 50 per cent of the exposed population but not all at the same time, some dying within a few days and others not for several weeks. In any litter of exposed rodent fetuses there is a wide range of response due, no doubt, to genetic variations in radiosusceptibility (see Figures 5–15, 5–16).

Second, there is no evidence of abscopal effects (i.e., effects from irradiation of distant areas). The embryo or fetus must be either in the direct line of exposure or in an adjacent area where scattered radiation and toxic by-products of direct exposure on adjacent tissues have an effect through diffusion. There is no evidence, for example, that localized treatment of a brain tumor even with high voltage X-irradiation could affect the fetus in the gravid uterus unless

by chance there were scattered radiations which reached the fetus. Likewise, a dental series could hardly affect the fetus if proper conditions prevail. Nevertheless, one hears that a dental series of X-rays in a pregnant woman could, or is likely to, induce an abortion; there is no evidence for this whatsoever.

Third, the term "low dose" has no significance unless we have adequate statistical data and specify the test organ. A dose which might cause lymphopenia could be 1/10,000 of the dose which can cause necrosis of the differentiated cortical neurons. Moreover, the term "threshold dose" cannot be used in the sense of causing an all-or-none reaction at certain levels of exposure, but rather is the dose at which a response to graded exposures first appears with statistical significance. It is unlikely that a threshold dose for any human congenital anomaly can ever be established, especially since the human is not a homogeneous and consistent entity. For this reason we can only refer to probabilities or possibilities, based upon extrapolations from animal experiments. For example, most experimental radiobiologists would agree that 25 rads to the human embryo or fetus during the period of organ differentiation (the first six weeks) would be sufficient to produce anomalous development. Evidence for such conviction is taken from statistics from animal experimentation. But Hammer-Jacobsen in Denmark (1959), on the basis

*Dose lethal to 50 per cent of X-irradiated animals within 30 days after exposure (see Chapter 9).

of observational data in humans, believes that the cut-off dose should be ten rads and that any fetus which gets this much or more during the first six weeks should be aborted in order to avoid the possibility of producing an anomalous child. The present author agrees, but there is no clean-cut "threshold." The Russians believe (U.N., 1969) that one rad can elicit retinal response, and possibly we should consider the effective amount of radiation to be a single ionization rather than the roentgen, as did Muller (1954) in discussing the cause of mutations. This is nonsense, of course, since all fetuses probably accumulate as much radiation as one rad from medical and environmental sources, and the consequences cannot be identified, much less measured. So the terms "low dose" and "threshold dose," if used, must be clearly delineated. Certainly the developing organism, whether embryo or fetus, must have a dose threshold for any particular anomaly which is much lower than that which produces a discernible effect on somatic tissues of the adult.

Fourth, there is certainly some difference between "chronic" or "fractionated" exposures when compared with "acute" exposures. When one divides the exposure in time, or uses a low level of constant exposure (chronic), the embryo or fetus will be less traumatized per R of radiation than with a single acute exposure, even though the total exposure in both cases is the same. This points up the fact that the developing organism is a mosaic of constantly changing organ radiosensitivities. An acute exposure at any instant can kill those organs differentiating at that moment, leaving others unaffected. Chronic or fractionated exposures, though lower per unit of time, will cover a longer period of time and will, therefore, affect more differentiating organs, many in their most susceptible period. The word "repair" as sometimes used in this discussion of embryonic effects does not mean that damaged cells can "recover" their prior condition, but rather that undamaged cells can replace cells, probably by cell division, that have been killed by radiation. Chronic or fractionated exposures of malignant somatic tissues are generally tolerated better than acute exposures because of the reduced effects on the surrounding normal tissue and the general body response (see

Chapter 6). When one discusses embryonic or fetal chronic or fractionated exposures, it is generally forgotten that the developing organism is different at any two consecutive moments, and that a human fetus exposed to X-rays on day 35 will respond differently from one exposed on day 36, or even on day 35.5. The genetic effects of a given dose of radiation in germ cells are the same whether accumulated in small fractions over a period of time or acquired from a single acute exposure. This cannot be the case with developmental effects.

Fifth, the physicochemical effects of ionizing radiations on any biologic system are immediate, but the biologic manifestations may appear soon or after delays of up to 35 or more years. The most immediate effects are on the chromosomes (DNA) and are best seen in fetal tissue within six hours after exposure. It is the DNA synthesis of the chromosomes that allows proliferation of fetal cells leading to differentiation. Squamous cell carcinoma has been known to occur 35 years after exposure of the skin to radium. Evidence is not available for man, but it seems likely, from rodent experiments, that embryonic and fetal X-irradiation can even cause the shortening of the life span. Some have tried to show an inverse relation of life shortening with linear increase in dose, but this is difficult for a phenomenon as complex as aging. In contrast to genetic mutational effects, which may not be evident for several generations, congenital effects may be evident at birth, shortly thereafter, or after many years. Exposure of the fetus during the third trimester cannot produce gross and demonstrable congenital anomalies because most of the organ systems are already structurally complete. However, owing to radiation damage to the widely distributed neuroblasts, there can still be functional or behavioral effects on the CNS following late fetal exposures (Figure 5–17). They may not be evident, however, until the individual has reached adolescence and refined behavioral tests are applicable. To say of a child at three months that he is totally free from any ill effects of a massive exposure to ionizing radiations while *in utero* is very unwise. He may not show structural anomalies that can be identified, but he may later show evidence of lowered visual acuity, immature EEG recordings,

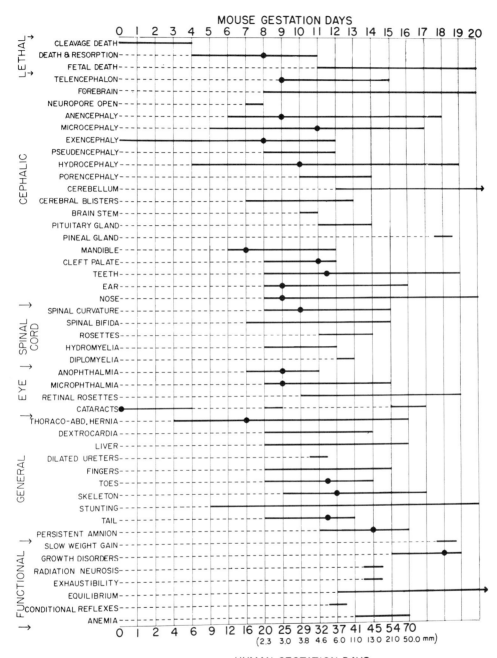

FIGURE 5–17 Table of congenital anomalies produced by irradiating the mouse embryo and fetus with X-rays at each of the 20 gestation days. Note the black spot, indicating gestation age at which the anomaly can most easily be produced by radiation; the black line shows the spread during gestation during which the anomaly could be produced, usually by a higher level of radiation. The comparable human gestation days are shown below. It is obvious that between 8 and 11 days for the mouse and probably between 20 and 32 days for the human is the period of greatest susceptibility to radiation-induced congenital anomalies of all categories. (From Rugh: Radiology, 82:917–920, 1964.)

and even low IQ tests, as well as behavioral peculiarities. The point is that there are short- and long-term sequelae of fetal irradiation, and that structural and functional evidence of damage may not all be manifest at birth. It has been reported several times in the literature that a third trimester fetus which accumulated over 1100 rads showed no *discernible* ill effects at birth. Later, however, defects in behavior appeared as the child matured.

Sixth, in contrast to the adult, the fetus, being a mosaic of differentiating cells and organs, reacts to ionizing radiations by having many of the cells destroyed (necrotized), then phagocytized and removed by the scavenging facilities of the organism; thus the fetus is left with inadequate building blocks for normal development. The embryo or fetus at any time consists of transforming cells of all types, particularly neuroblasts, all of which are hyper-radiosensitive. The necrosis of such cells results in hypoplasia which may or may not be lethal, depending on which cells were dynamically active at the time of exposure. Fetuses with hypoplasia can present a variety of appearances: topographically normal fetus, unbalanced stunting (Figure 5–18), the loss of parts or whole organs as in the retina or cortex of the brain, or the reduction in length of the appendages. These are all deficiencies which, if they do not kill the fetus, can leave it debilitated. There is no evidence of repair to the CNS, only the marshaling of the undamaged cells which try to do the major job of differentiation. This often results in rosettes in the retina and nervous system, in skeletal deficiencies, and in impaired functioning of certain organs. The suggestion has appeared in the literature that the time of day may alter the response of the fetus to X-irradiation. If so, this is because the embryo or fetus is not the same in the morning as it is the following evening, but this, to our knowledge, has nothing to do with time of day. Post-natal death resulting from fetal X-irradiation is not a simple phenomenon, but is most often complicated by many factors, the least of which could be the effects of the X-irradiation. The debilities brought on by fetal X-irradiation could be the difference between survival and death when other complications are involved, even late in life, so that one cannot always blame mortality or anomalies solely upon exposure to ionizing radiations unless all other variables are controlled.

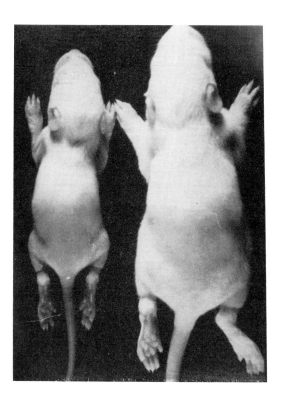

FIGURE 5–18 Two rats at 1 month of age. The control is on the right; the one on the left is a member of a litter exposed to 150 R of X-rays at 13 days gestation (equivalent to a 5 to 6 week human fetus), a time when the skeletal elements are actively differentiating. Note the topographical reduction that results in a well balanced but stunted rat.

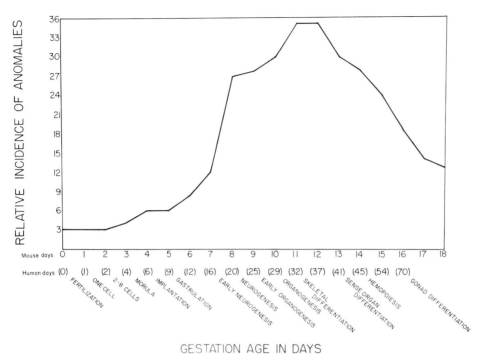

TERATOGENESIS IN MOUSE AND MAN DUE TO X-RADIATION

GESTATION AGE IN DAYS

FIGURE 5–19 If congenital anomalies are simply listed in relation to the gestation day when they are *most apt to occur*, it is seen in this graph that the peak for the mouse is at 11 or 12 days and for the human (*below*) 32 to 37 days. (From Rugh, 1971.)

Seventh, the question arises, what is the maximum dose that can be tolerated without any ill effects? Is there a "safe period?" In general it can be stated that if the pre-implantation embryo is exposed to ionizing radiations, it may be killed and absorbed and the woman would never know that she had conceived. X-radiation shortly after conception is likely either to be lethal or to allow the embryo to survive without evidence of anomalies. When the embryo consists of only a few cells at the time of irradiation, damage to even one cell is likely to be fatal to the whole embryo. From implantation (day eight or nine) through the first six weeks is the most radiosensitive period, known as that of major organogenesis. At this time X-radiation could cause any of a vast number of possible congenital anomalies of a structural nature. It is during this period that most of the embryonic cells are in their "blast" stage (erythroblast, myoblast, chondroblast, neuroblast, etc.), and it is precisely in this stage of transformation that all cells are particularly radiosen-

sitive, no matter what their destination. This happens to be the period in the human embryo during which the tranquilizer Thalidomide took its toll and rubella is so damaging. In the mouse it has been adequately demonstrated that the fetus at days 11 and 12 responds to ionizing radiations with the maximum variety of congenital anomalies, and this period corresponds in human development to days 32 to 37 (Figure 5–19). From six weeks to the end of pregnancy (about 224 days more) recognizable structural anomalies are much less likely to occur, but cell depletions resulting from radiation insult can cause functional disabilities. These are much more difficult to recognize and identify. If the nervous system of a fetus is affected so that the ultimate IQ of the child is drastically lowered, this might go undetected simply because there is no control, not even siblings, with which to compare. The author has such respect for the effect of ionizing radiations on biologic systems, and so much experience with embryonic and fetal reactions, that *it is inconceivable to him that ionizing radiation at any level is without some effect.* This would be difficult to either prove or disprove, but is based partly upon the demonstrated sensitivity of the lymphocyte to one to two rads, and the conviction that the differentiating cell is as radiosensitive as the lymphocyte. *There is probably no developmental stage which is "safe" in the sense of being entirely immune to some effects of ionizing radiations,* and this applies most particularly to the neuroblasts. Any cell which becomes anomalous but survives will pass on such anomalies to its cellular progeny. They are probably irrevocable and irreparable. It can be hoped that practicing radiologists will include in their history work-ups a question relating to the last menstrual period (LMP) so that they can schedule any pelvic radiologic surveys during the first ten days after the onset of the LMP. In this way, there is less chance that an unrecognized pregnancy could be involved, for in the normal 28-day cycle, ovulation occurs between 13 and 15 days, or two weeks *before* the onset of the next expected menstruation. However, it must be pointed out that in the interest of proper medical care a woman may require pelvic X-irradiation, radiograms, fluoroscopy, and so on, and a choice must then be made between the welfare of the mother and the

possibility of inflicting on the embryo or fetus congenital anomalies. In the event the dose to the fetus is ten rads or more during the first six weeks after conception, this author would strongly urge a therapeutic abortion with the advice, if asked, to initiate another pregnancy after a reasonable period of recovery from the abortion and the mother's malignancy.

5.13 HUMAN FETAL IRRADIATION

Without attempting to survey the literature on human fetal irradiation, let us cite a few studies which indicate rather definite results.

A. Growth Retardation

Growth retardation can result from X-irradiation of the early human embryo or fetus, and late exposures may all affect growth. Pre-implantation X-irradiation has no effect on growth, but exposure of the neonate does retard growth. The 86 children exposed to the atomic bomb radiations at Nagasaki while *in utero* showed reduction in head circumference, body height, and weight. The greatest growth retardation was observed in those children whose mothers showed symptoms of radiation

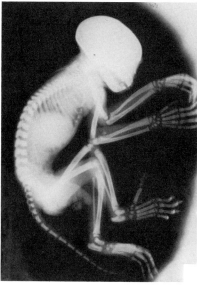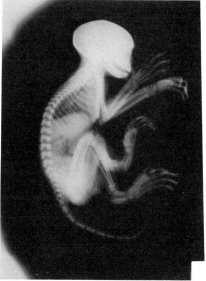

FIGURE 5-20 Radiograms of monkey at two weeks of age. Control (*left*) was delivered normally and had had no radiation. Experimental (*right*) had received 300 rads at 90 days gestation (complete gestation 150 days). This illustration shows topographical reduction, or stunting; without the control for comparison, it might not be recognized as showing any congenital effect of radiation. Both photographs are shown at the same magnification.

sickness, indicative of considerable exposure, who were closer than 1500 meters from the hypocenter and who were less than 15 weeks pregnant. It is now believed that such growth effects occur most frequently when the fetus is irradiated between the third and twentieth weeks. Figure 5–20 shows radiation-induced stunting in the monkey.

Testicular hypoplasia is more likely to follow late fetal exposure, and ovarian hypoplasia, or sterility, can follow neonatal exposure in animal experiments. It appears that the gametes of the adult rodents are more radioresistant than are the maturing germ cells of the neonate. This is probably true also of the human in which the sterilizing dose for the adult gonads (single doses of about 400 rads for females and more than 800 rads for males) is probably many times that sufficient to cause sterility when applied to the late fetus, newborn, or pre-adolescent.

Diagnostic exposures of the human fetus can be leukemogenic, and one to two rads of *in utero* radiation may increase the chances of leukemia in the offspring by a factor of 1.5 to 2.0. Such an exposure of the adult population would not cause a comparable increment in leukemia. As Lillienfeld (1966) reported, "When one considers the variety of control groups used and the sampling variability, the results are remarkably consistent in showing an excess of leukemia among children of radiation-exposed pregnant mothers."

B. Neurological Effects of Irradiation

It has been estimated that 80 per cent of the malformed children with a history of irradiation *in utero* are microcephalic. In experimental rats, as little as 20 rads produced discernible but subtle microscopic changes in the brain which persisted to the adult stage. The author has produced retinal and cortical rosettes in the monkey fetus (Figures 5–21 and 5–22) at 80 to 90 days gestation (normal complete gestation is 150 days), which persisted 23 months after birth, and in rodents 25 rads at 11 days caused such rosettes that persisted. These rosettes are the expression of attempts at repair from inadequate cellular reserve. A case

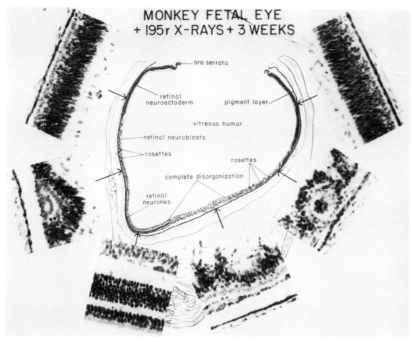

FIGURE 5–21 Radiosensitivity of the monkey fetal eye. Drawing (*center*) with corresponding photographs of the retina 3 weeks after the monkey fetus was exposed to 195 rads. Note that the retinal neurectoderm appears unaffected; lateral retinal neuroblasts are destroyed; and the posterior retinal neurones are resistant, having achieved differentiation. Maturation is from posterior to anterior, and irradiation by X-rays will select out for damage those cells in the neuroblast stage. (Rugh and Skaudoff: X-rays and the monkey fetal retina. Investigative Ophthal., 8:31–40, 1968.)

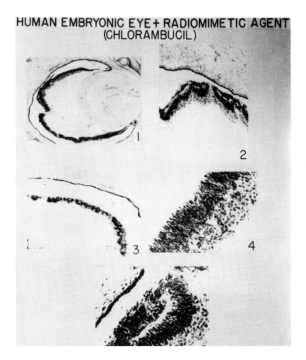

HUMAN EMBRYONIC EYE + RADIOMIMETIC AGENT
(CHLORAMBUCIL)

FIGURE 5–22   These are sections of a human fetal eye after being exposed to a radiomimetic agent, Chlorambucil, in the treatment of the mother for Hodgkin's disease. Note that the same type of retinal rosettes seen after irradiation with X-rays are seen here, so that this agent seems to be truly radiomimetic in this respect at least.

has been reported of a woman who was given radiotherapy for rheumatoid spondylitis and whose fetus received 900 rads in the third month of gestation. The child was severely microcephalic with hypoplasia of the brain and dilated ventricles. Among 26 human cases studied, mental retardation was a common sequela of fetal irradiation. In another case a child was exposed during its third fetal month in the course of maternal treatment for uterine myoma. It was later found to be microcephalic and was seriously uncoordinated. Therapeutic abortions and histopathologic studies of fetuses exposed to rather high therapeutic doses of radiation showed neuronal hypoplasia in both the cerebral cortex and cerebellum. There have been cases in which large exposures of the late fetus produced no overt neurologic sequelae. The difficulty with any of these isolated reports lies with the inability for anyone to be sufficiently accurate in estimating the dose delivered in rads. In animal experimentation irradiation between implantation and delivery is apt to cause abnormal neurologic symptoms. Rats exposed late in gestation manifested difficulty in learning. Cataracts have been produced by irradiating rodent fetuses with X-rays but no radiation-induced cataracts occurred in survivors of *in utero* radiation

in Nagasaki or Hiroshima. Among 27 infants who were exposed during development to therapeutic radiation of the mother, two developed cataracts. Other workers found 6 per cent incidence of eye anomalies, but no cataracts, among 184 patients who had histories of *in utero* exposure or whose parents had radiation prior to conception.

The clinical radiologist is in a vulnerable position because congenital anomalies are found among five to six per cent of the normal births and some of these anomalies *can* be caused by ionizing radiations. Three case histories will be briefly reported here to illustrate several major points that should be made:

First: Mr. and Mrs. H. had three children of adolescent age, all normal. Mr. H. developed a right testicular malignant tumor which was excised, and 800 rads were given to the remaining testis for prophylactic reasons since the couple expected to have no more children. He thought he was sterilized by this exposure. However, two years later his wife became pregnant by him, since they had not felt it necessary to take contraceptive precautions. They had not heard that *radiation sterilization of the testis is sometimes temporary!* The question arose as to whether the child might be abnormal. The couple was advised to undergo a therapeutic abortion (which, at that time, was difficult to justify) for the simple reason that a dose causing some sterility would, in all probability, induce the maximum load of genetic mutations in any surviving stem cells. The abortus did not show any gross anomalies, but no doubt had poor survival prospects and genetic potential.

Second: Mrs. DeC.'s first child was born anomalous, without arms or legs, and died within a few hours. She remembered having low back pains at what turned out to be about 27 days gestation. Not knowing she was pregnant, her physician prescribed an I.V.P., plus fluoroscopy, plus pelvic radiograms. *Her lawyer immediately jumped to conclusions* and screamed his displeasure at "all doctors, after the quick buck." He was calmed, however, with the question as to where he would go had he need of medical help, if his diatribe were legiti-

mate. He was told to ask to see the radiographs and to get the radiologist to estimate the dose delivered to the fetus. It developed that the radiologist, with proper precaution, had shielded the pelvic area with a triangular piece of lead of adequate thickness during radiologic examinations which completely shielded the fetus. There was no malpractice case.

Third: Another out-of-state woman with two adolescent children was suffering from low back pains of unknown origin. Numerous X-ray and fluoroscopic examinations were prolonged to no avail until she missed her next period and became suspicious of a previously unrecognized and unplanned pregnancy. Being of a religious background which frowned on abortions, the couple cautiously investigated whether an interruption could be secured anywhere else in the world. They were told by the radiobiologist to find out how much radiation

TABLE 5–7 POSSIBLE NEUROLOGICAL EFFECTS OF X-IRRADIATION OF THE HUMAN FETUS*

Post-Conception Age (Days)	Effects
8–14:	Encephalia; encephalocele, arrhinocephaly; spina bifida; death
18–20:	Forebrain disorganization, anencephaly, pseudencephaly; anophthalmia; thoracoabdominal hernia; mandible and digits abnormal; thyroid abnormal
±21	Anophthalmia, microphthalmia; microcephalia; ataxia, equilibration reflexes, and myoclonous motor reflexes; hydromyelia; dextrocardia; cataracts; liver involvement; rosettes in retina and brain.
±26	Very active organogenesis throughout: hydrocephalus, dorsal encephalocele, third ventricle, anencephaly; ear and nose involvement; cardiac anomalies
±28	Hypoplasia and disorganization, particularly of forebrain cortical neurons, absence of corpus callosum; conditioned reflexes and learning processes altered; spinal curvature; anophthalmia, microphthalmia; genitourinary anomalies
±36	Production of maximum variety of congenital anomalies: behaviour neurotic or slowly adapted in novel environment, increased non-directional motor activity and slower responses, restlessness, apprehensiveness, increased heart action; spinal nerves and sympathetic system altered; equilibration and auditory factors abnormal
±38	Hydrocephaly, subcortical areas involved, increasing shock-stimulated seizures; brightness discrimination impaired; deterioration of conditioned reflexes, appendages, and their control; cortex jumbled
±42	Completion of basic organogenesis: reflexes altered: ataxia, myoclonous spasticity, seizures; auditory threshold suppressed; cleft palate, microcephaly, and hydrocephaly; atrioventricular anomalies
±65	Abnormal thalamocortical fibers; disrupted cortex, with deficiencies and jumbling; olfactory discrimination reduced; diplomyelia; toes and skeleton affected; cerebellum and corpus callosum to be affected
±75	Electroencephalograms and electrocorticograms show high-frequency waves increased to spikes; outer cortex and thalamus affected; corpus callosum affected
±84	Cerebellum disrupted (from now through birth); delay in both + and − conditioned reflexes
3–6 months	Scattered neurological effects due to wide distribution of sensitive neuroblasts; anomalies largely functional
6–9 months	Reduction in amplitude of EEG and spike frequency; poor response to light stimulation; aberrant cortex even with low exposure levels; anomalies functional rather than structural, determined by EEG, ERG, and EKG examinations and later by IQ tests.

*From Rugh, R.: X-ray-induced teratogenesis in the mouse and its possible significance to man. Radiology, 99:433–443, 1971.

the fetus received and the exact dates. The time of embryo exposure was critical, about four weeks. The resident radiologist said, "Oh, the dose must have been about 40 rads." The couple was told by the radiobiologist that *IF* the dose estimate *AND* their timing of gestation were correct, an abortion should certainly be sought because the fetus had little chance of being normal. When confronted with this situation, the radiologist, upon proper investigation, revised his estimate down to three rads, whereupon all thought of an abortion was abandoned. The child was born in due time and is not only "normal" but exceptional in every way at four years of age. However, during an interval of several weeks the couple was frantically phoning London, Paris, Tokyo, and Puerto Rico trying to arrange an abortion because of *unnecessary X-rays and the snap and ill-considered judgment of an inexperienced resident radiologist.* Had the exposure been ten rads or more, an abortion would still have been recommended by the radiobiologist. Now that abortions are legal in some states, a woman may have her pregnancy terminated if she so wishes when there is a distinct possibility that an anomalous fetus has been induced by radiation or any other agent.

On the basis of what we know about the rodent embryo and fetus, and about the correlation in development of the mouse and human, we can predict what types of neurologic anomalies might follow X-irradiation of the human fetus at different post-conception times (see Table 5–7). There is, of course, no certainty, only a possibility of such correlations, and no dose data can be given.

5.14 SUMMARY

Every radiologist should determine whether his female patient of reproductive age could be pregnant before scheduling any radiologic examination of her pelvis. If, for purposes of the best medical diagnosis or therapy, she must have pelvic radiologic examinations which exceed ten rads to the fetus, she should be apprised of the possibility of having a child with congenital anomalies, particularly if she is in her first trimester. If agreeable, she should be aborted, her condition rectified, and then advised to become pregnant again if she so desires. On the basis largely of animal experiments and fragmentary information of reliable nature for the human, we estimate that congenital anomalies are most likely to follow X-ray doses of ten or more rads administered during the first six weeks of a pregnancy, but there is inherent danger of functional debilitation after irradiation of the embryo or fetus at any time.

References

1. Brent, R. L.: Effects of radiation on the fetus, newborn and child: Sex-different responses. *In* Fry, R. J. M., Grahn, D., Griem, M. L., and Rust, J. H. (eds.): Late Effects of Radiation. Cincinnati, Van Nostrand-Reinhold, 1970.
2. Dekaban, A.: Abnormalities in children exposed to X-irradiation during stages of gestation: tentative timetable of radiation injury to the human fetus. Part I. J. Nucl. Med., 9:471–477, 1968. See also J. Nucl. Med., 10:68–77, 1968.
3. Furchtgott, E.: Behavioral effects of ionizing radiations. Psychol. Bull., 60:157–200, 1963.
4. Hammer-Jacobsen, E.: Therapeutic abortion on account of x-ray examination during pregnancy. Danish Med. Bull., 6:113–122, 1959.
5. Hicks, S. P., and D'Amato, D. J.: Low dose radiation of developing brain. Science, 141:903–905, 1963.
6. Jacobsen, L., and Mellemgaard, L.: Anomalies of the eyes in descendants of women irradiated with small x-ray doses during age of fertility. Acta Ophthal. (Kobenhavn), 46:352–354, 1968.

7. Lilienfeld, A. M.: Epidemiological studies of the leukemogenic effects of radiation. Yale J. Biol. Med., 39:143–164, 1966.
8. Miller, H. J.: Damage to posterity caused by irradiation of the gonads. Amer. J. Obstet. Gynec., 67:467–483, 1954.
9. Miller, R. W.: Effects of ionizing radiation from the atomic bomb on Japanese children. Pediatrics (Suppl.), 41:257–264, 1968.
10. Report of the United Nations Scientific Committee on the Effects of Atomic Radiation. Suppl. No. 13 (A/7613), 1969.
11. Rugh, R.: X-ray-induced teratogenesis in the mouse and its possible significance to man. Radiology, 99:433–443, 1971.
12. Rugh, R., and Shettles, L. B.: *From Conception to Birth; The Drama of Life's Beginnings.* New York, Harper & Row, 1971.
13. Russell, L. B., and Russell, W. L.: Pathways of radiation effects in the mother and the embryo. Cold Spring Harbor Symp. Quant. Biol., 19:50–59, 1954.
14. Stewart, J., Webb, D., and Hewitt, D.: A survey of childhood malignancies. Brit. Med. J., 1:1495–1508, 1958.

The Effects of Radiation on the Fetus

Melvin L. Griem, M.D.

5.15 INTRODUCTION

This discussion will be limited to our understanding of the qualitative and quantitative effects of radiation on the embryo and fetus as reflected by those observable somatic changes seen as malformations and those changes which result in tumor induction.

5.16 MALFORMATIONS

Ionizing radiation is known to disturb rapidly dividing tissue. Very high doses of radiation to the gravid uterus during the first part of pregnancy will result in death of the fetus and resorption of the embryo. The effect is thought to result from direct injury to the fetus and not from indirect damage to the corpus luteum. Placental dysfunction caused by irradiation may play a minor role in fetal mortality.

Ionizing radiation can seriously affect the central nervous system of the embryo, which is extremely sensitive to ionizing radiation in contrast to the relatively insensitive, well differentiated central nervous system of the adult. Microcephaly has been observed in humans following high doses of radiation. At doses of approximately 50 rads, fetuses exposed during the sixth through the fifteenth week of pregnancy showed a five-fold increase in mental retardation in children. Experiments with rodents have shown that doses of 15 rads result in gross abnormalities of the nervous system including exencephalia. Abnormalities of the eye have been associated with exposure of human fetuses to diagnostic X-rays.

Skeletal malformations in rodents have been reported as a result of X-ray exposures of 100 R, 200 R, and higher. These changes were most pronounced when the exposure occurred during the first trimester of pregnancy and consisted of drastic changes in the long bones and pelvic girdle, scapula, clavicle, ilium, femur, fibula, ischium, and pubis. There were also changes in the vertebral column and ribs accompanied by anomalies such as cleft palate and various signs of lateral compression of the skull, fusion of the incisor-bearing portions of the premaxilla, loss of the incisor-bearing portions of the premaxilla and loss of the incisors, as well as domed forehead, shortening of the floor of the cranium or absence of the cranium, and spina bifida.

In irradiated rodents abnormalities of the tail have been demonstrated, as well as shortening of the tail, digital reduction in the forefeet, and an occasional overgrowth of the forefeet. In addition to the skeletal abnormalities, microphthalmia, coloboma, hydrocephalus, open eyelids, and bulging of the eye were also associated with exposure. Also observed was small anal opening or imperforate anus with changes of the ureters and kidneys, sinus inversus, and, in a few instances, shallow cloacal opening for the rectum and urethra. Radiation also resulted in reduction in birth weight.

Tissue doses of five rads can result in congenital malformations in rodents, particularly when the radiation occurs during the period of organogenesis. Below five rads there has been reported an increase in incidence of audiogenic seizures in rodents exposed to chronic small doses of ionizing radiation during fetal development. It has been suggested by some Russian researchers that nervous system function may be altered following doses below one rad.

In humans a dose of 50 rads has resulted in decreased head size and stature; there was no correlation of the effect with irradiation trimester.

5.17   TUMOR INDUCTION

The embryo and fetus are more sensitive than the adult to ionizing radiation. Exposure of the fetus to doses of diagnostic X-rays between one and two rads has been reported to increase the incidence of tumors in children who were exposed during pregnancy. A number of investigators have demonstrated increased frequency of leukemia in children exposed to X-rays *in utero*; however, other investigators have not been able to confirm these observations where tissue doses absorbed by the fetus have been approximately one to two rads, but an increased frequency of hemangiomas has been reported with this dosage. One investigation suggests that multiple factors, one of which is diagnostic X-rays during pregnancy, results in leukemia in the off-spring, and that these multiple factors play an important role.

5.18   RADIOACTIVE ISOTOPES

Radiation may also be received by the fetus if radioactive isotopes are administered to the mother. Radioactive strontium, plutonium, phosphorus, iodine, tritium and a whole series of other isotopes can cross the placental barrier and become incorporated in the fetal tissues. Administration of radioactive phosphorus can produce malformations and lethality in rodent embryos when introduced into the body of the pregnant mother. Radioactive iodine administered later in pregnancy to humans can concentrate in the fetal thyroid, producing radiation injury that results in cretinism. Injections of tritiated thymidine in pregnant mice have been shown to result in an increased frequency of tumors in offspring and in premature aging. When isotopes are injected or administered orally to the pregnant animal, the radiation dose to the fetus is more difficult to estimate because of the variable uptake and transfer of the material.

5.19   RECOMMENDATIONS CONCERNING DIAGNOSTIC X-RAYS AND PREGNANT OR POTENTIALLY PREGNANT WOMEN

Hammer-Jacobsen of Denmark has suggested that the following elective booking rule should be used routinely: fertile women (ages 12 to 50) should be exposed to abdominal diagnostic X-rays *only* during the first 10 days after onset of a regular menstrual period of normal intensity and duration. The examinations to be avoided include radiography and fluoroscopy of the abdomen, hip, lumbosacral spine, lumbar vertebrae, and pelvis, as well as all nuclear medicine examinations. Use of the elective booking method will greatly reduce the chances that an unsuspected conceptus will be irradiated as well as the chances of court action being brought against the radiologist and the attending physician because of such irradiation.

When these above examinations must be performed because of clinical urgency, or because conception has occurred during the first 10 days after beginning of menses, Hammer-Jacobsen has presented guidelines concerning termination of the pregnancy for reasons of possible developmental abnormalities. On the basis of experience, he recommends: "Foetal doses below about one r do not indicate abortion. Foetal doses between about one r and about 10 r indicate therapeutic abortion only in the presence of additional indications. Foetal doses above about 10 r presumably always indicate abortion." Among "additional indications" can be included possible genetic effects and delayed tumorigenic effects.

Bennett has outlined procedures for carrying out the elective booking method. In countering the argument that the procedure is burdensome, he states that it works very satisfactorily in a hospital with more than 300 beds. Brent has questioned the timing of these suggestions.

5.20   SUMMARY

A. Doses of ionizing radiation above five rads may result in gross congenital malformations. These malformations will vary with the stage of gestation at which the exposure to X-ray occurs.

B. Development of the central nervous system is very sensitive to ionizing radiation and doses above five rads will result in detectable abnormalities.

C. Doses of 1.5 to 3 rads may result postnatally in an increased frequency of tumors, either benign or malignant.

D. Below doses of one rad there seems to be little evidence that the fetus is injured.

E. Radioactive isotopes administered to the mother can cross the placental barrier and result in injury to the fetus.

F. Diagnostic X-ray exposures of the maternal pelvis should be avoided, especially during the first trimester of pregnancy.

G. Diagnostic chest X-rays and X-rays of the skull and extremities have not been implicated in radiation injury to the fetus.

References

1. Bennett, R.: Diagnostic radiology in relation to the menstrual cycle. Brit. J. Radiol., *41*:952, 1968.
2. Bennett, R.: Some aspects of radiation protection in a diagnostic department, emphasizing elective examination of females of reproductive age. Australas. Radiol., *13*:224–229, 1969.
3. Brent, R. L.: Effects of radiation on the foetus, newborn and child. *In* Fry, R. J. M., Grahn, D., Griem, M. L., and Rust, J. H. (eds.): *Late Effects of Radiation.* London, Taylor and Francis, 1970.
4. Brent, R. L.: Irradiation and pregnancy. *In* Rovinsky, J. J. (ed.): *Davis' Gynecology and Obstetrics,* Vol. 2. Hagerstown, Md., Harper and Row, 1972.
5. Gibson, R. W., Bross, I. D. J., Graham, S., Lilienfeld, A. M., Schuman, L. M., Levin, M. L., and Dowd, J. E.: Leukemia in children exposed to multiple risk factors. New Eng. J. Med., *279*:906, 1968.
6. Goldstein, L., and Murphy, D. D.: Etiology of the ill health of children born after maternal pelvic irradiation. Amer. J. Roentgen., *22*:322, 1929.
7. Griem, M. L.: Effects of radiation on the fetus. J. Reprod. Med., *1*:367, 1968.
8. Hammer-Jacobsen, E.: Therapeutic abortion on account of X-ray examination during pregnancy. Danish Med. Bull., 6:113–122, 1959.
9. Jablon, S., and Kato, H.: Childhood cancer in relation to prenatal exposure to atomic-bomb radiation. Lancet, *II*:1000, 1970.
10. Russell, L. B., and Russell, W. L.: Radiation hazards to the embryo and fetus. Radiology, 58:369, 1952.
11. Sikov, M. R., and Mahlum, D. D.: Radiation Biology of the Fetal and Juvenile Mammal. U.S. Atomic Energy Commission, Division of Technical Information, CONF-690501, December, 1969.
12. Wald, N., Thoma, G. E., and Broun, G.: Hematologic manifestations of radiation exposure in man. Progr. Hemat., 3:1, 1962.
13. Warren, S.: Radiation damage in utero. *In* Behrens, C. F., King, E. R., and Carpenter, J. W. J. (eds.): *Atomic Medicine,* 4th ed. Baltimore, Williams & Wilkins, 1969.

6 CELLULAR RADIATION BIOLOGY

G. M. Kollmorgen, Ph.D., and Joel S. Bedford, D.Phil.

6.0 INTRODUCTION

Biologic systems vary in their organization and complexity as well as in their response to ionizing radiations. For example, the same effect produced in cells of mammalian tissue by 50 R may require an exposure of 10,000 R in *E. coli*, 30,000 R in yeast, 100,000 R in amoebae, and 300,000 R in paramecia when exposure occurs during optimal growth conditions. In studying the changes brought about by radiation, one may begin with the whole organism and descend the organizational hierarchy to the level of molecules and organelles, attempting to explain changes at higher levels of organization in terms of lesions seen at the biochemical and microscopic levels. Alternatively, one may begin with lesions in molecules and organelles and attempt to predict and correlate changes at higher levels of organization produced by these perturbations. Hence, radiation effects on cells may be considered the basis for understanding changes at the level of tissues, organs, and organisms, or they may serve as the primary biologic system in which change is dependent upon alterations induced in subcellular systems. This chapter deals primarily with the cell as a unit in a complex system, the mammalian body.

6.1 REVIEW OF CELLULAR STRUCTURE

Figure 6–1 illustrates the major anatomical features of a typical mammalian cell.

Every mammalian cell is bounded by a cell membrane, usually referred to as the plasma membrane. This structure consists of two layers of protein molecules separated by phospholipids in such a manner as to form a flexible, semipermeable structure. Substances may pass through the membrane by simple diffusion, or in some cases active transport mechanisms (energy-dependent) are required to transport substances against a concentration gradient, from lower to higher concentrations. The plasma membrane is tied to a continuous intracellular membrane network which forms an interconnecting series of channels inside the cell. This network of internal membranes is referred to as the endoplasmic reticulum, and it is associated with a number of cytoplasmic organelles including ribosomes, mitochrondria, lysosomes, secretory granules, vacuoles, and Golgi bodies. Ribosomes are the site of protein synthesis within the cytoplasm. Mitochondria are the site of several important enzyme functions including the respiratory enzymes which couple with oxidation and phosphorylation reactions resulting in ATP formation. Lysosomes contain degradative enzymes which are released as the cell ages and degenerates. These enzymes autolyze and digest the dead and dying cell. Secretory granules store and subsequently release products of cellular differentiation (i.e., serotonin and heparin in mast cells).

The Golgi bodies concentrate and channel various materials rather than actively synthesize them. However, the Golgi mem-

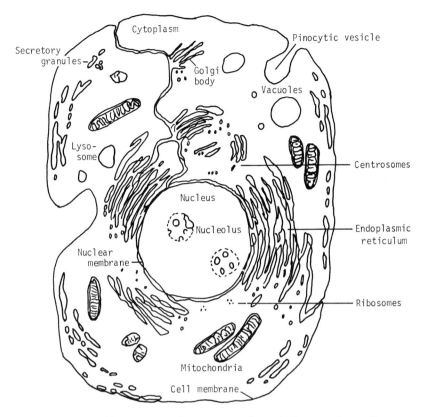

FIGURE 6–1 Characteristic ultrastructure of a typical mammalian cell.

branes may be engaged in some synthesis, particularly of mucopolysaccharides. Vacuoles containing various salts and organic molecules help to maintain the turgor or rigidity of the plant cell following uptake of water. Mammalian cells may contain vacuoles following pinocytosis. Food vacuoles are formed by evagination of the cell membrane surrounding food particles and enclosing the particles along with fluid within the cell.

The nucleus of the cell contains chromatin material which includes DNA, RNA, and protein; it also contains the nucleolus. Chromatin condenses into chromosomes during mitosis, by which time each chromosome consists of two separate but identical chromatids. The chromatids are connected at a constricted region called the centromere. After chromosomes are oriented on an equatorial plane, the sister chromatids are pulled to centrioles on opposite sides of the nucleus by contracting spindle fibers which connect the chromatid and the centriole. This process initiates cleavage of the nucleus and the beginning of cytoplas-

mic division. When the cytoplasm has divided, two daughter cells are formed and the chromosomes assume the pattern of interphase chromatin material.

The function of the genetic material, DNA, is partially mediated through RNA and protein. A detailed account of the function and relation of these three macromolecules is given in Chapter 4.

The nucleolus is the site of ribosomal RNA synthesis. After processing, this RNA is transported to the ribosomes. The nucleolus appears to be particularly susceptible to stimuli that alter RNA metabolism.

6.2 CULTURED MAMMALIAN CELLS

Mammalian cells which possess proliferative ability may be removed from the body and maintained in a suitable environment outside the body (*in vitro*) for prolonged periods of time. When these cells are provided with adequate nutrients, a suitable pH (about 7.0), and maintained near 37° C, they may proliferate for an

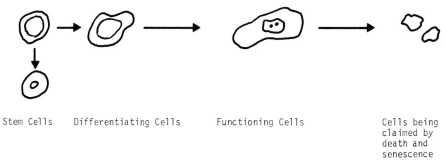

Stem Cells   Differentiating Cells   Functioning Cells   Cells being
                                                                      claimed by
                                                                      death and
                                                                      senescence

FIGURE 6–2 A schematic representation of cellular proliferation, differentiation, function, and death which is apparent in cell renewal systems. In some systems cell proliferation continues in early differentiating cells. Ultimately, differentiating cells fail to divide, complete their differentiation, and move into the functional pool. The rate of renewal is an inherent property of the tissue in question and is responsive to homeostatic factors which tend to inhibit or enhance cellular turnover.

indefinite period of time. Presumably, transformed (neoplastic) cells continue to proliferate for an indefinite period as long as suitable conditions are provided. Normal cells have a finite period of proliferative activity in cell culture. However, this latter point is currently being disputed by several investigators who believe that normal cells may also continue indefinite proliferative activity *in vitro* if provided with a suitable environment.

Various media exist for culturing mammalian cells. Unfortunately, nearly all these media require serum; hence, the nutritional requirement for most mammalian cells is not defined on a chemical basis. In addition, cell cultures are heterogeneous both with respect to the genotype and phenotype of individual cells; that is, cells in a given culture may differ in genetic information or in expression of the same genetic information. These character-

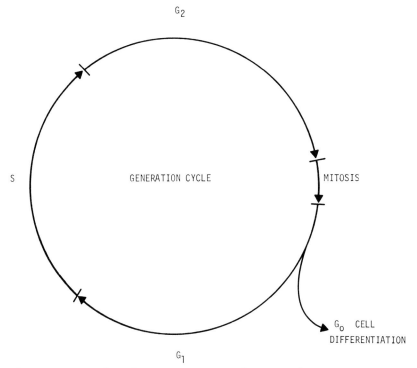

FIGURE 6–3 The generation cycle with respect to DNA replication and segregation as proposed by Howard and Pelc.

istics may be evidenced by differences in karyotypes, enzyme levels, inducible enzymes, and so on. These differences in genetic activity and the variation in environmental factors, such as differences in serum, are responsible for variations and alterations occasionally seen in cultured cells. In spite of these problems, well controlled cultured cells are considered an excellent test system for studying the effects of radiation or a variety of chemical agents on biologic structure and function.

6.3 CELL PROLIFERATION

The mammalian body contains a number of cell renewal systems in which cells live and function for a limited period of time. In order to maintain a steady state system, the death rate in these tissues must be offset by the birth rate. The birth rate in turn is dependent upon the per cent of the population in the stem cell compartment and the rate at which these cells divide and form new cells. A schematic presentation of cellular proliferation, differentiation, function, and death in renewing systems is shown in Figure 6–2. This illustration is applicable to such tissues as skin, gastrointestinal tissues, and blood.

Dividing cells (stem cells) traverse a generation cycle during which time there is a doubling of all cellular constituents (replication), followed by the separation of these constituents into approximately equal parts and the formation of two daughter cells. Replication of DNA is of paramount importance to the cell. Many microorganisms, such as bacteria, synthesize new DNA continuously from one cell division to the next. Proliferating cells of the so-called "higher" plants and animals, however, replicate their genome (DNA) only during a portion of the "interphase," the time between successive divisions. In accordance with the nomenclature introduced by Howard and Pelc, G_1 is the time interval between the end of cell division and the beginning of DNA synthesis, S is the time required for replication of DNA, G_2 is the time interval between DNA synthesis and the beginning of cell division, and M is the time required for chromosomal condensation, splitting, and segregation (see Figure 6–3). Cells which differentiate

leave this cycle in G_1 and enter a so-called G_0 phase. However, these events are not necessarily irreversible since some stimuli induce proliferative activity in previously differentiated cells. Table 6–1 lists some of the properties and characteristics of cells in different phases of the cell cycle.

The duration of the entire generation cycle ranges from hours to months in a variety of *in vivo* mammalian cell systems, whereas cultured mammalian cells usually have a generation cycle time measured in

---

TABLE 6–1 CHARACTERISTICS AND PROPERTIES OF THE VARIOUS STAGES OF THE CELL CYCLE*

G_1 Phase

Cells which lose proliferative ability (muscle, nerve) leave the cell cycle in G_1 and enter G_0.

Enzymes necessary for DNA synthesis (kinase, polymerase, synthetase, deaminase) are synthesized.

All species of RNA are made.

In renewing tissues, the rate of renewal is partially regulated by retention of cells in G_1.

Mammalian cells in embryogenesis as well as some protozoa, slime molds, and bacteria have no G_1.

Histone acetylation and phosphorylation are probably initiated.

Synthesis of regular protein(s) which initiate DNA synthesis probably occurs.

S Phase

Synthesis of chromosomal DNA occurs.

Maturation of daughter centrioles occurs.

Centriole reproduction begins.

Histone synthesis and other protein synthesis necessary to maintain DNA synthesis occurs.

Rate of RNA synthesis is about the same as during G_1 and G_2.

G_2 Phase

Centrioles separate into two pairs.

Proteins required for mitosis are synthesized.

RNA required to direct protein synthesis necessary for mitosis is synthesized.

M Phase

Cessation of RNA synthesis.

Decrease in protein synthesis.

Condensation and segregation of DNA along with associated RNA and proteins.

---

*A number of agents have been used to disrupt the metabolism of cells in various stages of the cycle. The reader is referred to reviews by Baserga and Prescott for a thorough analysis of age-dependent events.

hours or days. It is becoming more apparent that the length of the generation cycle is heavily dependent on the length of G_1. This phase is variable in duration, and it can be extended or contracted by regulatory molecules which are produced or activated by homeostatic mechanisms. On the other hand, the duration of S, G_2, and M phases are less susceptible to variation.

The duration of the individual phases has been measured by a number of different techniques, the most popular being the use of per cent labeled mitoses curves. This technique requires that cells are exposed for a brief period (pulsed) to radioactive thymidine, a specific precursor for DNA. The radioactive thymidine is incorporated into cells which are synthesizing DNA during the time of exposure (see Figure 6–4A). Following this procedure, cell samples are harvested at increasing intervals of time, and after appropriate fixing and staining, radioautographs are prepared. Later, mitotic figures from these radioautographs are scored as being either labeled or unlabeled. Cells harvested immediately after the pulse of radioactive thymidine have no labeled mitoses, but as the interval between pulsing and harvesting increases, there is a rapid increase in the percentage of mitotic cells which are labeled. This cohort of labeled cells passes into and through mitosis so that twice as many cells are labeled with approximately

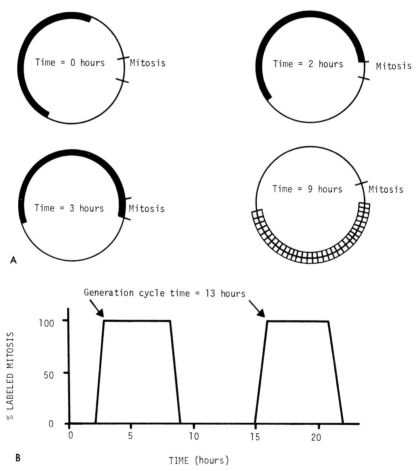

FIGURE 6–4 A, These figures illustrate the position of labeled cells after a brief exposure to radioactive thymidine. At time 0, labeled cells are in DNA synthesis; 2 hours later they have moved to the mitotic interface; 3 hours later they have filled the mitotic compartment; 9 hours later they have all moved through mitosis and into G_1 and S. B, A theoretical plot of per cent labeled mitoses as a function of time is shown for the data illustrated in Figure 6–4, A. These data indicate that the time for G_2 is 2 hours, the mitotic time is 1 hour, the time for DNA synthesis is 6 hours, and the generation cycle time is 13 hours. By subtraction, the time for G_1 is 4 hours.

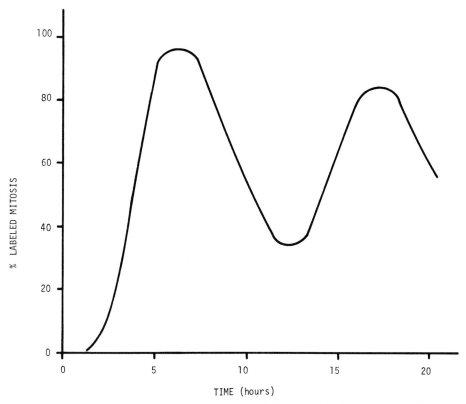

FIGURE 6–5 Per cent labeled mitosis as a function of time following a brief exposure to radioactive thymidine. These curves, obtained from neoplastic mast cells, are comparable to the theoretical curves shown in Figure 6–4, *B*. The duration of individual phases tends to vary and yields rounded shoulders, descending slopes which are less steep than ascending slopes, a brief interval of 100 per cent labeled mitosis, and a trough which does not reach zero.

one-half the original grain intensity. A diagrammatic illustration of this is shown in Figure 6–4B. The duration of G_2, M, and S phases is read directly from this curve. The length of the generation cycle (GC) is obtained by measuring the time difference of comparable points on the first and second waves of labeled mitoses. The duration of G_1 is obtained by subtracting the duration of G_2, M, and S from GC. While Figure 6–4B shows the theoretical per cent labeled mitosis curve, the data obtained using this technique with mast cells is shown in Figure 6–5. The difference in these curves is due to a mixing of cells at the G_2–S and G_1–S interfaces. Mixing occurs because there is some variation in the duration of individual phases for individual cells. A plot of the variations in the generation cycle time and the time for G_1 and M illustrates a skewed distribution around the mean (Figure 6–6).

While this technique gives information about the duration of individual phases and the length of the generation cycle, it does not necessarily indicate the doubling time of the population. The generation cycle time and the doubling time are equal only when all cells in the population are in the proliferative pool. As the percentage of the cells in the proliferative pool decreases, the duration of the doubling time increases with respect to the cell cycle time. In steady state systems in which there is neither an increase nor a decrease in the number of cells, there is equality in the number of cells retained as compared to those leaving the proliferative pool. An estimate of the percentage of population in the proliferative pool can be obtained by exposing cells continuously to labeled thymidine, as shown in Figure 6–7. As the length of the pulse increases, the percentage of labeled cells increases until all proliferating cells have incorporated labeled thymidine.

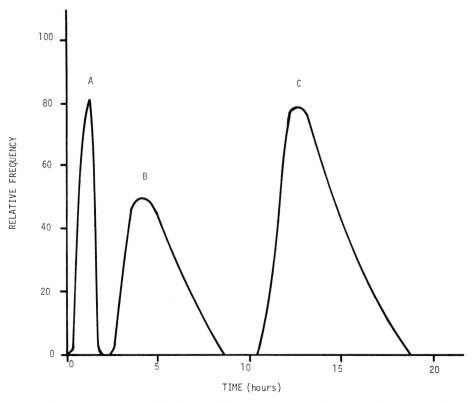

FIGURE 6-6   The duration of G_1 and M phases and the generation cycle time with respect to the relative frequencies in the population. Curve A indicates the variation in the mitotic time, Curve B indicates the variation in the G_1 time, and Curve C indicates the variation in the generation cycle time.

In addition to measuring the duration of individual phases, one may also ascertain the distribution of cells within the generation cycle. The per cent of labeled cells following a brief exposure to radioactive thymidine indicates the per cent of the population in the S phase. Likewise, the mitotic index can be used to ascertain the per cent of the population in mitosis. The per cent of cells in G_2 can be measured by blocking cells in mitosis with colcemide, after a brief exposure to labeled thymidine. Figure 6–8 illustrates that the mitotic index (considering only unlabeled cells) increases after a brief refractory period until all G_2 cells are in mitosis. These collected, unlabeled, mitotic figures represent the initial G_2 population. Cells not identified by these procedures as being S, M, or G_2 cells are considered as G_1 or G_0 cells. The per cent of cells in G_1 is easily determined after the per cent of the population in the proliferative pool has been measured.

6.4 CELL SYNCHRONY

The response of mammalian cells to ionizing radiation is partially dependent upon the position of the cell within the cell cycle at the time of treatment. Accordingly, it may be desirable to work with synchronous (unmodified) or synchronized (modified) populations of mammalian cells. A number of techniques have been devised, all of which have some limitations. Before selecting any technique, one needs to know the properties of the cells in question, the kinds of information which are desirable, and the advantages and limitations of the technique employed. While it is generally desirable to obtain a starting population of cells with a narrow age distribution, it is also necessary to retain the physiologic competence of these cells so that they are able to negotiate subsequent metabolic events with nearly uniform rates. Sinclair (1968), in a recent review, discusses

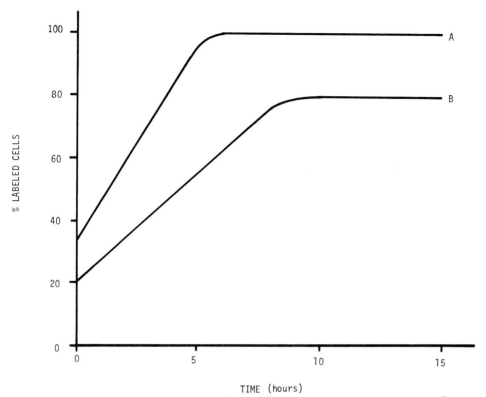

TIME (hours)

FIGURE 6–7 Per cent labeled cells as a function of time following a continuous exposure to radioactive thymidine. Curve A indicates a population of cells with an initial labeling index of 35 per cent, a flow rate from G_1 into S of about 9.3 per cent per hour, with all cells in the proliferative pool. Curve B indicates an initial labeling index of 20 per cent, a flow rate from G_1 into S of about 6 per cent per hour, with 80 per cent of the population in the proliferative pool.

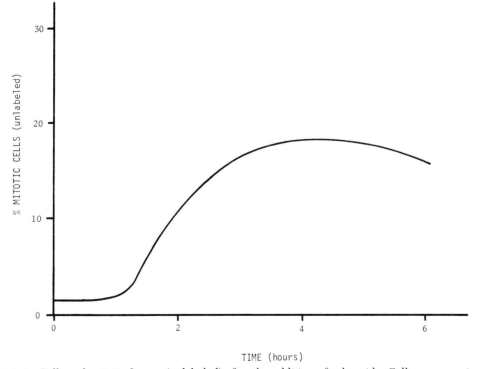

TIME (hours)

FIGURE 6–8 Collected mitotic figures (unlabeled) after the addition of colcemide. Cells were previously exposed to labeled thymidine for a brief period. The per cent of the initial population in G_2 is the difference between the final mitotic index (plateau portion of the curve) and the initial mitotic index.

methods for obtaining and evaluating populations of synchronous and synchronized cells.

6.5 METHODS OF ASSAY

One of the most important effects of radiation on mammalian cells is the reduction of viability in terms of reproductive potential. Several techniques have been developed to assay the viability of mammalian cells with respect to this function.

In search of a practical method of determining viability by a colony formation technique (*in vitro*) similar to that used in bacteriology, Puck and Marcus (1956) used large numbers of X-ray killed "feeder" cells (cells incapable of sustained division but capable of at least a limited amount of metabolism) to condition the medium to the point where it could support the unlimited growth of a small number of unirradiated cells. By means of this feeder cell technique, Puck and Marcus were able to grow colonies of HeLa cells with plating efficiencies up to 100 per cent. The development of this single-cell plating technique and variations thereof initiated a number of quantitative studies in radiobiology using cultured mammalian cells.

The first successful single-cell *in vivo* assay is the one developed by Hewitt and Wilson, who used a lymphocytic type of leukemia which arose spontaneously and is easily transferable in CBA mice. In mice with advanced disease, the liver sinusoids become extensively infiltrated with leukemic cells which can be "shaken out" in large quantities after mincing the liver. When appropriate dilutions of cells, harvested as above, are inoculated into leukemia-free CBA mice, a fraction of the recipients subsequently die of leukemia. For their system, an average of only two cells were required to transplant the disease. This permitted the development of a method for assaying competent leukemic cells. Competent cells are cells which are capable of producing the end point—in this instance, leukemia. For a radiation treatment which killed one-half the cells, an inoculum containing twice the number of cells would be required to transplant the tumor.

Till and McCulloch have developed a direct method of determining the survival response of isologous bone marrow (IBM) cells. This method is an *in vivo* counterpart of the colony formation criterion used in cell culture work. It is based upon the fact that a fraction of the nucleated IBM cells injected intravenously into a supralethally irradiated recipient will lodge in the spleens of these animals and produce nodules (clones) of progeny cells. A supralethal dose to the host drastically suppresses hemopoietic stem cell activity in the spleen, although the gross morphology of the host's spleen is maintained for some time after exposure. Presumably, sterilized spleen cells help maintain a nutritive environment since competent IBM cells proliferate in their midst to form nodules or "colonies." The latter, after appropriate fixation, can be counted readily by eye 10 to 11 days after the injection of IBM cells.

Withers and Elkind developed a technique for assaying dose survival characteristics of epithelial cells of mouse intestinal mucosa. A loop of small intestine is exposed to radiation and examined later (about 13 days) when discrete islands of regenerating epithelium may be seen in an area otherwise completely ulcerated. The assumptions are that each island of regenerating epithelium arises from a single proliferative cell surviving within a mucosal crypt and that these cells survive independently. Consequently, the dose-survival relationship determined from nodule counts represents the dose survival for single cells.

6.6 SURVIVAL CURVES

Cell reproductive death and hereditary changes in surviving cells are perhaps the two most important effects of ionizing radiation which are produced in biologic material. Cell reproductive death is defined as the loss of a cell's capacity for unlimited proliferation. By observing a population of cells exposed to ionizing radiation it can be seen that some of the cells lyse and disappear within a few hours or days following irradiation. However, many cells which are unable to proliferate remain in the population for some time. In a number of respects these cells are indistinguishable from reproductively viable cells. Even after massive doses of radiation, a large proportion of cells retain ability to carry out other functions. They may continue to metabolize nutrients, exclude certain dyes, or even synthesize virus particles. The majority of sterile cells are unable to complete more than one successful division, but a few may succeed in completing several divisions, producing abortive colonies containing as many as 20 or 30 progeny. In addition, sterile daughter cells may continue to grow and replicate their genome several times without dividing, thereby forming giant cells.

Generally speaking, a cell is considered to have survived treatment with a particular agent if it has retained its ability to proliferate indefinitely, or at least to produce a very large number of progeny. This is an operational definition, since surviving cells are distinguished from nonsurviving cells by allowing isolated single cells sufficient time to express their proliferative ability by forming discrete macroscopic colonies.

In order to obtain an accurate picture of the so-called radiosensitivity for a cell population, it is necessary to determine the proportion of cells surviving over a wide range of doses. The shapes of curves constructed through such a set of survival estimates can be very different. The shape of a survival curve may indicate a great deal about the nature of the cell population

irradiated and about the mode of action of various chemical and physical factors which affect survival. Survival curves also allow estimates to be made by interpolation (and, to a limited extent, by extrapolation) of the effects of doses not actually tested.

Two of the most puzzling observations concerning cell killing by ionizing radiation are: (1) a very small amount of absorbed energy is required to produce a drastic response and (2) dose-survival curves for many types of cell populations show either no threshold or relatively small thresholds. This form of response is in marked contrast to the type of dose response usually observed for heat inactivation or some types of chemical poisons which produce little or no effect up to a threshold dose, followed by a rapid increase approaching 100 per cent effect with only a small further increase in dose. The contrast in features of these types of survival curves is illustrated in Figure 6–9, in which the fraction of cells surviving is plotted on a linear ordinate against the dose on a linear abscissa.

In order to appreciate more fully the differences between these types of survival curves, it is necessary to consider what is known about differences in the general action of the agents themselves.

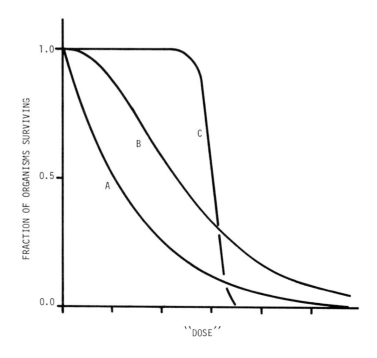

FIGURE 6–9 The fraction of organisms surviving is plotted as a function of dose. Curves A (no shoulder) and B (small shoulder) illustrate typical survival curves following exposure to ionizing radiation. Curve C illustrates survival which might be observed for some types of chemical poisons.

For ionizing radiation the sequence of events which leads to cell killing starts with the absorption of energy. This leads directly or indirectly to the disruption of molecules, which in turn leads to the expression of biologic damage. There is a great deal known about the initial absorption processes and their relationships to observed effects. Less is known of the production of chemical and biochemical damage, and the manner in which this chemical damage is expressed is not well understood.

Damage is initiated in biologic material as a result of ionizations and excitations which occur along the tracks of fast moving charged particles. These ionizations and excitations are discrete, very localized events which occur randomly along the tracks. For irradiation with energetic X- or gamma rays, the ionizations which occur in an absorbing material as a result of primary photon interactions is exceedingly small compared to the number of ionizations which occur along the tracks of the fast moving electrons set in motion following such interactions. Historically, this discrete and random nature of the occurrence of absorption events was the key to understanding (in principle) the general shape of cell survival curves and the remarkable efficiency of ionizing radiation in producing biologic effects. If these effects result from energy transfer to many very small volumes within the biologic material, rather than from a more uniform transfer of energy to the whole material, it is clear why dose-response curves for ionizing radiation are different from those observed in many cases for heat or chemical treatment. If a small amount of energy in the form of heat is absorbed by a body, the average kinetic energy of all the molecules comprising the body (i.e., the temperature) is increased by a small amount. This energy is not enough to strip tightly bound electrons from atoms or molecules. The same body exposed in a macroscopically uniform field of ionizing radiation, such that it absorbed the same amount of energy in ergs per gram, would contain on a microscopic scale many portions which would not be affected at all immediately following irradiation. Other areas would be drastically affected! Of course, much of the energy transferred to matter by ionizing radiation eventually becomes degraded to heat, but this is not the factor which effects biologic response. The temperature of a man irradiated to a dose of 1000 rads over the total body (which is lethal to 100 per cent of the population) would only increase by about 1/500 of 1° C.

6.7 TARGET THEORY

A very important concept was suggested nearly 50 years ago through the work of Dessauer (1922) and Blau and Altenburger (1922) which allowed a formal relationship between dose and effect to be derived. This so-called "hit" hypothesis considered the form of the dose response curve as being due to the discrete and random nature of the absorption process described above, and supposed that a biologic unit (cell, molecule, etc.) would react (die, become inactive, etc.) after some minimum number of absorption events or "hits" had been registered somewhere in this unit. Because of the statistical nature of this process, a relationship between the proportion of biologic units not affected and the radiation dose is easily derived. These ideas have been reviewed in detail by a number of authors, together with discussions of their extensions to practical applications. For the student who would like to gain a better appreciation of these concepts and their applications, the monographs of Zimmer (1961) or Elkind and Whitmore (1967) are highly recommended. Their importance has been concisely outlined by Zimmer as follows: ". . . the hit theory appears to offer an explanation of the dose-effect curve in radiobiology which seems at first sight so difficult to understand." Further development of these ideas (the target theory) ". . . opens the way to understanding the fact that irradiation is so efficient in inducing biological actions."

Figure 6–10 shows a "semi-log" plot of curve A taken from Figure 6–9 with the surviving fraction being plotted on a logarithmic scale against the dose on a linear scale. When the curve is presented in this way, it is apparent that dose is linearly related to the logarithm of the surviving fraction. A relationship of this kind can be expressed according to the formula:

$$f = e^{-D/D0} \qquad \text{Equation A (see Appendix 1)}$$

where f represents the fraction of cells sur-

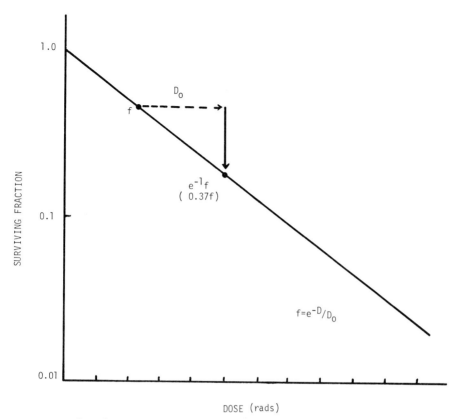

FIGURE 6–10 A semi-log plot of curve A taken from Figure 6–9, with the surviving fraction plotted on a logarithmic scale against the dose plotted on a linear scale. D_0, the reciprocal of the slope of this curve, is also referred to as the mean lethal dose or the D_{37}.

viving and D represents the dose. The constant, D_0, is the reciprocal of the slope of this curve. It may be defined as the dose necessary to reduce the survival from some value f to $e^{-1} \times f$ (approximately $0.37 \times f$) anywhere along the curve. D_0 is also called the mean lethal dose, or the D_{37}.[*]

Survival curves, which are truly simple exponential functions of dose, are consistent with the hypothesis that the organisms can be killed by a "single event" process, such as the occurrence of a single ionization or ion cluster in a critical volume within the cell. Equation A is sometimes referred to as the single-hit, single-target formula.

Figure 6–11 shows a similar semi-log plot of curve B from Figure 6–9. The similarities and differences between curves A and B are most easily seen when they are plotted in this way. While curve A shows a simple exponential function of dose, curve B displays a so-called threshold or shoulder region, only approaching a simple exponential at high doses. It is often described as a "sigmoid" type of survival curve. To a first approximation curve B may be described by the relations

$$f = 1 - (1 - e^{-D/D_0})^n$$

For high doses this relationship very nearly approaches the simple exponential

$$f = ne^{-D/D_0}$$

which is shown by the dashed line in Figure 6–11. The intercept of this line at zero dose corresponds to the number n. Since the two curves are practically coincident for surviving fractions below 0.1, the number n can be closely approximated by extrapolating the straight portion of the curve below 0.1 surviving fraction to its

[*]Many prefer to write the equation $f = e^{-\lambda D}$, where λ is the more conventional slope constant ($\lambda = 1/D_0$). Others prefer to use D_0, possibly as a carry-over from the hit and target theories in which D_0 is the dose required to result in an average of one hit per unit target volume. The unit of measure for D_0 is rads (ergs per gram) where the slope constant λ has units of rads^{-1} or grams per erg.

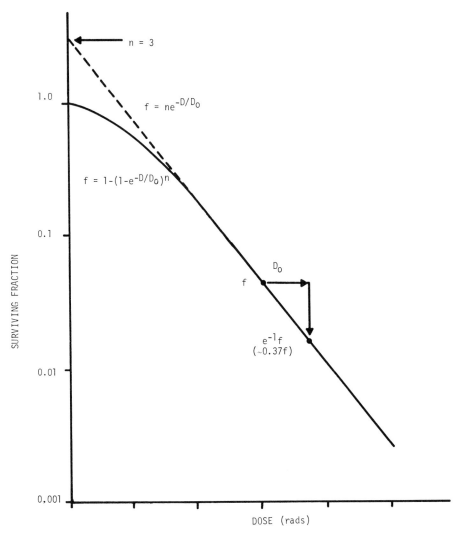

FIGURE 6-11 A semi-log plot of curve B taken from Figure 6–9, with the surviving fraction plotted on a logarithmic scale against the dose plotted on a linear scale. This curve has a "threshold" or shoulder region (extrapolation number = 3). It approaches a linear exponential curve at higher doses.

intercept on the ordinate at zero dose. The slopes of the two curves are nearly the same, and the parameter D_0 of curve B may be defined as the dose necessary to reduce the survival from some value f to $e^{-1} \times f$ *in the straight portion of the curve.*

Survival curves which have a shape similar to curve B imply, at least for a proportion of the cells in the population, that some sort of damage accumulation process is responsible for cell killing. Equation B is known as the single-hit, multi-target formula and describes a hypothetical type of cell killing in which an ionization or ion cluster must occur in two or more (n) separate

critical volumes within a cell in order to sterilize that cell.

In practice, these mathematical formulas are often used only as a first approximation to describe a set of experimental data, and both of these relationships can be derived by assuming certain mechanisms involved in cell killing. It should be kept in mind, however, that strictly speaking, survival curves are not determined experimentally. What is determined is a set of discrete points of statistically limited accuracy. The survival curve is a graphic representation of some particular continuous function whose parameters have been adjusted so that the curve will pass as closely as possible to all the survival estimates. An unlimited number of different functions are available, each of which would fit a given set of experimental data satisfactorily, and a very large number can be justified in principle by assuming various possible mechanisms of cell killing.

For example, one may allow for the possibility of inactivation by multiple hits on a single target, multiple hits on a multiplicity of targets, and even a biologic variability of hit and target multiplicity within a heterogeneous cell population. The satisfactory fit of a given curve to a set of data clearly is not sufficient in itself to establish the precise mechanism of cell killing. The possibilities may be narrowed, but a number of other independent considerations must be taken into account before the mode of cell killing by ionizing radiation can be established. Until these mechanisms can be worked out, it has become customary to characterize cell radiosensitivity in terms of the D_0 value for the straight line portion of the log-linear survival plot, and by using the intercept of this straight portion extrapolated to zero dose (i.e., the extrapolation number) as a measure of the shoulder. By convention we can remain uncommitted to the restrictions of any particular mathematical model.

At this point the student might be tempted to discard the hit hypothesis and the target theory since we frequently do not know how to apply them. There are many instances, however, in which the applicability of the target theory has been convincingly demonstrated for systems less complex than mammalian cells. Furthermore, within the framework of these general concepts much can be learned about the processes leading to cell killing, particularly through the use of different types of ionizing radiations.

6.8   MAMMALIAN CELL RADIOSENSITIVITY

It is appropriate at this point to examine in detail the radiosensitivity of mammalian cells and to attempt to put into historical perspective the important implications and ramifications arising from the determination of the first mammalian cell survival curve by Puck and Marcus in 1956. Before methods were available to assay the reproductive survival of single mammalian cells, the relative importance of major factors underlying the cause of tissue damage by ionizing radiations was not at all clear. Information could only be drawn from observations of physiologic and biochemical changes in tissues of irradiated animals, cultures of unspecified cell number, or from the quantitative survival estimates already available for such organisms as bacteria, yeast, and protozoa. It was not known whether changes in respiration, enzyme activity, nucleic acid metabolism, membrane permeability, blood pH, and viscosity were the cause or the effect of mammalian cell injury and death.

If the radiation sensitivity for mammalian cell killing was considered near that of microorganisms, then humoral effects must primarily account for the known high sensitivity of whole animals and their tissues. On the other hand, if mammalian cell reproductive function was much more sensitive than in microorganisms, physiologic and biochemical changes induced by the radiation, as well as changes in cell proliferation, could largely be attributed to secondary effects associated with cell injury and a failure of individual cells to maintain their role in tissue renewal. Since both these suggested mechanisms underlying tissue damage were tenable, a definitive test was needed.

Looking toward tissue culture experiments to provide an answer to the problem, however, did not appear very promising. To be sure, it was known that exposure to thousands of roentgens of X-rays would inhibit cell proliferation in a tissue culture. Exposure to hundreds of roentgens resulted in mitotic delay and the appearance of degenerate cells, but the extent of degeneration and its correlation with reproductive cell death could not be ascertained from available techniques.

Following the development of assay techniques which allowed a quantitative determination of the reproductive integrity of single mammalian cells, Puck and Marcus published the first mammalian cell X-ray survival curve. This curve, shown in Figure 6–12, demonstrated that the radio-

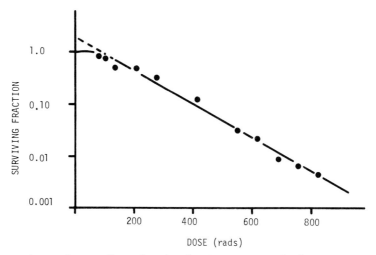

FIGURE 6-12   Survival curve for S3 cells irradiated with 230 Kvp X-rays. The dose in roentgens, which is known within a few per cent, has been multiplied by a factor of 1.35, which is known only approximately (1.20-1.50), thus converting the dose for glass-attached cells to rads.

sensitivity with respect to loss of reproductive function was enormously greater than had been observed for unicellular organisms, and was contrasted to the sensitivity of other cell functions such as the ability to concentrate or exclude dyes, synthesize virus particles, and metabolize nutrients. The latter were not appreciably affected in reproductively sterile giant cells that had received doses in excess of 10,000 rads.

The other important feature is the presence of a shoulder or threshold region on the survival curve, indicating that at least part of the cells in the population must be killed through some type of damage accumulation process.

The general features of this curve have now been confirmed for many different cell lines in laboratories throughout the world.[*] In addition, further confirmation has been obtained using techniques which allow survival assays to be made for cells *in vivo*. Under similar conditions, the D_0 values for different cell types may differ in some cases by a factor of two or three, but they are all of the same order of magnitude, and there is no indication that the radiosensitivity of normal cells is basically different from that of malignant cells.

A comparison of the radiation sensitivity

with respect to reproductive integrity of mammalian cells and various other microorganisms is shown in Figure 6-13. Curves 1 and 2 represent the extreme limits of mammalian cells' radiosensitivity that have been reported in the literature. The D_0 values are about 60 rads for the particularly sensitive strain of mouse leukemia cells and about 280 rads for the mouse "L" cells. For the vast majority of mammalian cells tested, the D_0 values range between 100 and 200 rads for irradiation in air with X- or gamma rays. Although these differences may indeed be important, it is the order of magnitude of sensitivity for these cells that is of greatest fundamental interest.

One important consequence of these results is that the underlying cause of acute tissue damage in mammals can be identified as cell reproductive death. In general, the different times of onset and degrees of damage in irradiated tissues can be explained in terms of differences in the kinetics of cell renewal in a tissue itself or in a tissue which supports it.

Although the radiosensitivity with respect to cell reproductive function is very similar for all mammalian cell types, there are a number of important factors which are known to alter their radiosensitivities. For purposes of discussion, these factors can be divided into three major categories: physical, chemical, and biologic, although the division is somewhat arbitrary.

[*]X- or gamma ray survival curves for one or two cell lines have been reported which appear not to have the shoulder (i.e., they are of the simple exponential type).

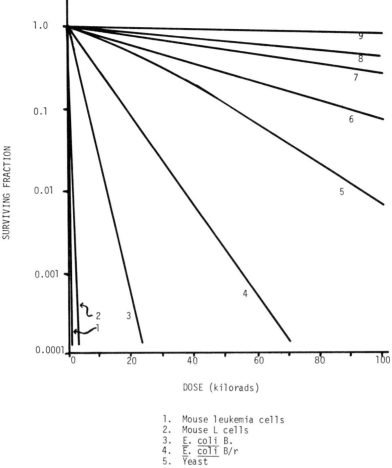

1. Mouse leukemia cells
2. Mouse L cells
3. E. coli B.
4. E. coli B/r
5. Yeast
6. Phage staph K
7. B. megatherium
8. Potato virus
9. Micrococcus radiodurans

FIGURE 6–13   The log of the surviving fraction is plotted as a function of dose (kilorads). This curve illustrates the relative radiosensitivity of several biologic systems.

6.9   PHYSICAL FACTORS AFFECTING RADIATION RESPONSE

Perhaps the most important physical factor affecting biologic response is the type and quality of radiation. The term relative biologic effectiveness (*RBE*) is used to compare the effectiveness of two different types of radiations in producing a given biologic effect. The definition of RBE suggested by the International Commission on Radiological Units and Measurements (ICRU) is shown at the top of the next column.

The standard radiation is usually taken to be X-rays generated at approximately 220 Kv. An example of the survival curves

$$RBE = \frac{\text{The dose (rad) from a standard radiation required to produce a given biologic effect.}}{\text{The dose (rad) from another radiation delivered under the same conditions which produces the same biologic effect.}}$$

which might be obtained for irradiation of a cell population with X-rays or fast neutrons is shown in Figure 6–14. In order to obtain the RBE for the fast neutrons according to the definition, a given level of effect corresponding to some particular surviving fraction is chosen (0.01 for the example shown in Figure 6–14) and the

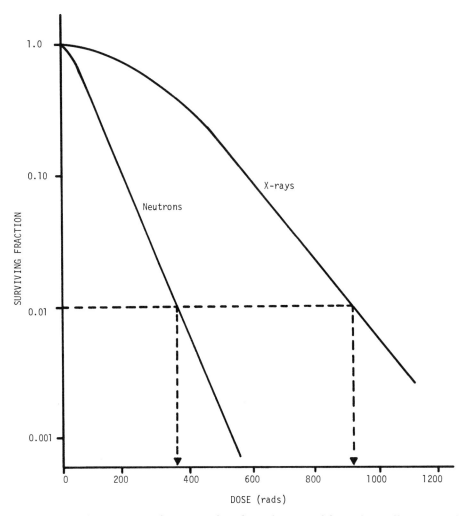

FIGURE 6–14 The log of the surviving fraction is plotted as a function of dose when cells were irradiated with X-rays or fast neutrons.

doses required to produce this effect are read off the dose scale for both curves. In this case the doses are 922 rads for X-rays and 369 rads for the neutrons. The RBE of the neutrons relative to X-rays is therefore 922 rads/369 rads = 2.50.

Since the survival curve for X-rays has a much more pronounced shoulder than for neutrons, it can be seen that the RBE depends on the level of effect chosen for comparison. In the shoulder region the RBE increases rapidly. This can be seen by referring again to Figure 6–14 and recalculating the RBE for survival levels of, for example, 0.2 and 0.8. For surviving fractions of 0.2 on both curves, the ratio of doses is 480 rads/140 rads = 3.43; for 0.8 surviving fraction the ratio is 155 rads/30 rads = 5.17.

It is important to note that RBE comparisons are made between radiation absorbed doses (rads) and not radiation exposures (Roentgens). Differences in relative penetration or depth dose characteristics in tissue are not the factors of direct concern here. The property associated with the radiations which is of concern is the spatial distribution of the ionizations and excitations along the path of incident charged particles or the charged particles set into motion by X-rays, gamma rays or neutrons. The term used to express this important parameter is the linear energy transfer (LET), which is a measure of the rate at which an ionizing particle loses energy along its track, usually given in units of thousands of electron volts per micron.

More than 90 per cent of the radiation

dose resulting from an exposure to X- or gamma rays is deposited along the tracks of electrons set in motion by these radiations. They are often called "sparsely ionizing," as are beta particles or energetic electrons produced by an accelerator. The LET's associated with these radiations for the most part range from about 0.1 to 20 KeV per micron. For a given particle, the higher its energy, the lower is its LET. Since a particle loses energy along its track, its LET is not constant but increases as the particle traverses the absorbing medium until it is finally stopped. LET values are normally quoted as "averages," being either "track average" or "energy average" LET's. Even these concepts are not very useful in many cases.

In contrast to the sparsely ionizing radiations, very dense tracks of ionizations are produced by heavy particles such as accelerated atomic nuclei, energetic recoil protons, which deliver most of the dose resulting from neutron irradiation, or alpha particles emitted during the decay of certain radioactive nuclides. The LET for some of these densely ionizing radiations may range up to 2000 KeV per micron or higher. Thus, a given absorbed dose for densely ionizing radiations is delivered in relatively small compact columns of ionizations, whereas for the same absorbed dose from sparsely ionizing radiations the ionizations are more widely distributed throughout the absorbing material.

For mammalian cell killing, RBE relative to 220 KVP X-rays increases from approximately 0.85 for ^{60}Co gamma rays where the associated average LET is about 0.3 KeV per micron to between 2 and 4 for alpha particles or accelerated atomic nuclei having average LET's of 100 to 200 KeV per micron. With further increase in LET, the RBE decreases.

The relationship between RBE and LET can be understood qualitatively on the basis of the target theory if it is assumed that cell killing requires a certain minimum number of absorption events or ionizations to occur within some specified small volume, or volumes, in the cell. If there are very few ionizations per unit track length (low LET), such that more than one ionizing particle must traverse the small critical volume before enough damaging events are deposited to inactivate, then the efficiency for inactiva-

tion per rad (i.e., on a macroscopic dose scale) will be less than optimum. When the average number of ionizations which occur along the particle track during its traverse through the small critical volume is near the minimum number necessary to inactivate, then this LET will be most efficient in killing the cell. If there are more ionizations deposited than necessary to inactivate as the particle crosses the volume (high LET), then some of the damaging ionizations are wasted. Since these wasted absorption events still contribute to the total absorbed dose, the radiation is less efficient in killing the cell. A rough analogy can be drawn to the duck hunter shooting into a thick flock of ducks with a sawed-off shotgun. The size of the shot he chooses will be very important. If the shot size is too small, a large number of "hits" may be required to bring down any one duck. If the size is just right, it may require only one "hit" per duck and this would bring down the maximum number from the flock. If the hunter chooses a very large shot size, one "hit" would be more than enough to kill any particular duck, but more ducks would be missed altogether.

For some systems, such as enzyme solutions or virus particles, a single absorption event is sufficient to produce the end point. In this case the RBE is maximum for the lowest LET used (gamma rays or high energy X-rays) and decreases continuously as the LET increases. This is in marked contrast to the situation we have described for mammalian cells, in which the RBE increases to a maximum for average LET's around 100 to 200 KeV per micron, then decreases as the LET increases further. In this case, the survival curve D_0 values decrease with increasing LET, and the curve shoulder also decreases until the curve becomes a simple exponential function of dose. For even higher LET radiations, the curve remains exponential or "single-hit," but the D_0 values begin to increase again. Typical relationships between RBE and LET for mammalian cell killing and virus or enzyme inactivation are shown in Figure 6–15.

The actual situation with respect to RBE and LET is far more complex than we have indicated. One of the principal difficulties is that no particle has a unique LET. As the particle loses energy to the absorbing

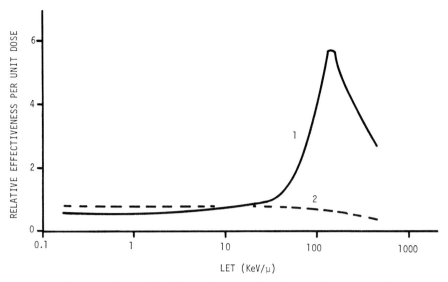

FIGURE 6–15 General aspects of possible relations between the relative effectiveness of ionizing particles and their LETs, concerning changes induced in different systems. Curve 1 is characteristic for various biologic effects on cells; curve 2 is characteristic for various effects on enzymes and phages.

medium its LET progressively increases until the particle is finally stopped. A more complete description can be found in the recent monograph of Elkind and Whitmore (1967). As will be discussed shortly, the RBE associated with various LET radiations also depends upon a number of other factors such as the chemical environment of the cell at the time of irradiation and the radiation dose-rate.

It should be noted in a discussion of physical factors influencing radiosensitivity that temperature and dose rate can affect the response of cells. Except for cryogenic temperatures and extremely high dose rates, these effects can be attributed to secondary changes in the metabolic state of cells or intracellular repair processes. They are therefore discussed in section 6.11.

6.10 CHEMICAL FACTORS AFFECTING RADIATION RESPONSE

The second category of factors influencing radiosensitivity is the chemical environment of the cell. Some chemical compounds, when present at the time of irradiation, can exert a protective effect; some can exert a sensitizing effect. Other compounds can alter radiosensitivity if cells are kept in their presence before, or in some cases after, irradiation.

For most biologic systems, radiation-induced changes do not follow directly on the deposition of energy, but instead the injury is developed in both radiochemical and biochemical stages before the effects become apparent. It is not surprising, therefore, that this chemical development might be subject to outside chemical influence at one or more of these stages.

About 20 years ago several groups of investigators reported that some compounds, when injected into mice immediately before irradiation, would protect them against the lethal effects of the radiation. It was found to be essential that the compound should be present at the time of irradiation. No protection whatsoever was obtained when the compound was given even seconds later.

The naturally occurring amino acid cysteine was the first protective chemical found. It belongs to a class of compounds known as sulfhydryl amines. Other effective chemicals of this class include cysteamine (2-mercaptoethylamine or MEA) and aminoethylisothiourea dihydrobromide (AET). In aqueous solution, AET rearranges to mercaptoethylguanidine (MEG) which is the protecting molecule. The chemical structure of these compounds is shown in Chapter 9. The sulfhydryl amines are the most effective class of chemical protectors. The three mentioned above are of approximately equal effectiveness, and although many other compounds of this class have been studied, none is more effective than cysteine, the first such substance found.

Most chemical protective substances act to reduce the effective dose to the cells, in which case the survival curves in the presence and absence of the compound are similar in shape and differ only in their final slopes. Such substances are known as dose modifying agents since the dose-survival curves obtained in their presence and absence can be made to superimpose exactly on one another by applying a dose scale factor or dose modifying factor to one of the curves. In other words, although the two curves plotted on the same scale will be separated, if one of the curves is plotted on a compressed dose scale or the other on an expanded dose scale, the two can be made to lie precisely on top of one another. The dose modifying factor for the three compounds described above is about 1.8; that is, in the presence of these protectors it takes about twice the dose to produce the same degree of cell killing as in their absence. The use of these compounds in whole mammals is further complicated owing to differences in their toxicity and the rate at which they are oxidized by the animal.

Several hypotheses have been advanced concerning the mechanism of action of the sulfhydryl amines. Among the less controversial are the "radical scavenger" hypothesis and the hypothesis of damage repair by donation of hydrogen atoms. The radical scavenger hypothesis proposes that when important biologic molecules are subject to indirect damage from free radicals produced nearby, then protection can take place if an appropriate substance is present which can compete for reaction with the free radicals. Many of the sulfhydryl amines are readily oxidized by free radicals to form relatively stable products. The second proposed mechanism suggests that if an important biologic molecule loses a hydrogen atom either as a direct or indirect result of irradiation, a sulfhydryl amine may donate a hydrogen atom to the damaged molecule in such a way that it would be restored to its original state.

From a practical standpoint, probably the most important chemical radiosensitizing agent is oxygen. It has been recognized for nearly half a century that the presence of oxygen during irradiation with X- or gamma rays greatly enhances the effect of the radiation. Like some of the radioprotective compounds, oxygen is known to act as a dose modifying agent. An effect produced by a given dose in the presence of oxygen requires a dose "r" times as great to produce the same effect in its absence. With oxygen, the dose modifying factor depends on the concentration of dissolved oxygen at the time of irradiation. The maximum dose modifying factor corresponding to the relative radiosensitivity for fully oxygenated conditions with respect to anoxic conditions is approximately 2.5 to 3.0 for sparsely ionizing radiations. This is often called the oxygen enhancement ratio. For example, if a mammalian cell survival curve obtained under fully oxygenated conditions were found to have a D_0 of 135 rads and an extrapolation number of 5, under fully anoxic conditions the survival curve would be expected to have a D_0 of about 405 rads with the extrapolation number, 5, remaining the same. The relationship between oxygen concentration and radiosensitivity is shown in Figure 6–16. For anoxic conditions the radiosensitivity is minimal, and as the oxygen concentration is increased, the radiosensitivity increases rapidly to a maximum. From Figure 6–16 it can be seen that for oxygen tensions between about 5 to 8 (mm Hg at 37° C) the radiosensitivity has already reached half its maximum value, and that above about 30 mm Hg there is very little further increase in radiosensitivity.

Several mechanisms have been proposed to account for the oxygen effect. It has been shown that oxygen increases the yield of certain oxidizing free radicals which may be more likely to damage other nearby molecules. In addition, it is possible that damage to critical biologic molecules may be reversible in the absence of oxygen, whereas in its presence the damage is permanent. Whatever the precise mechanism, it is clear that oxygen modifies radiation damage at the radiochemical level.

There are several lines of evidence to suggest that the mechanism of the oxygen effect is not physiologic in nature. For example, the state of the respiratory enzymes, as reflected by the respiratory rate of cells, is not an important factor. At an oxygen   concentration   corresponding   to

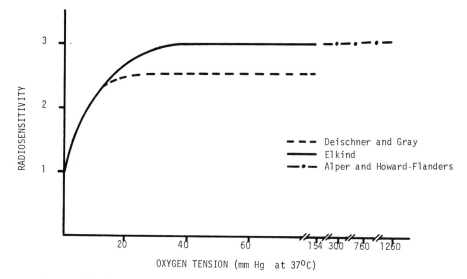

FIGURE 6-16 Curves of radiosensitivity as a function of oxygen tension at the time of irradiation. (Data from Alper and Howard-Flanders, 1956; Deschner and Gray, 1959; Elkind et al., 1965.)

half maximum radiosensitivity, cells still respire at maximum rate. Furthermore, the oxygen effect has been shown to be independent of temperature over a range in which metabolic rates are greatly altered. Another important observation is that oxygen must be present at the instant of irradiation to exert its effect. Oxygen introduced as little as 0.02 second after irradiation will not sensitize the cells. Finally, while radiosensitivity is strongly dependent on oxygen concentration for sparsely ionizing radiations, it is much less so for densely ionizing or high LET radiations.

Since the oxygen effect is LET-depend-

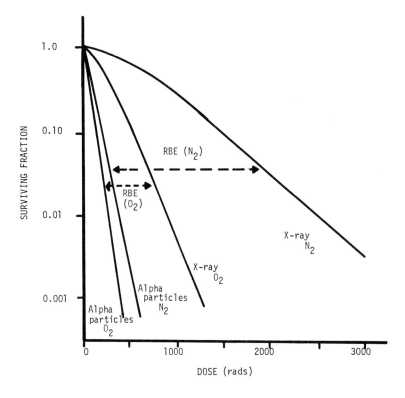

FIGURE 6-17 The log of the surviving fraction is plotted as a function of dose (rads). The curves illustrate survival of mammalian cells with X-rays or alpha particles in the presence or absence of oxygen.

ent, it is not surprising that the RBE may also be influenced by the presence or absence of oxygen. Figure 6–17 shows a set of survival curves which might be obtained for irradiation of mammalian cells with X-rays or alpha particles in the presence or absence of oxygen. With alpha particles there is very little difference between the anoxic and oxygenated survival curves, but there is a very pronounced change for irradiation with X-rays. The RBE is therefore greater under anoxic conditions. The manner in which RBE and the oxygen enhancement ratio vary with LET is shown in Figure 6–18.

The use of neutrons in radiotherapy has stimulated a great deal of interest over the past few years. The rationale behind this interest lies in the possibility that many tumors may contain viable hypoxic cells which are resistant to sterilization by X- or gamma rays. If only a small proportion of these resistant hypoxic cells remained in the tumor cell population over the course of treatment with sparsely ionizing X- or gamma rays, eradication of the tumor would be much less likely. This problem might be reduced if high LET radiations were used. Neutrons are very penetrating and transfer most of their energy to biologic material through collisions with protons, which then deposit energy along relatively densely ionizing tracks. The oxygen enhancement ratio for 14 MeV neutrons has been estimated to be about 1.7.

Of even greater interest is the possible

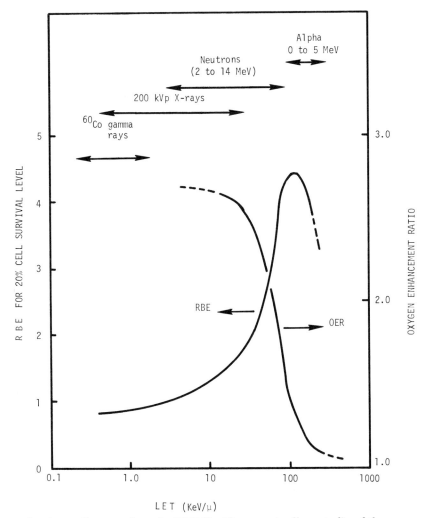

FIGURE 6–18 This figure illustrates how the RBE (for 20 per cent cell survival) and the oxygen enhancement ratio vary with LET. The range of LET's associated with various types of radiations is also shown.

use of negative pi mesons for radiotherapy. Most of the dose delivered by these particles is deposited in the Bragg peak region where negative pi mesons are captured by carbon, nitrogen, and oxygen nuclei. When captures are achieved the nuclei literally explode, sending fragments in all directions. These fragments have high LET values; therefore, the RBE is high and the oxygen enhancement ratio is low. If the oxygen effect is not a limiting factor in conventional radiotherapy, the greatly improved depth dose and high RBE for negative pi mesons in the region of the tumor would remain as a significant advantage. If the oxygen effect is important, the advantage would be even greater.

Another class of chemical agents which increase the radiosensitivity of cells is the halogenated pyrimidines. These compounds are of great interest because of their effect on the mode of action of cell killing by ionizing radiation. It is known that the pyrimidines 5-chlorodeoxyuridine (CUdR), 5-bromodeoxyuridine (BUdR), and 5-iododeoxyuridine (IUdR) are biologically active analogs of thymidine (TdR). Like thymidine, they are selectively incorporated into the cell's DNA. Following such incorporation cells become appreciably more radiosensitive, the degree of sensitization apparently depending on the extent of incorporation of these analogs into DNA. Experiments involving the use of BUdR indicate that with increasing incubation time of cells in the presence of the drug, both the D_0 and extrapolation number decrease. The halogenated deoxyribosides of cytosine such as 5-bromodeoxycytidine (BCdR) and 5-iododeoxycytidine (ICdR) are converted by the cell to BUdR and IUdR, thereby causing the cell to be more radiosensitive.

The fluoro derivatives, 5-fluorouracil (FU) and 5-fluorodeoxyuridine (FUdR) are not incorporated into DNA. Although they are biologically active in other respects, they will not be considered further in the present discussion.

The fact that the thymidine analogs are selectively incorporated into DNA and also sensitize cells to radiation strongly implicates DNA as a principal "target" molecule, damage to which can lead to cell reproductive death. Considerable circumstantial evidence has been accumulated on a number of grounds which implicate DNA as the prime "critical target" responsible for mammalian cell death following irradiation. Nevertheless, the complex interplay of all the processes subject to radiation damage which are important to the maintenance of cell reproductive function should be kept in mind. Cells may be killed in a number of different ways, each of which contributes to a greater or lesser extent to the observed overall effect. There is no doubt that DNA is damaged in many ways following irradiation. However, if DNA damage proves to be the most critical factor, which seems likely, many questions still remain regarding the nature of the damage itself and the way, or ways, in which it leads to cell death.

6.11 BIOLOGIC FACTORS AFFECTING RADIATION RESPONSE

Finally, there are several important biologic factors which are known to alter or modify cell radiation response. The two which will be discussed in some detail are the repair of radiation damage and the dependence of radiation response on the cell reproductive life cycle.

It has been recognized for about 30 years that in microorganisms certain treatments, such as holding the cells at reduced temperatures or in a suboptimal medium, can increase survival following irradiation. These treatments are thought to operate either by creating intracellular conditions which enhance a damage repair system or by suppressing processes which hinder or oppose repair. More recently, similar observations have been made using mammalian cells. It has been postulated that radiation produces damage which is potentially lethal and will kill a cell if it remains in such a state. If irradiated cells are maintained under conditions which are less than optimum with respect to cell division, the repair of potentially lethal damage is enhanced.

Another process, which may or may not be related to that just described, is the repair of sublethal radiation damage. To understand the features of this process it is necessary to recall two important features of the mammalian cell survival curve. First, a shoulder or threshold type of survival

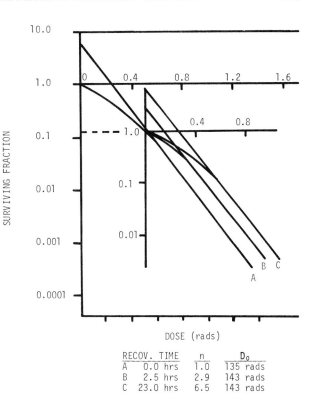

FIGURE 6-19 This figure illustrates survival curves when fractionated doses were given at intervals of 2.5 (curve B) and 23 hours (curve C). Curve A shows survival following a single dose given at time 0.

RECOV. TIME		n	D_0
A	0.0 hrs	1.0	135 rads
B	2.5 hrs	2.9	143 rads
C	23.0 hrs	6.5	143 rads

curve implies a damage accumulation process for cell killing. In other words, at least a portion of the cells in the irradiated population must accumulate damage in order to be sterilized. When they have accumulated all the damage they are able to tolerate, one further damaging event will be sufficient to kill them, and the survival curve subsequently approaches a simple exponential function of dose. Secondly, it follows that essentially all the cells which survive after irradiation to a dose corresponding to the exponential region of survival must be sublethally damaged.

Elkind and his co-workers performed a series of experiments, based on this line of reasoning, to see whether cells, sublethally damaged by a dose of radiation, could repair this damage. They found that if a survival curve was determined for cells which had survived a previous dose of radiation, the shoulder on the curve promptly returned with incubation time after the initial "priming" dose was given. After a time, the accumulation of sublethal damage was again required in order to sterilize sur-

viving cells, and therefore the sublethal damage accumulated by survivors of the priming dose must have been repaired. An experiment illustrating this effect is shown in Figure 6-19.

Further experiments have also been carried out to determine the time course of recovery as reflected by changes in survival for a particular total dose delivered in two approximately equal fractions with increasing incubation times being allowed between the fractions. Figure 6-20 illustrates the change in survival for one of the fractionation experiments. For this so-called "recovery period," it can be seen that survival increases rapidly to a maximum when the doses are separated by about 2 to 3 hours, then decreases to a minimum for a separation of about 6 hours, and finally increases again for longer incubation times between doses. The survival curve obtained 5 hours after an initial dose of 505 rads corresponding to the minimum in the recovery curve indicates that the shoulder is again lost, and that this minimum is therefore due to changes in the cell threshold tolerance.

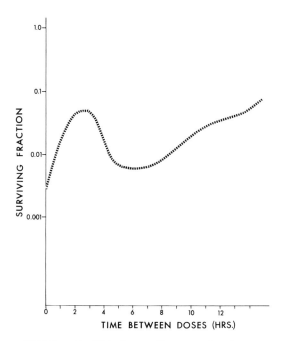

FIGURE 6-20 This figure illustrates the change in the surviving fraction as a function of time between two doses of 505 rads each.

Similar studies by other investigators have produced results which are qualitatively similar. Cell division is delayed after the first dose of radiation by an amount which is proportional to the magnitude of the dose. Repair of sublethal radiation damage begins without delay and is essentially complete before cell division resumes. The minimum in the recovery curve reflects the fact that radiosensitivity of cells differs appreciably as they progress through their life cycle.

Repair processes also apparently operate during continuous irradiation at low dose rate. A greater total dose is required to produce the same effect when it is delivered continuously over a longer period of time. Using Chinese hamster cells, dose rate effects can be clearly demonstrated for dose rates below about 30 rads per minute, and for HeLa cells below around 10 rads per minute. Dose rate effects are very pronounced in the range commonly associated with radiotherapy treatments using low activity interstitial or intracavitary radioactive sources (i.e., between about 0.1 and 1 rad per minute).

For high LET radiations, dose rate or dose fractionation effects are reduced or absent. This might be expected since survival curve shoulders are also reduced, indicating that cells exposed to them either will die or that there will be no sublethal damage to repair. Here again is another factor which affects RBE. Since cell killing is less dependent on dose rate for high LET radiations, the RBE for high LET radiations is increased as the dose rate used in the comparison is decreased.

Experiments involving dose fractionation and dose rate are very important from a number of different viewpoints. For one, an understanding of the repair process leading to the recovery of sublethal damage may facilitate understanding of lethal radiation damage itself. Also, these studies have obvious implications for radiotherapy. Tumor treatment regimens have been decided largely on empirical grounds. Fortunately, for some tumors these treatment regimens have been remarkably successful. For others, exactly the opposite is true.

Up to this point we have described various radiation survival responses which apply to cell populations in which cells are randomly dividing and are distributed in all parts of the life cycle. The pioneering work of Terasima and Tolmach led the way to an examination of the response of populations of cells which were synchronized with respect to their position in the life cycle. Observing monolayer cell cultures grown on glass surfaces, Terasima and Tolmach noted that, although most cells were stretched out and flattened, during mitosis the cells became rounded. These rounded mitotic cells were much less firmly attached and could be selectively removed by gentle agitation of the culture. In this way Terasima and Tolmach succeeded in collecting populations of cells which were essentially all mitotic. By plating replicate samples of these cells immediately after collection and irradiating different sets of samples after various periods of incubation, they were able to observe changes in radiosensitivity as the cells progressed together through their life cycle. Many workers have since adopted this elegant technique for the study of a variety of cell cycle related phenomena.

Other methods of obtaining synchronized cell cultures have also been developed. These include, for example, the use of drugs which reversibly block DNA synthesis but allow the remainder of cells to accumulate at the end of the G_1 period, incubation of cells for brief periods in high specific activity tritiated thymidine which selectively kills cells synthesizing DNA in its presence, and the use of agents such as hydroxyurea which for some cells both blocks the initiation of DNA synthesis, allowing an accumulation of cells at the end of G_1, and kills cells which are synthesizing DNA when the drug is added.

Fundamental differences between cell lines, along with differences in the method used to synchronize cultures, have made the interpretation of results somewhat difficult. It is also difficult to obtain purely synchronous cultures, particularly for the study of G_2 cells, since there is some variation in the rate at which cells of a given population progress through the life cycle. The synchronized starting population therefore becomes desynchronized rapidly. Nevertheless, several generalizations can be made and some of the ramifications of the results can be discussed.

In 1968, Sinclair reviewed the results obtained by about 10 different groups of investigators using a variety of cell lines and methods of synchronization. He summarized the findings in general which indicate that for cell lines with a short G_1 period, cells are most radiosensitive in G_2 and mitosis, less sensitive in G_1, and least sensitive (most resistant) toward the end of the S period. For cell lines having a

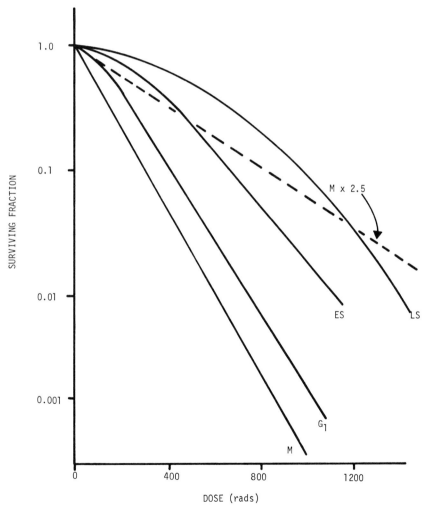

FIGURE 6–21 This figure illustrates that single cell survival following radiation is dependent on its position in the generation cycle at the time of radiation. A dose-modifying factor of 2.5, which might be expected for anoxic conditions, has been applied to mitotic cells as shown by the dotted line.

long G_1 period, there is a prominent peak of resistance in G_1 followed by an increase in sensitivity toward the end of G_1. The remaining changes in sensitivity are similar to those for short G_1 cell lines.

The magnitude of cell cycle-dependent radiosensitivity for a line of Chinese hamster cells, as illustrated by Sinclair, is shown in Figure 6–21. Survival curves for mitotic (M), G_1, early S phase (ES), and late S phase (LS) cells are plotted with a hypothetical anoxic survival curve (dashed line for M cells assuming a dose modification factor of 2.5). It is clear from this comparison that fluctuations in survival related to the cell life cycle can be as significant as the oxygen effect in dose modification. The reason that these fluctuations in radiosensitivity occur through the life cycle is not clear. For Chinese hamster cells it has been shown that the addition of sulfhydryl compounds to synchronized cultures protects mitotic and G_2 cells to a much greater extent than S phase cells. It may be that there are cyclic variations of intracellular sulfhydral groups during the life cycle. It does not appear, however, that this can fully account for variations in sensitivity.

The finding that cells differ in their sensitivities through the life cycle opened the way to understanding the cyclic recovery curves for split dose irradiations. Such recovery curves have been examined extensively in the light of cell life cycle responses, and can be satisfactorily accounted for on this basis. When an exponentially growing asynchronous population of cells is given a single acute dose of X- or gamma rays, the surviving cells will be predominated by those comprising the most resistant portion or portions of the life cycle. The progress of cells is temporarily halted, but repair of sublethal damage starts immediately and progresses rapidly as evidenced by the rapid increase in survival for the second dose. After a brief delay, surviving cells resume their progress through the life cycle. The majority of survivors, being in the most resistant phases, can only progress one way—toward a more sensitive phase. This is reflected in the recovery curve by a decrease in survival followed by a second increase.

Studies over the past two or three years have pointed to another possible aspect of radiosensitivity as related to the cell life cycle; that is, under certain circumstances a cell may temporarily leave the life cycle altogether. This state has, in some cases, been referred to as the G_0 state. Under the control of some outside stimulus, cells may be triggered into or out of a proliferative moiety of the population. Such situations are, of course, the rule rather than the exception in normal adult mammals where tissue stem cells may proliferate rapidly when there is an injury or loss of cells from the population. When the lost or injured tissues are replaced, the proliferation decreases and returns to its normal steady state. Study of normal tissues which are ordinarily nonproliferating, but which are capable of being stimulated to divide, would be very important. However, techniques for accomplishing this have not yet been developed.

In recent years, methods have been devised for culturing cells in a plateau phase, in which cell proliferation is inhibited either by nutrient depletion or by overcrowding. It has been suggested that cells in this condition may be a better model of a solid tumor than cultured cells under optimal growth conditions. After a certain cell density is reached in a culture, the population growth slows and finally stops altogether, but as in many mammalian tissues there is a limited degree of cell turnover. If the cultures are "fed" by frequently changing the medium, the cells can be kept for long periods of time in this plateau phase and yet immediately resume proliferation when they are diluted. Although there is only limited information on the response of these cultures, recently studied in detail by Hahn and by Little, it appears that survival curve D_0 values are somewhat lower. For some cell lines there is a reduced extrapolation number and little or no repair of sublethal radiation damage; for other cell lines this does not seem to be true. Also, in some instances it appears that for plateau phase cultures the repair of potentially lethal damage may be favored. If irradiated plateau phase cultures are stored for some time before replating for the colony survival assay, an increase in survival is observed.

In summary, there are a number of important biologic factors, such as damage repair and life cycle-related phenomena, which have been shown to have a very important influence on the survival of cells. They are of interest both with regard to the advancement of our knowledge of the nature of radiation-induced cell reproductive death and in their implications for radiotherapy.

6.12 SUMMARY

Cell reproductive death and hereditary changes in surviving cells are perhaps the two most important effects of ionizing radiation which are produced in biologic material. This chapter deals primarily with measurements of single cell survival following radiation using *in vitro* techniques comparable to those established by Puck and Marcus. Cell sensitivity is typically expressed in terms of the mean lethal dose, D_0, and the extrapolation number, n. Mammalian cells are generally more sensitive to radiation than bacteria, yeast, and virus particles. D_0 values for mammalian cells range from 60 rads for a particularly sensitive strain of mouse leukemic cells to about 280 rads for mouse "L" cells, when using X- or gamma rays. Extrapolation numbers range from 1 to 10 for most mammalian cells. Values for both of these parameters vary, depending upon the "age" of the cell at the time of irradiation.

Cells are more sensitive when radiations (particulate) with high linear energy transfer are used. The relative biologic effectiveness increases as the linear energy transfer increases until an optimal number of ionizations per unit of track length is obtained. Further increase in linear energy transfer (overkill) is associated with a reduction in relative biologic effectiveness.

Some radiation-induced injury is reversible and capacity for repair and recovery has been studied by using fractionated doses and by using suboptimal growth conditions following single acute doses. Cell survival generally increases as the interval between fractions increases or as the dose rate decreases. Dose rate and fractionation effects are reduced for radiations with high LET.

Radiosensitivity is increased when cells are irradiated in the presence of oxygen, as compared to irradiation in the presence of nitrogen. The oxygen enhancement ratio decreases as the linear energy transfer increases. Radiation damage can be reduced by using radioprotective agents. The sulfhydryl amines are the most effective class of chemical protectors. The dose modifying factor produced by this agent is about 1.8. Generally these agents need to be present during radiation in order to exert their effect. Some agents, such as halogenated pyrimidines which are selectively incorporated into DNA, also sensitize cells.

References

1. Baserga, R.: Biochemistry of the cell cycle; a review. Cell Tissue Kinet., *1*:167–191, 1968.
2. Casarett, A. P.: *Radiation Biology.* Englewood Cliffs, N.J., Prentice-Hall, 1968.
3. Elkind, M. M., and Whitmore, G. F.: *The Radiobiology of Cultured Mammalian Cells.* New York, Gordon and Breach, 1967.
4. Hahn, G. M.: Failure of Chinese Hamster cells to repair sublethal damage when irradiated in the plateau phase of growth. Nature, *217*:741–742, 1968.
5. Hewitt, H. B., and Wilson, C. W.: A survival curve for mammalian cells irradiated *in vivo. Nature, 183*:1060–1061, 1959.
6. Howard, A., and Pelc, S. R.: Synthesis of deoxyribonucleic acid in normal and irradiated cells and its relation to chromosome breakage. *Heredity,* 6:261–273, 1953.
7. Powers, W. E., and Tolmach, L. J.: Demonstration of an anoxic component in a mouse tumor-cell population by *in vivo* assay of survival following irradiation. Radiology, 83:328–336, 1964.
8. Prescott, D. M.: Composition of the cell life cycle. *In* Fry, R. J. M., Griem, M. L. and Kirsten, W. H. (eds.): *Cancer Research: Normal and Malignant Cell Growth.* New York, Springer-Verlag, 1969.
9. Puck, T. T., and Marcus, P. I.: Action of X-rays on mammalian cells. J. Exp. Med., *103*:653–666, 1956.
10. Sinclair, W. K.: Cyclic X-ray responses in mammalian cells *in vitro.* Radiat. Res., 33:620–643, 1968.
11. Sinclair, W. K.: Methods and criteria of mammalian cell synchrony. *In* Fry, R. J. M., Griem, M. L., and Kirsten, W. H. (eds.): *Normal and Malignant Cell Growth.* New York, Springer-Verlag, 1968.
12. Terasima, T., and Tolmach, L. J.: Variations in several responses of HeLa cells to X-irradiation during the division cycle. Biophys. J., 3:11–33, 1963.
13. Till, J. E., and McCulloch, E. A.: A direct measurement of the radiation sensitivity of normal mouse bone marrow cells. *Radiat. Res., 14*: 213–222, 1961.
14. Withers, H. R., and Elkind, M. M.: Radiosensitivity and fractionation response of crypt cells of mouse jejunum. *Radiat. Res.* 38:598–613, 1969.
15. Zimmer, K. G.: Studies in Quantitative Radiation Biology. (Trans. by H. D. Griffith.) Edinburgh, Oliver and Boyd, 1961.

7 CLINICAL RADIATION THERAPY

Carl R. Bogardus, Jr., M.D.

7.0 INTRODUCTION

Three-quarters of a century ago Röntgen's discovery of a "new kind of ray" together with the Curie's discovery of radium became the preface of an interminable volume of interrelated discoveries that were to change man's entire existence from the conquest of the atom and space to a key role in the eventual conquest of cancer.

The beginning of radiation therapy was fraught with endless frustrations, problems, and some surprising cures. Shortly after their discovery, radium, and X-rays became the chief treatments for practically every known illness. As a result, during the following years there were many tragic examples of radiation injury to both patients and physicians until the hazards of the indiscriminate use of these powerful modalities were eventually realized.

It was soon discovered that the use of radiations had a markedly deleterious effect on the growth of cancer. Indeed, it was found that cancer could even be cured by the judicious application of radium and X-rays. From these early discoveries arose a complete new armamentarium for the treatment and cure of what had been, up to that time, practically an incurable condition.

Many cancers and benign conditions totally unsuited for radiation therapy were irradiated by physicians who had practically no understanding of the tool they were employing. Unfortunately an early evaluation of the results of indiscriminate irradiation was not possible owing to the long-term effects that often resulted. Many times these mistakes in judgment were not recognized until years later.

Physicians and researchers continue to strive for the final cure of all cancer. A fact often not realized is that we now possess the knowledge, ability, and equipment to effect a permanent cure of one-half the cancer patients that we subject to a curative attempt by radiation therapy. New treatment schemes, new therapy machines, and imaginative combinations of treatment modalities will continue to raise this already impressive cure rate.

7.1 CELL SYSTEMS

The human body is composed of an almost endless variety of cell systems each with its own specific purpose. All of these systems have their own individual cell turnover rates with various biological properties associated with them.

This vast array of systems may be separated into four basic categories, based upon cell turnover time and potential for replacement.

A. Static Cell Population

The prime example of a static cell system is the neuron population of the central nervous system. Shortly after birth this cell system has reached its maximum number. Beyond this point there is only a decline. As these cells die and are replaced by scar tissue the total cell population continues to dwindle. Any action which destroys or removes cells from this system will result in a decrease in the number of cells and thereby loss of the functions which these cells were supporting. Radiation damage to the brain is basically irreparable. Under some circumstances alternate pathways may be established and some minor improvement might be noticed. However, major radiation damage cannot be repaired.

Striated muscle and some of the major connective tissues of the body are other examples of systems which do not achieve significant repair once they have been damaged.

The individual cells of a static population show a rather high degree of radioresistance owing to the fact that they are not capable of division. In the absence of mitosis one of the most radiosensitive phases of the cell cycle has been removed as a lethal target for radiations. This is not to say that the cells are immune to radiation damage; they are not. The amount of radiation required to destroy individual cells is high; however, the amount of radiation necessary to disrupt the combined functioning system is not as high as one would think. The sole reason lies in the inability of the cells to replace functional components once they are lost.

B. Renewing Cell Populations

The majority of the systems in the human body undergo a continuous renewal process. Skin, bone, glandular tissue, the vascular system, and many other systems have a specific cell turnover time. Basal, or precursor, cells are continuously producing progeny to replace the older cells which are being destroyed and removed by the normal life processes. An example is the skin, which has a turnover time from basal cell layers to the final shedding of the upper layers of the epidermis in approximately 21 days.

C. Rapid Renewal Populations

These cells must be replaced almost continuously owing to the high demands either for an enormous number of adult cells or by being exposed to excessive trauma. The hemopoietic system is in a continuous state of rapid replacement with the life span of some of the mature blood elements being no more than a few hours or days. The mucosal lining of the small bowel is another example in which the cells pass through their entire life cycle from production to shedding in an extremely short period of time.

Cells in this rapid renewal system are extremely vulnerable to radiations. These cells have a high mitotic rate, making them much more susceptible to radiation damage than cells with a lower mitotic rate. This will often lead to a high radiosensitivity of tumors that arise from these systems—for example, leukemias—but not necessarily to radiocurability. Cancers that arise from these systems may have a very high proliferation capability and may be able to outgrow the radiation damage and make up for lost numbers faster than the normal supportive tissues are able to.

D. Neoplastic Cell Populations

Neoplasia, or new cell growth, is generally considered to be synonymous with malignancy. Malignant tumors may arise from practically any tissue within the body. A great deal of the radioresponsiveness and ultimate radiocurability of malignant tumors is determined by their tissue of origin. In general, malignant tumors that arise from the renewing cell population group will not necessarily be the most radiosensitive but will comprise the majority of radiocurable lesions. Those that arise from the rapidly renewing cell populations will tend to be more radiosensitive but often less radiocurable. Tumors that arise from the static cell population have a tendency to respond very poorly to radiation therapy.

Most neoplastic cells grow without any response to the normal cell regulation mechanisms. Except for a few examples of hormone-dependent tumors they can be neither speeded up nor slowed down by the control systems that regulate normal cell growth and division.

The selective destruction of tissues forms the basis of radiation therapy. Neoplastic cells are almost invariably more easily destroyed by radiations than their normal precursor cells. This is not due to inherent differences in radiosensitivity but rather reflects differences in repair and recovery between normal and neoplastic tissues.

It should be re-emphasized that radiosensitivity does not necessarily lead to radiocurability. The two terms are not synonymous. For example, the tumor cells of leukemia are extremely radiosensitive yet the disease is not radiocurable. In contrast a well differentiated squamous cell carcinoma of the tongue is often very slow to respond to radiation therapy yet the tumor may eventually be cured.

Perthes first noticed the correlation of reproductivity and radiosensitivity of cells in 1903. Later, in 1906, these basic experimental facts were expressed in the form of a general radiobiologic law (the law of Bergonié and Tribondeau). In essence this law states that the intensity of the effect of radiations on living cells is increased (1) the greater the cells' reproductivity, (2) the longer their mitotic phase lasts, and (3) the less their morphology and function are differentiated.

This law is often modified in various ways. In its general application this law has often been found to be inaccurate. However, its relative value is confined to the explanation of the different radiosensitivities of cells with different mitotic rates. It is useful as a historical concept rather than as a theoretical means of establishing a guide of radiosensitivities for different tissues.

If neoplastic tissue is observed microscopically immediately following a given dose of radiation, all cells in mitosis will disappear after a very short period of time. This will be followed by an abnormally large number of degenerative mitoses, which is followed by death of these cells. This sequence of cell death can be brought about repeatedly by new doses of radiations. Eventually the complete destruction of the tumor may be expected. There are many situations, however, in which destruction of the tumor does not occur. Under these circumstances, the tumor cells are able to continue multiplication at a rate faster than their destruction, or else the cells themselves possess some degree of resistance to radiation death and continue to grow in spite of the repeated irradiation.

7.2 FRACTIONATION AND PROTRACTION

A definition of fractionation and protraction is necessary for a complete understanding of the various principles involved. Establishing separate definitions for this pair of terms is often difficult for the clinician, and the cell biologists have their own specific concepts of the terms.

Clinically, fractionation-protraction is often used as a coupled term, the two words being almost synonymous. However, there is a distinction between them.

A radiation treatment may be given in a single dose and as such is neither fractionated nor protracted. If this treatment dose is broken up into two or more components, it may then be said to be fractionated. If a course of treatment is broken up into fractions and distributed over an interval of time, then the course of treatment may be said to be not only fractionated but also protracted. Protraction usually implies the extension of a course of treatment over a relatively long period of time. This may be a matter of days, weeks, or even months. If a course of treatment is protracted over a long period of time, the amount of radiations necessary to achieve the same effect as a shorter course should be increased. The concept of NSD, or nominal single dose, to be discussed later, relates to this factor.

In a situation in which a given total dose of radiations is divided into increments and these increments are then delivered over a period of hours, days, or weeks, the biologic effect is always different than if these radiations had been delivered as a single dose. Invariably the biologic effectiveness is less under these circumstances. It is felt that the decreased response with fractionation and protraction is probably related to cell recovery. The effect works not only for the cancer being treated but also for the normal supporting tissues. This dependency of biologic effectiveness upon the fractionation-protraction is usually referred to as "the time dose relationship." These effects are easily shown in cell cultures and are observable in clinical situations. Repair and recovery have been mentioned in Chapter 6.

Coutard first noted the possibility and

advisability of protraction over many weeks, as related to more rapid treatment, for squamous cancers of the upper airways and the cervix. It is extremely important in the field of radiation therapy that the dose of radiations delivered be expressed not only as a total dose, but also over the time of delivery. The classic example of time-dose relationship relating cure of cancer versus radiation complications was presented by Strandqvist in 1944.

The physiologic and morphologic changes that radiations induce upon normal cells and cell systems will be covered very completely in later chapters. The effects of radiations upon cancerous tissue are basically the same as upon normal cell systems, but the chief difference lies in the ability of the normal supportive cell system to repair itself even under the influence of a course of radiation therapy. The normal cell system is more likely to be able to repair radiation damages between treatments than is the cancer cell system.

It is generally accepted that radiation-induced cell death initiates a feedback mechanism that activates a reparative process. Malignant cells are theoretically uneffected by this stimulus. During the period of time when no radiations are being applied, the normal tissues may proceed unhampered with their reparative processes. There is evidence that the cancer cells also recover and multiply, but at a much slower rate.

Scanlon (1965) and others have attempted to take advantage of the reparative interval between courses of radiation therapy to allow the normal tissue to recover. This has resulted in the concept of "split course" technique. A rapid, intense course of radiation therapy is followed by a rest interval, after which the course is again repeated. This method gives good tumor response combined with a recovery phase for the normal supportive tissues.

The advantages of fractionation and protraction are many. The following are a few of the more important reasons for their use in clinical radiation therapy.

1. Large tumors are almost invariably composed of a high percentage of hypoxic cells. Fractionation will reduce the mass of the tumor and the absolute number of cancer cells in the mass. If the total oxygen supply of the area remains constant, there will be fewer cancer cells; therefore the available oxygen per cell will be increased. Blood vessels which were compressed by the large bulk of the tumor will be decompressed as the mass shrinks, thereby increasing the availability of oxygen to the tumor. Finally, the distance the oxygen must diffuse through the mass of tissue is significantly reduced as the bulk of the tissue shrinks. All of these factors will contribute to better oxygenation of the tumor as the radiation therapy progresses.

In "split course" therapy, if the cancer has been responsive to the treatment, there will be considerable shrinkage between courses. This theoretically will allow for better oxygenation of the remaining cells and thereby make the cancer more susceptible to repeated courses of irradiation which will follow.

2. As mentioned earlier, there is a differential recovery rate between normal tissue and neoplastic tissue. The tumor, not being under any regulatory controls, receives no more stimulation than it initially possessed. The repair process contributes to a regrowth of the normal cell population as the cancer tissue dies out. Clinically, we will commonly see re-epithelialization of damaged areas of skin, even as the radiation therapy progresses. Islands of normal cells will spring up in the midst of a treatment field and proliferate rapidly to replace the cells being killed by the treatments.

3. The initial treatment often reduces hemorrhage and infection, and allows an improvement in nutrition with the result that normal tissues are better able to withstand a full course of treatment.

4. High dose-low fraction radiation therapy can create local edema which may produce its own complications and sequelae.

5. Rapid treatment of an extremely radiosensitive tumor will release a large amount of toxic by-products from the dead and dying tumor cells into the system. These must be handled by the patient's liver and kidneys. High intensity radiation therapy of an extremely radiosensitive tumor can cause renal failure from nitrogen breakdown products overloading the patient's already compromised renal system. Low dose–long-term treatment will minimize or eliminate this problem of treatment.

7.3 NOMINAL SINGLE DOSE

For many years it has been customary to express the dosage of radiations delivered to a tumor volume in terms of total dose delivered, the number of treatments, and the total elapsed time of treatment. The concept of integrating these three sets of factors into a single, universally understood unit has always intrigued both the theoretician and the clinician. The very nature of fractionation and protraction, with its tissue recovery factors, as well as the changes within the tumor and the patient's general condition markedly limit the validity of most methods of comparing radiation dosage schedules.

A concept known as nominal single dose (NSD) has been developed, in the absence of any more meaningful concept, to express the effects produced by a given treatment course related to the same effects produced by a single dose. The concept of NSD allows the comparison of the tumor effects resulting from different dosage and fractionation-protraction techniques. By integrating these three factors we can arrive at a nominal single dose which would, in theory, produce exactly the same effects. This, then, allows us to interrelate a variety of different courses of radiation therapy back to a single specific number, namely the NSD.

The following empirically derived equation for normal tissue, suggested by Ellis, may be used to arrive at an equivalent nominal single dose for any resonable course of fractionated-protracted radiation therapy:

$$NSD = Dose \times F^{-0.24} \times T^{-0.11}$$

where Dose = total dose in rads, F = total number of treatments (fractionation), and T = total number of elapsed days (protraction).

The NSD is usually expressed in rets or rad equivalent therapy units. This unit is similar to, but more precise than, the rem.

A table which eliminates the calculations with negative exponents and makes the determination of NSD a simple procedure is located in the appendix of this book. The expression ($F^{-0.24} \times T^{-0.11}$) is calculated for some of the more common values of F and T. This decimal from the tables may then be multiplied by the dose to give the NSD. The following are a few examples.

1. The classic 6000 rads in 6 weeks is usually delivered at the rate of 200 rads per day, five days a week, for a total of 30 fractions in a time of 40 days.

$$\left. \begin{array}{l} F = 30 \\ T = 40 \end{array} \right\} \text{Table Value} = .2946$$

$$NSD = 6000 \times .2946$$

$$NSD = 1768 \text{ ret}$$

2. A skin cancer is treated to 3000 rads with treatments of 1000 rads every other day for 3 fractions in 5 days.

$$\left. \begin{array}{l} F = 3 \\ T = 5 \end{array} \right\} \text{Table Value} = .6435$$

$$NSD = 3000 \times .6435$$

$$NSD = 1930 \text{ ret}$$

3. An oral cavity lesion is treated to 8000 rads in 53 fractions over 73 days.

$$\left. \begin{array}{l} F = 53 \\ T = 73 \end{array} \right\} \text{Table Value} = .2405$$

$$NSD = 8000 \times .2405$$

$$NSD = 1924 \text{ ret}$$

It should be pointed out that in any of these time-dose studies, the endpoints for different tissues and tumors are markedly different. The endpoints for tissue tolerance levels for cervix tissue is obviously markedly different than that for brain tissue. One must always remember the specific parameters which surround the total dosage tolerances for various organs and organ systems. The total tolerance levels are covered in the following chapter. The reader should be aware that most of these values are related to the classic five equal fractions per week over a protracted course of therapy.

The tremendous variability of the human subject will often invalidate all but the broadest of "laws" regarding the radiobiologic responses of tissues, and NSD is no exception to this rule. It is the awareness of this fantastic complexity of the human patient that makes us cautious of any allegedly simple relationship. The single number attached to NSD may be valid only when appropriate limits are established and observed.

7.4 THE OXYGEN EFFECT IN RADIATION THERAPY

A vast amount of work has been done over the past 20 years utilizing oxygen as a modifying agent for radiation changes in molecular systems. The ability of oxygen to potentiate radiation response is called the oxygen effect and has been well documented in all phases of radiobiologic experimentation.

Large cancers have a tendency to outgrow their blood supply with a consequent development of hypoxic but viable tumor cells. Such hypoxic foci are less sensitive to radiations than surrounding well oxygenated tissues, and may give rise to local recurrence following radiation therapy.

Many studies, both *in vitro* and *in vivo*, confirm the fact that for a given lethality, anoxic cells require two to three times the dose required for well oxygenated cells. The first applications of hyperbaric oxygen were made in 1954 by Churchill-Davidson, Sanger, and Thomlinson. In 1957, they reported their preliminary results of high pressure oxygen radiation therapy. Later, considerable work was done utilizing experimental tumor systems, relating the effects of anoxia, normal air breathing, 100 per cent atmospheric oxygen breathing, and hyperbaric oxygen.

A ratio is established relating the dose of radiations required for a given effect under anoxic conditions as related to the amount of radiations required for a similar effect under well oxygenated conditions. A ratio of these doses is known as the oxygen enhancement ratio (OER). This also has been referred to as the oxygen effect ratio. Most of the work utilizing mouse tumor systems indicated an OER of approximately 2.3 to 2.7. It was felt that the results of these experiments showed the upper limit of the OER for mammalian cells to be approxi-

mately 3 (see Figures 6–16, 6–17, and 6–18).

It has been postulated that cell clusters more than even a few millimeters in diameter will contain some hypoxic cells because rapid tumor growth exceeds the nutritional supplies of the area. Owing to their decreased radiosensitivity, these hypoxic tumor cells could account for a proportion of local cancer recurrences. If the oxygen levels in different areas of the tumor remain reasonably constant during the course of irradiation, then there could be a relative sparing of the anoxic fraction of cells. Even though this fraction may be small initially, it may eventually comprise a large portion of the surviving cells as the better oxygenated cells are destroyed by the irradiation.

It has been shown that it is possible to alter the partial oxygen pressures of tumors and other tissues by varying the composition and pressure of the respired gas. The radiosensitivity of tumors and other tissues is a function of these oxygen partial pressures.

Most experimental work has demonstrated an increase in the radioresponsiveness of normal oxygenated tissues when irradiated under hyperbaric oxygen conditions. Many people have suggested a dose reduction factor of at least 25 per cent to account for the increase in sensitivity of the normal supportive tissues.

Churchill-Davidson reported on 12 years' experience utilizing hyperbaric oxygen in connection with radiation therapy. It was his feeling that the results of therapy were improved when the patients were treated with hyperbaric oxygen, compared to a similar group of patients treated under normal conditions and breathing atmospheric air. A reduction in total radiation dosage was found to be necessary because of the increased effect on normal tissues. They found that the most favorable tumors to treat were those of moderate size which had a relatively good blood supply and were surrounded by healthy supportive tissues.

Induced normal tissue hypoxia has been found to be useful for protection in radiation therapy. This utilizes the hyperbaric principles in reverse. Normally oxygenated tissue is reduced to hypoxic levels to decrease its sensitivity to radiations. The oxygen content of the already hypoxic tumor cells changes very little. Various methods have been attempted with lesions of the extremities utilizing tourniquets, vaso-constrictors, or other methods of decreasing blood supply. Some workers have attempted induced anoxia by means of total body hypothermia. This is extremely hazardous and has not found wide acceptance.

For many years we have been utilizing local hypothermia in the form of rapid chilling of the skin prior to irradiation of deep-seated tumors. We have found this useful in giving a reasonable degree of protection of the skin in locations where even normal radiation reactions might present a serious dose-limiting problem.

It is recognized that the chilling of mammals during irradiation will protect them against radiation injury. This protection by hypothermia is not due to the temperature depression, but rather to the resultant reduction in partial pressures of oxygen in the tissues and to the oxygen effects.

Hibernation delays the radiation response but does not apparently decrease the lethal effects of irradiation. When the animals' normal temperature is regained, they show the same sequence of radiation syndromes as non-hibernating animals irradiated under similar conditions. The circulatory and respiratory systems function normally during hibernation and the tissues are apparently well oxygenated, but the metabolic rate is markedly decreased. Under induced hypothermia the metabolic rate exceeds the decreased oxygen supply, thereby creating an hypoxic situation. This has been found to be true also by increasing the body temperature of animals during irradiation. The respiratory and circulatory systems are not able to keep up with the elevated metabolic demands, and a moderate degree of hypoxia and protection results during hyperthermia.

7.5 LINEAR ENERGY TRANSFER

A wide variety of energies and types of radiations are available. These range from extremely large and heavy particles, such as alpha particles, to X- and gamma rays, which have no mass at all, to the nebulous neutrino, which has the smallest cross section of probability of interaction of any

of the radiations studied. This wide variety of radiations creates a marked difference in biologic responses which may be produced in the system being irradiated. Ionizing radiations transfer their energy to the irradiated medium by the formation of ion pairs and by excitation. Ionization is the most important of these phenomena for producing biologic changes. Heavy particulate radiations, such as alpha particles, have a short path and release a vast amount of energy over a very short distance with the production of many ion pairs per unit of track length.

Radiations of smaller mass, such as beta particles (electrons), may release the same total amount of energy; however, it will be distributed over a much longer path.

Electromagnetic radiations such as X- or gamma rays will have an even longer path of travel, and although a similar amount of energy may be released, it will be distributed over an even greater length.

Radiations may be compared on the basis of the average number of ion pairs formed per unit track length. The average energy release per unit track length is called the linear energy transfer, or LET. The LET is an average value based upon both the energy of excitation and the energy of ionization, but it does not necessarily imply a knowledge of the number of ionizations produced. An LET value is usually expressed in units of keV per micron (thousands of electron volts of energy released per micron of path length).

The LET of an ionizing radiation depends in a complicated way upon the mass, energy, and charge it possesses. The greater the mass and charge, and the smaller the velocity, the greater is the LET. This is illustrated in Table 7–1.

The biologic effect of radiations depends upon the LET. It would be preferable in radiobiologic experimentation to use monoenergetic radiations of a single type, all possessing exactly the same LET. A phenomenon which alters the quality and the energies of the radiations takes place whenever radiations interact with tissue. As the irradiating particle or beam interacts with tissue, it releases secondary radiations or particles which have considerably different LET values from the original primary beam. Consequently the LET of a given beam of radiations changes as it advances

TABLE 7-1   SOME MORE COMMONLY ACCEPTED
LET VALUES FOR SEVERAL DIFFERENT
TYPES OF RADIATIONS

Radiation	Energy	LET (keV/μ)
Fission Fragments	Very high	5000.00
Alpha	5 meV	100.00
Alpha	Low	250.00
Proton	10 meV	4.00
Proton	2 meV	16.00
Proton	Low	100.00
Neutron	19 meV	7.00
Neutron	2.5 meV	20.00
Electron	1 meV	.25
Electron	100 keV	.42
Electron	10 keV	2.30
Electron	1 ke V	12.30
X-ray	3 meV	.30
^{60}Co	1.17, 1.33 meV	.30
X-ray	250 keV	3.00

into a biologic system. Even if a purely monoenergetic beam is utilized initially to bombard a system there will be a spectrum of LET values present once the beam has penetrated to a significant depth within the system.

The LET gives the average energy loss of a particle per unit length of travel. Far more relevant, however, is the amount of energy that will be deposited in the critical volume or the target of the biologic system. Methods have been worked out to measure the distribution of energy release in extremely small volumes of tissue. This methodology is beyond the scope of this book, and we will discuss the broad overall concept of linear energy transfer as it relates to the primary irradiating beam.

Isolated ion pairs are very likely to recombine immediately after they are created following a radiation incident. In situations in which the LET values are low, the isolated ion pairs allow molecular repair to take place readily. When the LET values are high there are many ion pairs created within a given region. The chances of these ion pairs recombining correctly becomes much less as the number of ion pairs increases.

The presence of oxygen also interferes with repair processes by combining with radiation-induced lesions at the molecular level. This phenomenon explains why oxygen enhancement is more effective when using radiations with a low LET value.

7.6   RELATIVE BIOLOGIC EFFECTIVENESS

The many different types of ionizing radiations have been found to produce effects in biologic systems which are qualitatively similar. There are other situations, however, in which important qualitative differences occur. One type of radiation may be far more efficient in creating an effect in a given system than is another type of radiation in producing changes in the same system. The expression "relative biologic effectiveness" (RBE) is commonly used in radiobiology to compare the effectiveness of two radiations in producing a given change.

RBE is an expression based upon the dose of baseline radiation needed to produce a given magnitude of effect in a specific system as related to the dose of another radiation needed to produce exactly the same magnitude of effect in the same system.

To a great extent the RBE of various radiations depends upon the rate of energy loss (LET) along the paths of the individual ionizing particles or photons. Radiations with low LET values produce diffuse ionization throughout the media. In contrast, the individual tracks of particles with high LET values will be short and dense so that the effects will be much more pronounced over the same given track length and will demonstrate a higher RBE.

7.7   THE USE OF RADIOACTIVE MATERIALS FOR RADIATION THERAPY

A. Radium

In 1898, Marie and Pierre Curie isolated a naturally occurring radioactive element which they named radium. Radium-226 is a decay product of the uranium-238 series. Radium decays to radon-222, which decays rapidly through a series of steps to lead-210. During this rapid decay process many different types of radiations are released. Among these are a number of high and low energy gamma rays as well as multiple beta and alpha particles. In clinical utilization the radium salt is sealed inside a capsule of either gold or platinum whose wall is of sufficient density and thickness to stop all of the heavy particulate radiations, but thin enough to transmit the majority of the high energy gamma radiations.

Radium has been used for many years for the treatment of cancers which are in accessible locations, such as the skin, oral cavity, uterus, and cervix. The radium is inserted into the area to be treated and left there for a specified length of time while delivering the prescribed dose of radiations to the area under treatment. Radium implantation is often done in conjunction with external beam therapy. Radium may be used as a supplementary form of high intensity local irradiation for cancers of the skin, oral cavity, uterus, and cervix.

The radioactivity present in one gram of radium was defined as 1 Curie, with 1 milligram of radium being equal to 1 milli-Curie. Early radium dosimetry was expressed as milligrams administered for a period of hours, or, as is commonly stated, milligram-hours. Statements of dose in this unit are meaningful only when the geometric arrangement of the sources is reproduced exactly from one patient to the next. The expression of radium dosage in milligram-hours is giving way to the more accurate dosage expression in rads to specific areas as calculated by high speed computer dosimetry.

B. Radium Substitutes

Many institutions have recently replaced or augmented their existing radium supply with artificially produced radioisotopes. Various objections to the use of radium have been made over the years. Chief among these were the cost of radium and its serious contamination hazards. Cobalt-60 and cesium-137 have both been extensively used to replace radium for interstitial and intracavitary Curie-therapy. These sources may be made physically as small or smaller than radium, are much less costly, and have the advantage of a marked reduction in contamination probabilities.

Tantalum-182, iridium-192, and gold-198 have also been utilized for Curie-therapy.

All of these radioisotopes require a decay correction owing to their relatively short half-lives as compared to radium.

There is a difference in gamma energy between radium and some of the radium substitutes mentioned earlier (see Table 7–2). The difference in RBE which results from this slight variation in gamma energy is of very little clinical significance. All of these radioisotopes have a gamma energy of greater than 400 keV with the average energy of radium being approximately 1 MeV. The only exception is the neutron emitter, californium.

C. Californium-252

In 1969, about 50 milligrams of californium-252 were produced by the Atomic Energy Commission and released in small quantities to qualified individuals and institutions for research and evaluation. This material is available either uncapsulated as the chloride salt, deposited on

TABLE 7–2 PHYSICAL CHARACTERISTICS OF SOME OF THE MORE COMMONLY USED INTERSTITIAL AND INTRACAVITARY RADIOISOTOPES*

Radioisotope	R/Hr/mCi @ 1 cm	Average Gamma Energy (MeV)	HVL (mm Lead)	Half-life
^{60}Co	13.4	1.172 1.333	12.5	5.2 y
^{137}Cs	3.3	.662	5.5	27. y
^{182}Ta	6.1	.05 →1.23	9.8	115 d
^{192}Ir	5.5	.136→ .613	2.5	74.5 d
^{198}Au	2.5	.412	3.0	2.69 d
^{226}Ra and equilibrium products (.5 mm Pt Wall)	8.25	.053→2.43	12.0	1622 y
^{222}Rn and equilibrium products (.5 mm Pt Wall)	8.25	.053→2.43	12.0	3.8229 d

*Adapted from Johns: *The Physics of Radiology*, 2nd Ed., 1961. Courtesy of Charles C Thomas, Publisher, Springfield, Illinois.

platinum foil, or doubly encapsulated in platinum-iridium capsules. It should be pointed out that californium-252 is an extremely expensive limited-production radioisotope which is in an evaluation phase at the present time.

Californium-252 is the only known radioisotope that can be fabricated into small-sized sources that emit neutrons intensely over a practical period of time. Californium-252 has a half-life of 2.625 years. This radioisotope decays by both alpha emission and spontaneous fission. Its principal route of decay is by alpha emission of 6.12 meV energy 97 per cent of the time. There is a 3 per cent spontaneous emission of fission neutrons at the rate of 4.4×10^9 neutrons per second per Curie, and this emission of fission neutrons has aroused interest in the utilization of californium as a source for Curie-therapy. The neutron energy spectrum reaches a maximum at approximately 1 million electron volts; the average neutron energy is 2.3 million electron volts. There is also approximately a .01 per cent release of 100 keV gamma photon.

Californium-252 sources now give the radiation therapist an intense but tiny neutron source for interstitial Curie-therapy. The implantable sources of californium-252 may be used to deliver a highly localized radiation dose of neutrons into the cancer. There is evidence that would suggest that the fast neutrons from californium-252 may be more effective in treating some types of cancer than the gamma radiations from radium.

The high linear energy transfer of neutrons make them more effective than gamma radiations in overcoming the radiation resistance of anoxic cells. The RBE of californium-252 is approximately 2.9 with respect to the protracted irradiation with radium.

D. Gold-198 and Phosphorus-32 Colloids

During the last 20 years colloids of gold-198 or phosphorus-32 have been injected into the peritoneal and pleural cavities for the control of malignant effusions. Some cancers have a tendency to seed throughout the pleural or peritoneal cavities and implant upon the walls. These implants exude fluids which are difficult for the body to reabsorb. A solution of radioactive colloid may be injected into the cavity and distributed throughout the area. The distribution of a radioactive material in this fashion will permit high intensity irradiation of small surface implants. Very often this form of irradiation will be quite effective in completely eliminating the fluid production from these cancer implants.

Table 7–3 summarizes the more important physical characteristics of these two radioactive colloids (and iodine-131).

The beta particles released from these radioactive materials give a very high radiation dosage to the cells lying near the surface, with a relatively lesser amount of radiations delivered to deeper structures. The significant penetrating power of this form of treatment is no more than a few millimeters. This form of therapy allows intensive radiation of the surface lining of the cavities, and the malignant cells implanted on the surface, with a relative degree of protection afforded to the bowel and other structures which are a greater distance from the surface.

E. Iodine-131

There are some organs in the body which, owing to the physiology of their function, are able to selectively take up chemical elements or compounds. The most notable of these is the thyroid gland, which selectively takes up iodine. The affinity of the thyroid gland for iodine has long been utilized both as a functional tracer study and as a therapeutic modality. Radioactive iodine, either in the form of iodine-131 or iodine-125, will be taken up by the thyroid in exactly the same fashion as the non-

TABLE 7–3 RADIOISOTOPES USED FOR CANCER THERAPY

Radioisotope	Form	β-Energy	γ-Energy	Half-life
Gold-198	colloid	.962 MeV	.412 MeV	2.7 d
Phosphorus-32	colloid	1.7 MeV	none	14.5 d
Iodine-131	NaI solution	.608 MeV	14.5 d	8.1 d

radioactive elemental iodine-127 found in the diet.

Well differentiated follicular carcinoma arising from the thyroid gland often will continue to carry out the physiologic functions of its precursor cells. Well differentiated cancers of the thyroid will take up radioactive iodine in small amounts. If all the normal thyroid tissue is removed or destroyed, these cancers will then take up even larger amounts.

Patients with metastatic thyroid carcinoma may be treated by having their cancer stimulated by thyroid-stimulating hormone and then given a large amount (100 mCi) of iodine-131. Functioning sites of metastatic cancer will selectively take up the radioactive iodine and will receive an intensive internal irradiation from it. Successful palliative treatment over long periods of time of well differentiated follicular carcinoma of the thyroid has been carried out utilizing large doses of iodine-131. Often lung and bone lesions may be managed for years by this form of treatment.

The more poorly differentiated papillary carcinoma is less responsive to iodine-131 therapy. Anaplastic carcinoma of the thyroid seldom demonstrates iodine uptake function and is never treated with radioiodine.

F. Phosphorus-32 for Bone Metastasis

Metastatic cancer in bone, notably from carcinomas of the prostate and breast, may be treated by the administration of relatively large doses (10 to 20 mCi) of ^{32}P given in divided doses over a period of one to two weeks. Phosphorus normally concentrates in growing bone and the radioactive phosphorus will follow the same metabolic pathways. The radioisotope tends to concentrate in areas of increased bone destruction and re-formation such as are found in metastatic lesions. This method is quite useful in treating widespread painful metastasis from these cancers. This is not a curative procedure but is only palliative.

In metastatic cancer of the thyroid the malignant cells themselves take up the radioactive iodine. In metastatic cancer in bone the re-forming bone in and around the metastatic sites selectively takes up the radioactive phosphorus as the calcium salt and thereby irradiates the cancer cells which are creating the bone destruction by

their presence. The cancer cells take up a small amount of the phosphorus as a constituent of the cell's DNA and RNA.

G. Fractionation-Protraction

The laws of fractionation and protraction are somewhat difficult to interrelate with the use of radioactive materials for radiation therapy. These radiations are delivered at a relatively low dose rate, but are delivered continuously over a period of hours or days or even longer. There are some radiobiologic theories that would tend to favor a slow but continuous deliverance of radiations as more effective than the routine intensely delivered but interrupted treatment commonly found in most radiation therapy schedules.

The average course of radiation therapy delivers an effective amount of radiation only during the few minutes that the machine is directed at the lesion each day. A radioactive substance left in place will deliver a much slower dose rate in terms of unit time but will deliver the radiations continuously over the hours or days that the application is in place. The total elapsed treatment time is far less; therefore, the total dose to be delivered to the cancer is usually decreased as related to conventional fractionated external beam therapy.

7.8 HISTOLOGIC DEPENDENCY OF CANCER RESPONSE TO IRRADIATION

It is understandable that different histologic types of cancers arising from different sites of origin should display differences in radiosensitivity and radiocurability. It is also reasonable to postulate that the degree of differentiation of the cancer, whether it is well differentiated or poorly differentiated, will play an important role in its overall responsiveness to radiations. The differences in radiosensitivity of various malignant tumors is primarily attributed to their cells of origin. Many tumors are composed of a variety of cell types. These different cell types may represent a widely different spectrum of susceptibility to radiations. A particular cell type may be extremely radiovulnerable and as such may be easily destroyed by the radiations. Another cell type may not exhibit the same degree of radiosensitivity and at the completion of a course of therapy may be the predominant and surviving cell fraction.

One of the most frustrating aspects of clinical radiation therapy arises when dealing with almost identical cell types which show a marked difference in radioresponsiveness because of either variations in tissue of origin or site of spread. An excellent example is the squamous cell carcinoma of the lip. The average well differentiated squamous cell carcinoma of the lower lip exhibits approximately a 90 per cent cure rate under ideal circumstances. A histologically identical cancer arising in the same patient but on the upper lip exhibits no more than a 50 per cent cure rate under the very best of circumstances. Both of these cancers show no more than a 30 per cent control rate if they have spread to adjacent lymph nodes. In all three situations the cancers may appear absolutely identical in their morphology and growth patterns. The theories behind these differences are many, but the reasons remain obscure—the answers still lie hidden in the radiobiology of the tumor-host relationship.

The early reactions and the ultimate late effects of radiations on organs depends to a large extent upon the tissues themselves. The wide range of variability between animal models and the human patient, as well as the inconsistency within the human species, has lead to considerable controversial experimental findings. This great range of variability must always be considered by the student when he reads in the literature of an attempt to translate animal and cell line experiments directly to the human patient. He must also consider the great range of variability within human subjects when he considers new "treatment regimens" which are producing astonishing results in a limited number of cases.

7.9 NUTRITIONAL DEPENDENCY OF CANCER RESPONSE TO IRRADIATION

The patient's general health and nutritional status play an extremely important role in his overall chances for cure. Growing cancer, even a small one, requires a tremendous amount of nutritional support. Often in the patient's initial phases of cancer growth he will exhibit a normal or increased appetite but with a progressive weight loss. If this is allowed to continue unchecked, the patient will become markedly debilitated and exhibit signs of a malnutritional state.

Such a patient, obviously, is a much poorer candidate for surviving the radical treatments which will be necessary to eradicate his cancer whether this be radical surgery, radiation therapy, or chemotherapy. A declining nutritional status with anemia is a very common early finding in cancer patients. Under these circumstances normal tissue tolerance is decreased and wound healing is slow. If anemia and a negative nitrogen balance are allowed to continue, patients will exhibit a marked impairment of healing of radiation-induced injuries. In a patient of good nutritional status these injuries correct themselves very promptly with the completion of therapy.

It has been reported that a severe decline in general nutritional status may precipitate late changes within the treatment field even months or years following the completion of a course of radiation therapy. Many of these changes are probably based upon an accentuation of vascular damage which appears to progress at a much faster rate within previously irradiated fields.

7.10 PRINCIPLES OF CANCER THERAPY

There are many different ways of treating cancer. Two methods are particularly effective for inducing remissions or eliminating cancer. These methods are surgery and radiation therapy. A third method, chemotherapy (the use of systemic drugs to treat cancer), has gained considerable impetus over the past 20 years. A few isolated cases have been reported cured by chemotherapy. Its main use, however, is for palliation following failure of the primary method of treatment. Cautery and escharotics are occasionally used against minor skin lesions but have failed to gain any degree of recognition for major systemic cancer. From time to time, unorthodox "cancer cures" come onto the scene only to be disproven in the final analysis. Krebiozen, Laetrile, and other "miracle drugs" are good examples of this category.

A. Surgery

Surgery is generally considered as the treatment of choice for the majority of early cases of cancer. Surgery almost invariably is necessary for the initial biopsy to establish proof of cancer. This often will be followed by a total removal without further treatment being necessary. Many situations arise in which surgery is not successful in the removal of all of the cancer, then radiation therapy is usually necessary as a follow-up procedure. Other situations arise in which radiation therapy may be used in a pre-operative fashion to be followed by curative surgery. These various indications will be taken up in more detail later in a discussion of specific cancers. There are many cases in which surgery is not applicable and radiation therapy will be used as the primary mode of treatment.

B. Chemotherapy

Chemotherapy is heavily relied upon for palliative treatment of far advanced or recurrent cancer. It is very seldom used as a curative measure. It may be employed either before, in combination with, or following either radiation therapy or surgery or both. The indications for chemotherapy are many and varied. These will be covered in greater detail in the section on chemotherapy.

C. Radiation Therapy

Following surgical biopsy of a cancer, radiation therapy may be elected as the treatment of choice. There are many cancers which cannot be successfully removed surgically. Often the decision will be made to treat the patient with curative radiation therapy. Other situations will arise in which the radiation therapy may be given either in a pre-operative or a post-operative fashion.

In many instances the final selection of treatment modality will be based on a multitude of variable factors including histology of the tumor, duration of symptomatology, extent of spread of disease, fears and desires of the patient, and, finally, the medical judgment of the physican in charge of the case.

7.11 THE TREATMENT OF MALIGNANT TUMORS

The following discussion will deal primarily with malignant tumors which may arise from any of the various organ systems under discussion. Tumors may be either benign or malignant. Cancers are always malignant. These terms are often used interchangeably, but the reader should be aware of these degrees of distinction. Most of the following discussions will center about the various aspects of malignant tumors. Benign tumors will be mentioned only if they are pertinent to the discussion. The majority of benign tumors are surgical problems and present only the technical difficulties of removal. Unless a benign tumor creates a mechanical problem in a vital area it usually does not cause death. Malignant tumors have the capability of invading from their local site of origin into the surrounding tissues. They also have the capability of metastatic spread, by means of which cells or groups of cells break loose from the parent tumor and are distributed through either the circulatory or the lymphatic systems. These cells have the capability of lodging at a distant site, flourishing, and creating a new tumor growth.

Untreated malignant tumors almost invariably lead to the death of the host. There have been isolated instances of malignant tumors maturing into benign forms; however, this is extremely rare. This probably accounts for the apparent spontaneous regression and occasional "miraculous cure" of proved malignant tumors.

In theory, no tumor should be able to withstand irradiation indefinitely. However, neither can normal tissue withstand these repeated onslaughts of irradiation, and eventually death and degeneration of supportive structures would take place. In many situations this would be incompatible with life.

Considerable time will be devoted in Chapter 8 to the radiation tolerance levels of normal structures. The data that is quoted relates to experimental work with animals as well as to the results of clinical treatment schedules. I will not go into the sequential changes that take place during a course of radiation therapy, nor attempt, in "cookbook" fashion, to cover all parameters of clinical radiation therapy. In the following section organs and organ systems and the cancers which may arise from them are discussed. Some of the interrelationships between the sensitivity of the cancer and the tissue of origin will also be discussed, and some general ranges of radiation dosages for control are given and some of the responses that one might expect are indicated.

A. Skin

Two very common lesions which the physician may be called upon to treat will be squamous cell carcinoma and basal cell carcinoma of the skin. These lesions were among the first cancers to be treated and cured by X-ray and radium therapy in the early days of this specialty. Skin cancer is one of the most common and curable forms of cancer seen today. In spite of its high degree of sensitivity and curability this cancer should not be taken lightly. Improperly treated, skin cancer can lead to death just as surely as can the most malignant cancer described anywhere in the body. Cancer of the skin may be treated with many different schedules of total dosage and fractionation. Strandqvist utilized cancer of the skin as his model for the construction of his original treatment schedules.

The major precaution that must be observed in treating cancer of the skin is the avoidance of previously irradiated areas, skin grafts, scars, or areas which might have an impaired vascular supply. The chances of curing cancers arising in these areas are reduced, and the chances of complications following treatment are increased.

If a skin cancer is small and on a mobile area of skin, it should be surgically excised with wide margins. This will give an adequate chance of cure and not be inconvenient to the patient. If the area is large but cannot be treated with radiation therapy owing to poor skin condition, the surgical excision and skin graft will still be the treatment of choice.

Very small basal cell carcinomas may be successfully treated by electrocautery. Squamous cell cancer should never be treated in this fashion because of the more aggressive nature of this lesion.

Skin cancer is generally treated with orthovoltage irradiation. The skin-sparing effects of supervoltage would be contrary to the desires of delivering a high dose within the substance of the skin and its infiltrating cancer.

Small lesions may be treated with a high daily dosage and limited fractions, whereas large lesions are better treated by a greater accumulated dose over a longer period of time. The larger fields require a better quality of radiations. Skin cancer is occasionally treated with radium implants or applications.

Malignant melanoma, arising in the skin, presents an entirely different picture from squamous and basal cell carcinomas. Malignant melanomas are usually considered radioresistant and as such are better treated by wide surgical removal. There have been instances in which these tumors have been irradiated and have shown some degree of radiosensitivity, even a few isolated cases of cure have been reported.

B. Oral Cavity and Upper Airways

The epithelium lining this area is moderately radiosensitive. Most of the tumors arising within the oral cavity and upper airways are squamous cell carcinomas.

These cancers present an interesting, challenging, and frustrating phase of radiation therapy. Although histologically, most of them appear quite similar, their behavior characteristics under radiation therapy are markedly different. There is a wide difference in radiosensitivity within the same cell type depending upon its site of origin. A squamous cell carcinoma confined to the true vocal cord is highly radiocurable, while a squamous cell carcinoma arising in the pyriform sinus is very difficult to control by irradiation. A carcinoma confined to the true vocal cord is nearly twice as radiocurable as one that has spread only a few millimeters away to adjacent muscle and mucosa.

Eighty per cent of the cancers arising in the oral cavity will be squamous cell carcinomas. Transitional cell carcinomas and lymphoepitheliomas will make up most of the remainder.

Cancers arising from the tongue show marked differences in radiosensitivities and radiocurabilities, depending upon the portion of the tongue in which they originate.

Cancers of the anterior two thirds of the tongue and the floor of the mouth are not highly radiosensitive, yet in early cases they demonstrate cure rates as high as 60 per cent five-year survival.

Carcinomas of the base of the tongue usually infiltrate deeply into the substance of the tongue and metastasize to lymph nodes very early. The average cure rate for even early lesions arising in this area is no greater than 30 per cent. High total dosage is required for control of carcinoma of the tongue, and doses as high as 8000 rads in a period of 10 to 12 weeks delivered by means of external radiation, radium implants, or both, are not uncommon.

The tonsils are composed primarily of lymphoid tissue covered by a stratified squamous epithelium. Cancers may arise from both of these tissues of origin. Their behavior and treatment are quite different, however, depending upon the tissue of origin.

Cancer of the tonsil behaves in a very aggressive fashion, usually spreading very early to the base of the tongue, the soft palate, and metastasizing to lymph nodes. The average cure rate for carcinoma of the tonsil is about 30 per cent. High doses of radiations in the range of 6000 to 8000 rads in a period of 6 to 10 weeks have been recommended for squamous cell carcinoma. Lymphosarcomas, like lymphomas arising in other portions of the body, are much more radiosensitive, and doses of 5000 rads in five weeks have yielded very good results.

Surgery alone may be used as the primary treatment modality for most of these lesions. The cure rates in early cases are about the same as with radiation therapy. Surgery has little to offer in the far advanced cases. Surgery may result in serious and often debilitating deformity unless good reconstructive treatment is carried out early. Surgery and radiation therapy combined have given an increase in control rate for most of the lesions of the upper airways.

C. Alimentary Tract

The mucosa of the gastrointestinal tract does not tolerate irradiation well owing to the rapid turnover of cells, making the normal tissues much more susceptible to radiation injury.

Paradoxically as it may seem, cancers arising from this system are, as a rule, relatively resistant to radiations. The reason lies in the fact that most gastrointestinal tract cancers are adenocarcinomas, arising from the mucus-producing cells and not from the columnar epithelium which lines the gastrointestinal tract. The mucus-producing cells have been shown to be very radiation-resistant.

The radioresistance of adenocarcinomas combined with the high degree of radiosensitivity of the lining cells of the alimentary tract, make radiation therapy a very unsatisfactory primary curative treatment for gastrointestinal tract malignancy.

Lymphosarcoma and lymphomas comprise approximately 5 per cent of the gastric cancers. By virtue of the radiosensitivity of the cells of origin, lymphosarcoma and lymphomas arising in the stomach can be successfully treated by radiation therapy. Four thousand to 5000 rads in 6 to 8 weeks can cure these tumors and at the same time still be tolerated by the gastric mucosa.

The small bowel presents a different set of problems for the radiation therapist. It is very rare that he is ever called upon to treat either a primary or recurrent cancer of the small bowel. Very often, however, he will treat segments of small bowel while irradiating abdominal or pelvic cancers of other origin. Injury to the small bowel is always a prime concern in any patient receiving this type of treatment.

As mentioned earlier the epithelial lining of the small bowel is extremely radiosensitive, and gastrointestinal death can result from irradiation of a large amount of small bowel. The widespread destruction of the epithelium can result in a serious loss of fluids and electrolytes.

If a large amount of the small bowel must be treated, the radiation therapy should be delivered on a long-term, low-dose, protracted basis. The moving strip technique is a very useful means of irradiating the entire abdomen to reasonably high doses (4000 to 5000 rads) while still maintaining the integrity of the small bowel.

The high degree of motility and mobility of the small bowel prevents it from remaining within a localized field of irradiation for any successive series of treatments unless the field is unduly large. This gives time for mucosal recovery between treatments. Serious injury to the small bowel can result if a loop or segment is bound down by adhesions. Such a loop of bowel may be irradiated to a high level, far beyond its normal tolerances. This can result in interruption of the treatment and often death of the patient unless corrective measures are taken. If the patient has a past history of major abdominal surgery or infection, this possibility always exists.

Cancer of the colon is one of the most significant causes of cancer death in the United States. Nearly all the cancers that arise in the colon are adenocarcinomas and as such are rarely radiocurable. Pre-operative irradiation and palliative irradiation have been attempted with variable success.

Usually doses of 5000 to 6000 rads in 5 to 8 weeks are required to even attempt control of these cancers. This dose level still stands a greater chance of causing bowel necrosis than tumor death.

Except for the lymphomas, all gastrointestinal tract lesions are better treated by surgical means. Radiation therapy has some limited use as a palliative treatment. At present a number of studies are being conducted to determine the value of pre-operative radiation therapy followed by definitive surgery. These studies as yet have not provided conclusive results.

D. Salivary Glands

Malignant tumors occasionally arise in the salivary glands. These are generally adenocarcinomas, although occasionally a squamous cell cancer will arise from the lining of the ducts. These cancers exhibit a moderate degree of radiosensitivity. This factor combined with the proximity of the cancer to the surface of the skin and the absence of any crucially radiosensitive structures in the immediate area allows high doses of radiations—6000 to 7000 rads in a period of 6 to 8 weeks—to be delivered.

The salivary glands are often included in treatment fields when head and neck lesions are being treated. The serous secretory glandular components are more affected than the mucous glands. This creates very thick tenacious secretions which often lead to associated complications with the teeth owing to loss of the flushing and buffering action of the saliva.

E. Liver

Primary hepatomas are occasionally seen arising from the substance of the liver. These tumors are generally extremely anaplastic and quite radioresistant. This fact coupled with the normal liver tolerance levels to radiation of 3500 to 4500 rads creates an impossible situation for primary radiocurability of cancer of the liver.

Metastatic cancer to the liver is more frequently seen than primary tumors. The substance of the liver makes an excellent bed for the growth of metastatic cancer cells. For this reason the liver is one of the most common sites of metastatic cancer with involvement often seen from cancer of the gastrointestinal tract, breast, kidney, and lung.

F. Kidney

Radiation nephritis will be discussed in Chapter 8. Radiation dosages in the range of 2000 to 3000 rads with routine fractionation almost invariably produces this picture. It is the feeling of most radiation therapists that if the kidney must be included in the irradiated volume owing to the necessity of treating cancers of other than renal origin, then the maximum dosage delivered to the kidney should not exceed 2300 rads in five weeks (or its biologic equivalent) if the kidney is to be saved. Irradiated above this level, the patient runs a serious risk of late renal damage. Renal irradiation should be avoided when at all possible. This implies accurate definition of tumor extent and recognition of the presence of any anatomic variation in the position of the kidney. If renal irradiation is unavoidable, the maximum dosage should be limited to 2000 rads in a period of two weeks, with an upper limit of tolerance of 3000 rads in six weeks.

In many situations it is necessary to treat all or part of both kidneys because of massive lymph node involvement from lymphoma, seminoma, or other intra-abdominal neoplasms. If these tumors are quite radiosensitive and regress well under the initial course of treatment, it is often possible to re-define the field borders and move the field off the renal areas early in the course of treatment. If this is not possible, the kidneys must then be blocked for part of the treatment. Some physicians have recommended selective infusion of the renal arteries with vasoconstrictors to produce local ischemia and anoxia during the treatment times. This should give some degree of protection to the kidney during the crucial period of irradiation. This, however, is still in the experimental stage.

Primary cancers of the kidney are divided into three major categories:

1. Adenocarcinomas of the renal parenchyma
2. Wilms' tumors
3. Carcinomas of the renal pelvis

Adenocarcinoma of the kidney probably arises from glandular elements of the epithelium of the renal tubules. The normal tubule epithelium is reasonably resistant to radiation; therefore, cancers arising from this tissue are also very tolerant of irradiation. Radiation doses in the range of normal kidney tolerance have very little effect on carcinomas arising in this area. It is impossible to salvage normal kidney function and treat a primary adenocarcinoma of the kidney simultaneously.

Nephrectomy is usually the treatment of choice. In many instances this is followed by postoperative radiation therapy to the kidney bed. Preoperative radiation therapy has been advocated by some radiation therapists, although this is still in the investigation stage.

Wilms' tumor occurs only in children, is extremely malignant, and metastasizes early. These tumors are thought to represent embryonic renal tissues and are often termed embryoma or nephroblastoma.

These tumors are composed of malignant epithelial elements and malignant connective tissue or sarcoma elements.

The epithelial element responds less well to irradiation than does the sarcomatous element. These cancers often regress remarkably well with the initial course of radiation therapy. In spite of their apparent radiosensitivity, these tumors are not often radiocurable.

Radiocurability is definitely enhanced in children under two years of age, in patients with small tumors, and in the absence of local infiltration or vessel invasion. Most authorities feel that if these patients survive over two years free of disease, they probably are permanently cured.

Preoperative irradiation in Wilms' tumor is the recommended form of treatment. The generally accepted dose is 3000 rads tumor dose delivered in about 3 weeks. A recent series, reported from Boston Children's Hospital on patients who received surgery, postoperative irradiation, and Actinomycin D, showed an 89 per cent two year survival. Some of the cases developed metastasis which were successfully treated with combinations of irradiation and Actinomycin D.

Cancers that arise in the renal pelvis are usually transitional cell or epidermoid carcinomas. These behave similarly to the same cancer in the urinary bladder. They are best treated by surgery.

G. Bladder

The urinary bladder is often irradiated unavoidably during radiation therapy for lesions located in and around this area, the most common of these being carcinoma of the cervix.

Carcinomas commonly arise from the mucosa of the bladder. These are generally squamous cell or transitional cell carcinomas. One sees a great variety of differentiation from highly anaplastic, invasive, early metastasizing lesions to very benign-appearing, extremely curable papillomas.

Approximately 80 per cent of the cancers are transitional cell carcinomas; about 10 per cent are squamous cell carcinomas. Transitional cell carcinomas are more radiosensitive and more radiocurable than squamous cell carcinomas. As is true in many other sites within the body, the anaplastic cancers are more radiosensitive than the better differentiated types; however, generally they are less radiocurable. The normal bladder shows a moderate degree of radiation tolerance, with doses of 6000 rads in six weeks being well tolerated. This is the lower limit of curability for carcinoma of the bladder, and most radiation therapists will carry these lesions to 7000 rads in 6 to 8 weeks. This level gives some increase in late radiation sequelae, but the additional cure rate warrants the higher dose.

The average five-year control rate may be expected to be about 50 per cent in early cases, ranging down to approximately 20 per cent in the later stages.

H. Prostate

The prostate tolerates radiation quite well. High doses of radiations can produce complete atrophy and replacement of the gland with scar tissue. Total radiation destruction of the gland seldom results in any symptomatology to the patient.

Cancers which arise in the prostate gland are almost exclusively adenocarcinomas.

Initially it was felt that carcinoma of the prostate was insensitive to radiations. This was based on the histology and the general behavior of adenocarcinomas arising in other parts of the body. J. A. del Regato has demonstrated that carcinoma of the prostate can be cured with high doses of radiation. With proper treatment planning high doses of radiations may be delivered to the gland and still spare the nearby rectum. An average course of treatment would be 7000 rads tumor dose in 6 to 8 weeks. The normal supportive tissues in this area are relatively insensitive to radiations; therefore, these doses can be delivered with only minor problems of the nearby base of the bladder and rectum. Such treatments will result in an approximate 50 per cent control rate of the cancer at the primary site.

Growth and function of normal prostatic tissues are partially regulated by the androgen hormone levels in the adult male. For this reason, cancers arising from this tissue are often sensitive to stimulation by androgen. Biologically this cancer appears to be quite dependent upon hormonal regulation. As a result, orchiectomy (removal of normal androgen production) and administration of estrogens result in a suppression of normal prostatic tissue and at the same time can result in marked suppression of cancers arising from the prostate. This method is not curative but often results in good palliation.

I. Testicle

The testicle has long been a favorite organ for study among radiobiologists because of its accessability and the variety of tissues present. The germinal epithelium presents a wide variation of radiosensitivities. The interstitial and sertoli cells present a still different picture of radiosensitivity.

As noted in Chapter 8 sterilization in the adult male may result with doses as low as 450 rads. Most radiation therapists feel that a dose of at least 1000 rads should be delivered to assure permanent sterility. Radiation sterilization may result in some slight decrease in androgen production; however, this is of little noticeable consequence in the average patient. Radiation sterilization is not synonymous with castration. It should be noted that although an irradiated testicle is incapable of reproduction, it is still capable of androgen production and as a result sex drives and secondary sexual characteristics are unaffected. The interstitial cells of Leydig are much more radioresistant than the spermatogonia. This is in direct contrast to irradiation of the ovaries, which causes not only sterilization but also castration.

Most of the significant carcinomas of the testicle arise from the germinal epithelium. An occasional tumor will arise from the interstitial cells which, by virtue of its origin, will be a relatively radioresistant tumor. There are five basic groups of histologically identifiable tumors of any consequence which arise from the testicle. These are arranged in order of increasing malignancy and decreasing radiocurability:

1. Pure seminoma
2. Embryonal cell carcinoma with or without seminoma
3. Teratoma with or without seminoma
4. Teratoma with or without seminoma, embryonal carcinoma, or choriocarcinoma
5. Choriocarcinoma with or without seminoma or embryonal carcinoma

Seminoma is by far the most sensitive of these tumors and is easily radiocurable even in metastatic sites. The choriocarcinoma is the most resistant to irradiation, metastasizes early, and is almost incurable by any means.

It is interesting to note the tumors of the testicle in ascending order of malignancy; the more malignant ones will often be mixed with less malignant tumors, which therefore seem to have little consequence on the final outcome of the primary lesion.

Seminoma is quite radiosensitive, doses as low as 1000 rads having been reported as being cancerocidal. The average treatment course is approximately 3000 to 3500 rads in a period of 3 to 5 weeks. This is associated with minimal radiation sequelae and results in an excellent control of this tumor. Embryonal cell carcinoma responds less well and as a consequence requires dosages to approximately 5000 rads in 5 to 7 weeks.

The radiocurability of terato-carcinomas is considerably less and is completely dictated by the malignant tissue of origin. It should be remembered that teratomas are often composed of a multiplicity of histologic cell types. Any of these cells or any combination of them may be the eventual malignant element in a terato-carcinoma. The origin of the malignant cells will dictate the radiosensitivity and ultimate radiocurability of this cancer.

All testicular tumors are treated by surgery initially. The testicle is removed to make the diagnosis, and an abdominal lymph node dissection may be done for the more malignant tumors. Radiation therapy alone to the abdominal nodes is recommended in seminoma and embryonal cell carcinomas.

J. Cervix

The majority of cancers that arise from the cervix are of the squamous cell type, most of these being well differentiated. A small percentage of adenocarcinomas and undifferentiated carcinomas arise from the cervix.

Because of the continuous shedding of cells from the surface of the cervix and consequently from a cancer which may arise from it, this cancer may be discovered at a much earlier stage by exfoliative cytology (Papanicolaou smear test).

This cancer has a tendency to invade the rich lymphatics of the cervix quite early; many authors have reported from 20 to 30 per cent lymphatic involvement with clinical stage I carcinoma of the cervix.

In cancer of the cervix the histology and site of origin, the route of spread, and the radiation tolerance of neighboring structures all play important roles in the treatment choice.

Surgery may be used as the primary form of treatment in very early (stage 0 or stage I) cases. If the patient is young, surgery is often preferred to preserve the ovaries, since radiation therapy always results in the loss of all ovarian function. If the patient still has a long life expectancy, it is of theoretical value to remove the uterus and cervix to prevent the possibility of a second cancer arising in the area at a much later time. The cure rate for Stage 0 or Stage I cancer is the same for surgery or radiation therapy. Surgery often is used to treat the occasional post-radiation therapy recurrence.

A small cancer that is still confined to the cervix and has not invaded the adjoining structures presents a situation in which the cancer is still well oxygenated and the supporting structures have not been appreciably distorted by tumor growth. These factors contribute toward increased radiocurability.

The tissues that make up the cervix can tolerate an extremely high dose of radiation. Routinely the cervix will receive between 10,000 and 20,000 rads during a course of radiation therapy, and some authors have reported the tolerance to be as high as 30,000 rads in two weeks. This high tolerance level permits a high dose of radiations to be delivered, which leads to the complete control of cervical cancer in practically all early cases. The normal epithelium of the cervix, uterus, and vagina have a remarkable ability to recover from radiation injury. The supportive connective tissues and smooth muscle structures of the uterus are also little affected by these high doses. It should be borne in mind that the cervix will not be called upon to carry out its normal functions following irradiation. Severe fibrotic changes and scar replacement that would be extremely symptomatic in other areas of the body pass unnoticed in the cervix.

Although the cervix will tolerate extremely high doses of radiation, these levels are usually not required for treatment. Most radiation therapists feel that 10,000 rads delivered to the cervix in a period of 6 to 8 weeks is cancerocidal. Indeed, metastatic cancer of the cervix in the pelvic lymph nodes can be sterilized by 6000 rads in six weeks. This amount of radiation is commonly delivered to the entire pelvis, with a more concentrated treatment being delivered to the cervix either by means of radium or transvaginal irradiation.

The ureters and the uterine arteries pass close to the cervix through an area which is commonly designated as "Point A." Routinely about 8000 rads may be delivered to this area, but this dose should not be exceeded if at all possible.

The control rates for carcinoma of the cervix range from approximately 85 to 90 per cent for Stage I, 65 per cent for Stage II, 45 per cent for Stage III, and 15 per cent for Stage IV.

Pregnancy is present in approximately 2 per cent of all patients diagnosed as having carcinoma of the cervix. This presents a problem for the radiation therapist as well as for the patient. The literature reflects a considerable difference of opinion as to the overall relationship between carcinoma of the cervix and pregnancy. The majority of reports state pregnancy accelerates the growth of carcinoma of the cervix. More recent reports have suggested that this may not be true. Delay in treating the cancer is probably of greater significance than the hormonal influence of the pregnancy upon the cancer.

An invasive carcinoma of the cervix discovered in the first trimester is usually treated as if the patient were not pregnant. The intensive irradiation of the early embryo usually results in abortion within 4 to 6 weeks. If this does not occur, then the pregnancy should be interrupted surgically.

If a carcinoma is discovered during the second trimester, hysterotomy followed by routine treatment is usually indicated.

If the cancer is discovered in the last trimester, treatment is often delayed until a viable baby may be delivered by Caesarean section. Delivery through the involved cervix should never be allowed because of the overwhelming chances of dissemination of the tumor by the mechanics of cervical dilation and delivery.

In some situations vaginal radium has been used with the fetus in place. Approximately 20 per cent of the viable babies delivered after such therapy show some damage to the head. This has been covered elsewhere in this book.

The cervix, uterus, and paracervical tissues tolerate high doses of radiations. Squamous cell carcinoma of the cervix is a moderately radiosensitive disease. The combination of these two factors leads to control of the cancer in a high proportion of cases.

K. Uterus

The tissues of the uterus tolerate high doses of radiations. The smooth muscle and fibrous tissues which make up the body of the uterus show atrophy following intensive irradiation but no other significant effects. Radiation necrosis of the surface epithelium may occur at points of very high dose from radium; however, this is usually not clinically significant.

The majority of the cancers that arise from the endometrial lining of the uterus are adenocarcinomas. Adenocarcinoma of the endometrium can spread to lymph nodes, the ovaries, the adjacent cervix, and upper vagina.

Complete surgical removal of the uterus is the recommended form of treatment. Recurrence at the surgical margins, most commonly the vagina, may occur.

Preoperative irradiation has been recommended to render nonviable the malignant cells that might be implanted in the operative site, disseminated into the circulatory system, or extend beyond the surgical margins. In far advanced cases, surgery may not be practical, and radiation therapy is the treatment of choice.

The advanced cases are generally treated with radiation therapy alone, and the earlier cases are treated with preoperative irradiation followed by surgery. Cure rates range from approximately 90 per cent for the early stages treated by the combination therapy to approximately 25 per cent for the later stages treated by radiation therapy only.

Adenocarcinoma of the endometrium arises from the glandular tissue of the lining of the endometrial cavity. These cells comprise the most hormone-dependent tissue in the body. The lining of the endometrial cavity normally undergoes atrophy during pregnancy. This fact has been capitalized upon in the treatment of carcinomas arising from this tissue. Patients may be given extremely high doses of progestational agents with a remarkable regression of both the primary cancer and its metastatic sites. In some cases there has reportedly been complete remission and cure of advanced cancer of the endometrium with this method. Most authors have found it to be extremely successful in the control of recurrent or metastatic disease for long periods of time.

L. Ovary

The ovary is made up of a variety of cell types with a wide range of sensitivities. Not only are there many different cell types within the ovary, but there are also a variety of stages of maturation, which affects the radiosensitivity of the cells.

The following is a histologic classification of the common primary tumors of the ovary:

a) Serous cystadenomas, benign and malignant
b) Mucinous cystadenomas, benign and malignant
c) Teratoma, benign and malignant
d) Dysgerminoma
e) Granulosa cell tumor
f) Endometrioid tumors, benign and malignant
g) Unclassified carcinoma

Malignant tumors may arise from any of the cells comprising the ovary. The majority of the carcinomas however arise from the germinal epithelium. Most ovarian carcinomas are poorly radiosensitive with the exception of dysgerminoma.

The clinical characteristics of ovarian carcinoma vary widely, and as a result the prognoses are markedly different. Surgical removal of the primary tumor is the desired form of treatment. If this fails, or if tumor is left behind, then radiation therapy should be used in an attempt to effect a cure.

The benign tumors of the ovary should be removed surgically, after which no further treatment is necessary. Malignant tumors of the ovary are often of enormous size and frequently will be ruptured or show evidence of tumor seeding at the time of surgery. These patients must be treated with postoperative irradiation either by intracavitary colloids (radioactive gold or radioactive phosphorus) or with external irradiation.

The follicle is the most frequently studied of the ovarian structures. The ovum in a young follicle is far more susceptible to direct radiation damage than is the ovum of a mature follicle. In contrast to this the granulosa cells become more sensitive as the follicle matures. The radiation changes seen with the various stages of development of ovarian follicles have been covered elsewhere in this book.

The overall effectiveness of radiation therapy for carcinomas of the ovary is extremely dependent upon the cell type.

Dysgerminomas and some of the malig-nant granulosa cell tumors are sufficiently radiosensitive to be frequently radiocurable.

Ovarian cancers are difficult to treat in that they have a tendency to seed throughout the pelvis and the abdominal cavity. The radiation therapist is dealing with a cancer that in most instances is reasonably radioresistant but has been disseminated among many radiosensitive organs and structures. At best, the treatment is usually palliative, although some of the more sensitive cancers may be cured by irradiation of the total abdominal cavity. The maximum tolerable dosage ranges from 2500 to 4500 rads, depending upon the patient and the method of delivery of the radiation. The average survival for carcinomas of the ovary ranges from approximately 50 per cent five-year survival with surgery and irradiation in early cases to less than 5 per cent in late stages. The highly radiosensitive dysgerminoma shows a survival rate which has been reported as high as 95 per cent.

M. Lungs

For many years the lungs were regarded as radioresistant organs. They were indiscriminately irradiated when other surrounding areas such as breast, the lung itself, esophagus, and mediastinum were treated. No thought was given to attempting to protect or observe the response on the underlying lung tissue. Eventually therapeutic radiologists began to look at the long-term changes that were occurring in the lungs following irradiation. Today we are well aware of the many physiologic changes which even small amounts of radiations will induce in the lung tissue. Some of these are due to the direct effects of the radiation on the lung parenchyma, while others are an indirect effect of the secondary radiation reactions followed by infection and the healing processes which follow all of these changes. Most of the acute changes that can occur will be covered later in this book.

The epithelium which comprises the lining of the trachea and lungs is moderately radioresistant. The majority of cancers of the lung arise from the bronchial epithelium or the mucus glands in the epithelium. Approximately 65 per cent of the tumors will be squamous cell carcinoma, 25 per cent will be an undifferentiated or Oat cell carcinoma, and approximately 10 per cent adenocarcinoma.

Carcinoma of the lung is one of the most formidable problems the radiation therapist faces. There is a steady rise in the incidence of cancer of the lung—approximately 60,000 cases were reported in 1968. This continued increase has resulted in the most extensive series of clinical, epidemiologic, and laboratory investigations ever attempted. The final verdict is yet to be decided; however, there is overwhelming evidence that would suggest that the cause, or causes, of carcinoma of the lung are environmental by-products of modern civilization. The high incidence of carcinoma of the lung coupled with the relative ineffectiveness of even our best methods of treatment presents a rather dismal outlook for the average patient.

Surgery is still regarded as the treatment of choice for localized carcinoma of the lung. However, its control rate is no more than 5 per cent of all cases. There have been some recent reports in the literature of radiation therapy being utilized as the primary treatment of choice in "resectable" carcinoma of the lung, with improvement of the cure rates. Both modalities generally fail because of the tendency of the cancer to metastasize very early.

Radiation therapy for carcinoma of the lung should be delivered with doses high enough to effect a cure of the local lesion and any known immediately adjacent spread.

The undifferentiated and Oat cell carcinomas are more radiosensitive than are the well differentiated squamous cell carcinomas. Unfortunately, the undifferentiated carcinomas have a much higher incidence of early metastasis and as a result present a diminishing chance of cure. If the patients do not present clinical evidence of metastasis at the beginning of radiation therapy, then intensive high-dose treatment should be given to the primary lesion with prophylactic treatment being delivered to the immediate areas of potential early spread, such as the mediastinum and supraclavicular areas.

We need to bear in mind that normal aerated lung tissue transmits more ionizing radiations than a comparable volume of fat, muscle, or bone. A solid tumor situated within a field of normal lung will receive a higher radiation dose than a similar tumor embedded in an equal volume of muscle or solid tissue. Treatment under such conditions results in the tumor actually receiving a higher radiation dosage than one might calculate from a depth-dose table, while the lung will receive a lesser dose of radiations owing to decreased absorption. There is no simple or accurate method for calculating the dosimetry around these tumors.

Some radiation therapists have advocated a rapid split course technique for management of carcinoma of the lung. This consists of 2000 rads tumor dose delivered in five fractions in a period of one week, a three week rest period, and a repeat of the course of therapy. The fields for the second course of therapy should be adjusted for shrinkage of tumor volume. We have found that this gives excellent palliative results and also results in approximately the same five-year, disease-free control rate that a more routine 6000 rads in six weeks accomplishes. The rapid split technique is well tolerated by the patient, gives a more rapid decrease in symptomatology, and, if the treatment is unsuccessful, has at least resulted in a shorter hospitalization for the patient. It carries the same or perhaps slightly better radiobiologic factors than the routine course of treatment.

N. Larynx

Radiation therapy has long been advocated as a primary means of treatment for squamous cell carcinoma of the larynx. Approximately 98 per cent of carcinomas arising within this area will be of the squamous cell type. Radiation therapy is the treatment of choice for carcinoma of the larynx in its early stages owing to its ability to cure the lesion and yet preserve the function of the larynx.

Although the great majority of cancers that arise in the endolarynx and hypopharynx are squamous cell and appear absolutely identical histologically, there is a wide variety of success in controlling these lesions. Carcinoma limited to the true vocal cord is extremely curable. A lesion of approximately the same size and with the histology found on the false cord is less likely to be cured. On the aryepiglottic fold it is even less curable, and in the pyriform sinus it will have an even poorer prognosis. The five-year control rates range from approximately 90 per cent for an early carcinoma of the true cord to approximately 30 per cent for an early pyriform sinus lesion.

O. Bone

Bone is made up of a variety of histologic structures, all of which have malignant tumors associated with them. The more common tumors are chondrosarcomas which arise from cartilage, osteosarcomas, which arise from the bone, and reticulum cell and Ewing's sarcomas, which arise from the bone marrow elements.

Tumors originating from the bone marrow elements are the most sensitive, as one might suspect. These tumors respond well to irradiation. Tumors that arise from the cartilage or the bone-forming elements are more radioresistant; this would be anticipated from the radiation tolerance level of normal adult bone and cartilage.

The highly cellular, anaplastic bone tumors are usually radiosensitive, but at the same time less radiocurable owing to distant metastasis.

Surgery with amputation of the involved limb is the usual treatment for malignant bone tumors except those that arise from the marrow elements. Radiation therapy is often used preoperatively to hold the primary lesion in check, meanwhile delaying the observation of distant metastasis.

Radiation therapy for the primary bone tumor is carried to high doses—6000 to 8000 rads mid-tumor dose in 6 to 12 weeks. This dose level is generally followed by amputation after "a reasonable length of time." Often the operative specimen is found to be free of cancer at the time of surgery. Should the patient develop metastasis prior to amputation, naturally the limb will be spared. In these situations, local tumor recurrence in the primarily irradiated area seldom occurs.

Normal bone is continuously being changed by the destruction of certain areas of bone and the reconstruction of new layers. The osteoclasts dissolve bone and then disappear. Osteoblasts appear to reconstruct the bone. This well-balanced process of destruction and reconstruction can be disturbed by high doses of radiations.

Normal adult bone is quite tolerant of radiations in the megavolt ranges. Six to seven thousand rads delivered in a period of 6 to 9 weeks apparently has little effect on adult bone unless the bone becomes infected or is subjected to great stress. The most common adult bone to become involved in radiation complications is the mandible owing to the ease of infection of this area.

Volumes of information have been written about the differences of radiation absorption in bone with a variation in energy of the irradiating beam. With low kilovoltage the majority of the absorption occurs by the photoelectric process which is based upon the fourth power of Z (the atomic number). With megavoltage, the majority of the absorption is by Compton interaction with energy absorption based upon the first power of Z. The probability of Compton interaction per atom depends upon the number of electrons present. In the neutral atom, this number is the same as the atomic number of the material (Z).

This difference in absorption may be graphically illustrated by comparing radiographs taken at megavoltage energy with radiographs taken at conventional diagnostic or low kilovoltage energies. The megavoltage films will show an almost complete lack of bone detail, with the bones appearing transparent. This clearly demonstrates the lack of significant differential absorption between bone and soft tissue.

Considerable optimism is expressed over the bone-sparing characteristics of megavoltage radiations. There is ample physical and biologic data to justify this optimism. For a given dose to soft tissue and adjacent bone, the inner oseous cellular structures of bone near the surface will always receive a higher dosage with low voltage X-ray beams than with megavoltage beams. The deeper areas of bone can be shielded from low energy X-ray beams by the overlying layers of surface bone. This effect is almost nonexistent with megavoltage.

The irradiation of the epiphyseal areas in children is very damaging. Doses as low as 500 rads will cause significant reduction in bone growth in the long bones. Doses over 1000 rads to the vertebral bodies will almost invariably cause scoliosis.

Adult bone is considerably more resistant

to severe changes following irradiation. The growth centers of the bone are closed and nonfunctioning in the adult, eliminating one of the more sensitive areas of treatment.

Ewing's tumor of bone is a very radiosensitive lesion. This tumor often infiltrates the soft tissues and extends throughout the shaft of the bone. The spread of this tumor dictates that the entire bone and a generous margin of adjacent soft tissue should routinely be irradiated. Ewing's tumor is highly radiosensitive and is frequently radiocurable. Five thousand rads in five weeks has been considered a curative dose for this disease.

Reticulum cell sarcoma of bone arises from the reticulum cells of the hemopoietic tissues of the marrow. This tumor is relatively radiosensitive and locally radiocurable. The entire bone may be treated to a dosage of 3500 to 4000 rads in approximately four weeks with excellent results, provided the disease has not metastasized.

P. Central Nervous System and Brain

Nerve tissue classically has been regarded as radioresistant. However, as with other radioresistant tissues, very often the results of irradiation and the subsequent damage are very slow to appear. Damage which occurs to nervous tissue is often very serious because once it has manifested itself little or no repair ever takes place and the damage is permanent.

Most of the normal adult neural elements are quite resistant to radiation damage, however when the damage does occur, repair is almost nonexistent. As a consequence of this relative radioresistance, tumors that arise from the primary neural tissues are equally radioresistant and seldom radiocurable.

Unfortunately, unless a brain tumor is located in an extremely accessible area, surgery is seldom successful in completely removing the tumor. Radiation therapy is often advocated postoperatively because tumor tissue has been left behind. With very few exceptions, radiation therapy seldom offers more to these patients than a palliative slowdown of the ultimate regrowth of the tumor.

Brain tumors are commonly subdivided into gliomas and nongliomas. The gliomas are subsequently divided into four groups— astrocytomas, ependymomas, oligodendrogliomas, and medulloblastomas. The astrocytomas are further subdivided into four grades of malignancy, depending upon their mitotic activity.

Astrocytomas, grades I through IV, comprise about two-thirds of all malignant brain tumors. Grades I and II are relatively benign tumors and as a result do not respond well to radiation. Grade III astrocytomas show a better response to radiation, and glioblastoma multiforme, or grade IV astrocytomas, responds to radiation therapy but is seldom cured. Tumor doses between 5000 and 7000 rads with concentrically constricted fields have been recommended.

In well-differentiated gliomas the cells of origin are quite distinct and the tumor is extremely radioresistant, whereas in glioblastoma multiforme the cells are extremely anaplastic, show a greater degree of radiosensitivity, but continue to be reasonably radioincurable. The low-grade tumors tend to have sharp margins and grow slowly, whereas the highly anaplastic lesions have diffuse margins, grow rapidly, and infiltrate the adjoining brain tissue.

Ependymomas and medulloblastomas have a tendency to seed through the spinal canal because of the shedding of cells from the surface of the tumor. Patients with this condition should be treated not only with total brain irradiation, but their spinal circulation should also be treated. These tumors show a moderate degree of radiosensitivity and radiocurability—a combination of surgery for the primary lesions and approximately 4500 rads tumor dose results in about a 50 per cent five-year survival.

Oligodenrogliomas are relatively infrequent lesions but are radiosensitive and can be radiocurable. Five to six thousand rads in a period of 6 to 7 weeks is recommended.

When brain tumors are treated in either a palliative or curative fashion, some degree of tolerance, based upon a combination of radiosensitivity of the area in question and functional importance, must be considered.

The brain stem is as radiosensitive as the spinal cord. Approximately 5000 rads in 5 to 7 weeks has been considered the dose limit for palliation with 6000 rads in six weeks being the maximum recommended dosage under curative circumstances.

Some of the areas of the brain which are of less functional importance, such as the frontal and occipital lobes, may have a higher dose given with an acceptable increase in sequelae. The dose limit is still between 5000 and 7000 rads in 5 to 9 weeks.

Lesions of the spinal cord have the same histologic classification as the brain lesions. The spinal cord also shows about the same degree of radiotolerance as the brain, the upper limits being between 5000 and 6000 rads in 5 to 7 weeks, depending upon the severity of the tumor being treated and the necessity for treatment.

Neuroblastomas. Neuroblastomas, as a definitive histologic type, behave somewhat differently than other tumors of neural origin. These tumors usually arise from the adrenal medulla or similar tissue found along the aorta. They are often seen in the posterior portions of the mediastinum. They are composed of malignant neurons and appear almost exclusively in children. The lesions grow rapidly and metastasize early. These tumors are extremely radiosensitive and radiocurable. Low doses of radiations have resulted in permanent control and even though widespread metastasis may be present, the patient should still be treated as completely as possible. In infants and small children a dosage of approximately 2000 rads in 3 to 4 weeks almost invariably controls the lesion being treated. There have been reported cases of these tumors spontaneously maturing to a benign ganglioneuroma. Control rates as high as 88 per cent have been reported for early lesions treated with surgery and radiation therapy.

Q. Eye

Carcinomas that arise on the conjunctiva are generally of the squamous cell type and are treated with the same general factors as cancer of the skin. The only significant factors that must be considered here are the closeness of the lens and cornea and subsequently protective measures should be taken with these areas to prevent excessive radiations from reaching them.

The major tumor of significance that arises within the eye is retinoblastoma. This arises from both the inner and outer nuclear layers of the retina and expands into the eye. These tumors can extend down the optic nerve and metastasize in this fashion.

This tumor has a hereditary tendency. Patients who have been cured of retinoblastoma are very likely to pass this disease tendency on to their children. The incidence is reported between 60 and 80 per cent chance of retinoblastoma developing in the offspring of a treated retinoblastoma patient. Surgical removal of the eye is the usual form of treatment. If there is an attempt to salvage the vision of the eye, radiation therapy can be used. The beam should be directed in such a fashion as to spare the lens and cornea if at all possible. A single lateral portal with the lens shielded is the preferred technique. The ultimate in precision of beam definition and dosimetry is necessary.

These lesions are relatively radiosensitive, with small lesions demonstrating as high as a 90 per cent control rate. Even large lesions demonstrate 20 to 30 per cent permanent control with a tumor dose of 4500 rads in five weeks.

R. Hemopoietic System

The various acute and subacute changes that can occur throughout the bone marrow have been previously described. The sensitivities of lymphatic and lymphoid tissue likewise have been adequately covered.

The only tumors of any significance that arise from the bone marrow are the leukemias. The leukemias vary biologically from chronic diseases with life expectancies of many years to the acute forms with a life expectancy of no more than a few weeks from the time of discovery until death. It is felt by many people that these are actually different forms of an overall disease category rather than phases of a single disease.

Acute leukemias are seldom a radiation therapy problem as their management is almost exclusively chemotherapeutic. Radiation therapy offers very little from either an immediate or long-term palliative standpoint.

In contrast, chronic leukemias are often controlled for long periods of time with either localized or total body irradiation. The treatments are usually directed to specific areas of involvement or organs which are infiltrated with the leukemic cells. The effects of irradiation of large leukemic infiltrates is astoundingly rapid. Low doses in the range of 500 to 1000 rads tumors dose in a period of 5 to 10 days usually results in a complete regression of the symptomatic area. This prediction is based upon the sensitivity of the cells of origin. Lymphatic leukemia is more sensitive than granulocytic leukemia, as would be expected.

Patients with a markedly elevated white count and a depressed platelet count can often be put into clinical remission of their disease with total body irradiation. The dosage ranges from 25 to 50 rads total body in a period of 1 to 3 weeks.

Patients with chronic leukemia can often be controlled for many years with a relatively stable white and platelet count by weekly low-dose total body irradiation. We have had a number of cases who have survived for over five years with this method of treatment and have accumulated in that period over 1000 rads total body irradiation with little or no untoward side effects.

Splenic irradiation is often quite effective in the treatment of leukemia. We have found that the treatment of a large spleen will often result in the abscopal reduction of the patient's white count and lymph nodes in other untreated areas of the body. Usually 1200 to 1600 rads tumor dose to the spleen will result in a complete reduction of splenomegaly. The field should be concentrically reduced as the spleen decreases in size.

S. Lymphatic System

Tumors that arise within the lymphatic system are termed lymphomas. These include lymphosarcoma, reticulum cell sarcoma, Hodgkin's disease, and giant follicular lymphoma.

Most lymphomas are extremely sensitive to radiation therapy, as one would predict, owing to the marked radiosensitivity of lymphatic tissue in general. Lymphomas are generally radiocontrollable and radiocurable if the disease is relatively localized. One can even expect long-term cures in advanced cases of Hodgkin's disease (Stages III and IV) with judicious application of "total nodal" type of radiation therapy, which includes treatment of all of the major lymph node areas in the body.

The lymphomas and lymphosarcomas are treated on a localized or a regional node group basis. Hodgkin's disease has recently been treated by the "total nodal" technique.

The average radiation dose for control of lymphomas is generally 4500 to 5000 rads tumor dose delivered over 5 to 7 weeks.

With the more favorable forms of histology such as lymphocytic predominant Hodgkin's and with localized Stage I disease as high as a 90 per cent five-year control rate might be expected, whereas with far advanced lymphosarcoma we can at best expect only a temporary palliation of immediate problems. In general, however, the high sensitivity of lymphoid tissue leads to a high sensitivity of tumors that arise from it and, as a consequence, a reasonable chance of radiocurability.

Surgery plays no role in the treatment of lymphomas except for a biopsy as proof of the lesion.

Chemotherapy is often used in the advanced cases both in combination with radiation therapy and as a palliative modality.

7.12 RE-IRRADIATION

Patients who have received radiation therapy in the past will occasionally be seen with cancer within the previously treated field. These patients fall into a very unfortunate category. The previous irradiation will have markedly altered the radiosensitivity of the residual cancer such that cure by further radiation therapy will be almost impossible. This is due to a number of factors, chief of these being that the previously radiosensitive portions of the lesion will have been destroyed, and the remaining cells will be the more resistant cell lines. These will have flourished and caused the cancer to regrow. It is also suggested that part of the decrease in radiosensitivity of recurrent cancer may be due to radiation-induced mutations with the production of resistant cell lines.

Other important changes that will have occurred in and around the tumor-bearing area are primarily related to changes within the tumor bed. The blood supply to the surrounding supportive tissue has generally been decreased with fibrosis developing throughout the previously treated area. These changes contribute to a decrease in availability of oxygen and nutrition. This will lead to further radioresistance, the cells being protected through the decrease in oxygen tension so that they are resistant to any further radiation therapy.

This emphasizes the fact that if a cancer is being considered for radiation therapy, it is the first course of treatment that stands the only chance of curing the lesion. If the initial course of radiation therapy is inadequate due to failure to carry the dose high enough, meager margins surrounding the cancer, or a general degree of resistance of the cancer, any further attempt at radiation therapy following a recurrence will almost invariably be fraught with failure. Surgery and chemotherapy are usually the selected modes of treatment for post-radiation recurrence. The exact choice will depend upon the circumstances of the case.

7.13 CHEMOTHERAPEUTIC AGENTS

There are five classes of chemotherapeutic agents now in use. These are (1) alkylating agents, (2) antimetabolites, (3) hormones, (4) antibiotics, and (5) plant alkaloids.

These agents may be used in combinations with each other and with schedules that often interrelate with radiation therapy and surgery.

A. Alkylating Agents

Alkylating agents act chiefly upon already formed nucleic acids. These drugs are directly cytotoxic, and the more drug that can be delivered to the area of the cancer, the better is the response rate and the cell killing capacity of the drug. It should also be noted that these drugs are almost equally as toxic to normal cells.

The most useful drugs among the alkylating agents are nitrogen mustard, Thiotepa, Chlorambucil, Cytoxan, Myleran, and Alkeran.

These drugs range in toxicity from nitrogen mustard, the most toxic, to Thiotepa, the least toxic. Cytoxan is probably the safest and most useful of the alkylating agents.

An additive toxic effect often exists between these drugs and radiation therapy, and care must be exercised when they are used in combination.

B. Antimetabolites

Antimetabolites act by interfering with the synthesis of chromosomal nucleic acid, which is necessary for new tumor cell production. This synthesis occurs only during the mitotic phase of the cell cycle, which results in the concept of "cycle active" for these drugs. These drugs seem to be most effective when given over long periods of time so that they may effect many tumor cycles.

Most common among the antimetabolites are the folic acid antagonist, methotrexate, the antipyrimidine, 5-fluorouracil, and the purine antagonist, 6-mercaptopurine.

Methotrexate is often used in combination with radiation therapy with very few additive side effects. Because methotrexate is not normally detoxified by the body, but is excreted in an unchanged form through the kidneys, it cannot be used in the presence of renal disease. Methotrexate seems to be most effective against squamous cell cancers, especially those arising in and around the oral cavity and upper airways. Overall improvement in therapeutic results have been difficult to demonstrate, but many clinical trials are still in progress.

Fluorouracil has been found to be of considerable value in treating patients with adenocarcinoma of the gastrointestinal tract and breast. Biochemically this drug interferes with the synthesis of thymidine, which is a major precursor of chromosomal DNA. Reduction of dose is necessary to avoid toxicity when used in combination with radiation therapy. Improper dosage can result in severe bone marrow depression.

C. Hormones

The most commonly used hormones in cancer chemotherapy are estrogens, androgens, and adrenal corticosteroids.

The addition or subtraction of female hormones is often used in the treatment of various malignancies related to the breast, uterus, and prostate.

Castration, either by surgery or by radiation therapy, is usually the treatment of choice in the premenopausal woman with metastases from carcinoma of the breast. Often androgens are utilized after castration in an attempt to reduce the activity of metastatic lesions. In older women who are well past the menopause, treatment *with* estrogens often results in a decrease in activity of metastatic breast cancer. Older women often show significant objective improvement, particularly with soft tissue metastases, when treated with estrogen.

Androgens are sometimes used in premenopausal women with bony metastases from carcinoma of the breast.

The adrenal glands are a source of many steroidal hormones, chiefly the corticosteroids, although there is also a significant level of androgenic and estrogenic hormone production. In patients with carcinoma of the breast who have become refractory to other forms of hormonal manipulation, adrenalectomy is often helpful. The patient most likely to benefit from this procedure is the woman who has demonstrated the hormonal dependency of her cancer by remission following castration.

Hypophysectomy has been employed in addition to, or in place of, adrenalectomy, but it is not widely used because of its undesirable side effects.

An alternative to adrenalectomy or hypophysectomy that has been used is the administration of high doses of adrenal corticosteroids. This has the advantage of avoiding the morbidity of the surgical procedure and the necessity of subsequent hormonal replacement therapy. High doses of steroids cause almost complete suppression of adrenal function, including the production of estrogenic and androgenic compounds.

In the patient with advanced carcinoma of the prostate, orchiectomy has been shown to be useful. Orchiectomy is the initial therapy of choice for the patient with widespread metastatic disease from carcinoma of the prostate. The improvement is often dramatic, immediate, and long-sustained. Estrogens may be used in conjunction with orchiectomy and maintained indefinitely. Estrogens have also been utilized in those patients who refuse orchiectomy.

Adrenalectomy has been advocated in the patient with carcinoma of the prostate, based on the same rationale and criteria as those for carcinoma of the female breast. The adrenal cortex does produce some androgenic steroids and as such its removal will decrease the level of these hormones. The undesirable effects of adrenalectomy make this form of treatment unsatisfactory in many cases.

Many of the well-differentiated adenocarcinomas of the endometrium have demonstrated sensitivity to the administration of progestational agents. The regression of metastatic lesions from endometrial carcinoma has often been marked, and many of these patients have remained in sustained remission for many years. The most common drugs utilized are Delautin and Provera.

Corticosteroids have been utilized widely in the treatment of malignant lymphomas and leukemias. They are routinely used in the treatment of acute childhood leukemia. Steroids are often used in conjunction with many of the other chemotherapeutic agents for the treatment of lymphomas.

The various steroidal compounds have a definite role in the palliation of many types of malignant diseases, achieving temporary and, occasionally, striking and prolonged remission in a small but significant percentage of patients. These agents are extremely useful singly or in combination with other drugs to produce prolonged remissions in patients suffering from widespread metastatic disease.

D. Antibiotics

The anti-tumor antibiotics are among the more recent additions to the chemotherapeutic armamentarium. Among the drugs included under this category are actinomycin D, daunomycin, and mithramycin.

Actinomycin D has been used with some degree of benefit in Wilms' tumor and choriocarcinoma. In combination with vincristine it is useful against carcinoma of the lung in adults and against rhabdomyosarcoma in children.

Actinomycin has an additive or synergistic effect with X-ray therapy. This is noted in the production of skin erythema as well as an increased effect on irradiated tissues, either normal or malignant. Daunomycin has been used in acute leukemia with some success. Embryonal cell carcinoma of the testis is sometimes responsive to mithromycin.

E. Alkaloids

Some of the most useful chemotherapeutic agents are the alkaloids. Vinblastine and vincristine are derived from the common garden periwinkle. Vinblastine is useful in Hodgkin's disease and other lymphomas, particularly in cases which are resistant to other forms of chemotherapy.

Vincristine is effective in the treatment of lymphomas and leukemias. Vincristine is toxic to the central nervous system; however, it has very little effect upon the bone marrow and as a result may be used with radiation therapy without untoward side effects.

Vinblastine does cause bone marrow depression and should be used with caution if radiation therapy is included as part of the treatment protocol.

Colchicine has long been known as a mitotic inhibitor and is a drug commonly utilized to synchronize cell cultures. This drug has been used in combination with radiation therapy, although the effects have been variable.

F. Combination Therapy

Recently many of these drugs, listed earlier, have been combined in a variety of studies. An example of combination drug therapy is MOPP, which is a combination of nitrogen mustard, vincristine (Oncovin), procarbazine, and prednisone. This combination is often administered over a two-week course with a two-week rest period between cycles. Another combination of the same general nature is COPP in which Cytoxan is substituted for nitrogen mustard. This combination is given on eight-week cycles—four weeks on the drugs and four weeks' rest. The results of these combined courses of chemotherapeutic agents have usually shown longer remissions and often with a decrease of overall toxic symptomatology.

COPP and MOPP can be used prior to

TABLE 7–4 SOME OF THE MORE COMMON CHEMOTHERAPEUTIC AGENTS IN CURRENT USE

Drugs	Tumor Indications	% Response	Toxicity
Actinomycin-D	Wilms' tumor	80	Nausea, vomiting, bone marrow
	Carcinoma of lung (with vincristine)	60	depression, stomatitis
	Choriocarcinoma (female)	80	
Alkeran	Multiple myeloma	30	Bone marrow depression
Androgens	Carcinoma of the breast	25	Masculinization
BCNU	Lymphomas	—	Delayed bone marrow depression
COPP	Lymphomas	—	Bone marrow depression
Cytoxan	Lymphoma	70	Leukopenia, nausea, vomiting,
	Neuroblastoma	—	alopecia
	Myeloma	30	
	Leukemia	30	
Estrogens	Carcinoma of the breast (post-menopausal)	50	Feminization
	Carcinoma of the prostate	60	Hypercalcemia
5-Fluorouracil	Cancer of the breast	20	Bone marrow depression, nausea, vomiting, diarrhea
	GI adenocarcinoma	20	
	Ovarian carcinoma	15	
Leukeran	Leukemia	—	Bone marrow depression
Methotrexate	Squamous cell head and neck	80	Bone marrow depression, GI ulceration, renal failure
	Choriocarcinoma	80	
	Leukemia (contraindicated with androgens)	20	
Mithromycin	Testicular tumors	40	Bone marrow depression, liver damage
MOPP	Lymphomas	—	Bone marrow depression
Myleran	Leukemia	—	Bone marrow depression
Nitrogen mustard	Lymphoma, leukemia	60	Nausea, vomiting, bone marrow depression
Prednisone	Lymphomas	40	Cushings' syndrome
	Leukemias	40	Osteoporosis
	Carcinoma of the breast	30	Susceptibility to infection
Progesterones	Endometrium	75	Masculinization
Thiotepa	Adenocarcinoma	—	Bone marrow depression
Velban	Lymphoma	40	Bone marrow depression
Vincristine	Lymphomas	60	Neurotoxic

radiation therapy to induce remissions in advanced lymphomas, after which the patients are carefully treated with radiation therapy.

Vincristine and actinomycin may also be utilized in combination. After the patient has shown some improvement on chemotherapy, radiation therapy may be instituted. Methotrexate is often given prior to radiation therapy to decrease the bulk of a tumor and to hopefully improve the geometry for the following radiation therapy. Combinations of fluorouracil and nitrogen mustard with radiation therapy have been tried, but considerable care in adjustment of the dose is required to avoid unacceptable toxicity.

Actinomycin D and X-rays have been used in the treatment of Wilms' tumor with a moderate degree of success.

Many attempts have been made to demonstrate some degree of synergism between radiation therapy and chemotherapy. Most of these efforts have ended with the conclusion that the toxic effects are markedly synergistic, whereas the increased overall curative or palliative effects on the tumors have been rather meager.

Table 7–4 lists many of the more common chemotherapeutic agents being used at the present time, the tumors against which they are often effective, and some indication of possible responses and toxicity.

7.14 SUMMARY

Since the discovery of X-rays and radium 75 years ago, our knowledge of radiation therapy has progressed through the years to the modern utilization of these modalities as one of the leading forms of treatment of cancer. At the present state of our knowledge radiation therapy has the potential for curing at least one-half of all the cancer patients that are accepted for curative therapy.

The human body is composed of an almost endless variety of cell systems, all of which may be separated into four basic categories. These are the static, renewing, rapid-renewing, and neoplastic cell populations. Radiation therapy is the utilization of different forms of radiations in an attempt to destroy cells that are found in the neoplastic cell population. Cells in this popula-

tion group will have arisen from one of the other three groups. The degree to which malignant cells will be responsive to radiation therapy is dependent upon the radiosensitivity of their cells of origin, as well as other characteristics of these neoplastic cells.

Many of the basic radiobiologic laws were expressed in the early part of the twentieth century; modifications were made over the years as our state of knowledge improved. The present basic laws of radiobiology serve as guidelines to the radiosensitivity of a given tumor system. The reader must be aware that radiosensitivity does not necessarily indicate radiocurability.

There are many factors which surround the relationship between the patient, his cancer, and the radiation therapy which will be utilized to treat it. The wide variability of the human subject will often invalidate all but the broadest "laws" regarding the radiobiologic responses of tissue. The effects of radiations upon cancerous tissue are basically the same as upon normal cell systems. However, the repair and recovery potential of normal tissue is much greater.

Most courses of radiation therapy are delivered over a period of time to allow the supportive tissues time for repair. The concepts of fractionation and protraction, with the total dosage of radiations to be delivered distributed over a period of time and broken up into multiple fractions, are very important. The concept of nominal single dose (NSD) has been suggested as a means of integrating these factors back to a single value so that various schemes of radiation may be compared.

Oxygen, either in increased or decreased amounts, has long been utilized as a modifying agent for radiation changes in molecular systems. The ability of oxygen to potentiate radiation response is called the oxygen effect. Large cancers tend to be anoxic; as a result, there can be foci of cells within these lesions which may survive a course of radiation therapy because of local anoxic conditions. Hyperbaric oxygen has long been utilized in an attempt to overcome this effect. A ratio relating the dose of radiation required for a given effect under anoxic conditions as compared to the amount of radiation required for a similar effect under well-oxygenated conditions is known as the oxygen enhancement ratio.

The wide variety of energies and types of radiations available for treating cancer has necessitated the formation of a basis of comparison. The concept of linear energy transfer relates to the amount of energy deposited from a given beam of radiations while passing through tissues. The linear energy transfer depends upon the mass, energy, and charge of the radiation. The greater the mass and charge, and the less the velocity, the greater is the linear energy transfer. An increase in tissue oxygen tension will increase the effective linear energy transfer for a given beam of radiations.

The many different types of ionizing radiations have been found to produce effects on biologic systems which are qualitatively similar in some situations and qualitatively different in other situations. The expression, relative biologic effectiveness, is used to compare the effectiveness of two radiations in producing a given change in a biologic system. To a great extent the relative biologic effectiveness depends upon the linear energy transfer.

Cancers of different histologic types arising from different sites of origin will display considerable differences in radiosensitivity and radiocurability. Different cancers arising from the same tissue will also show differences in radiosensitivity, depending upon their degree of differentiation. The differences in radiosensitivity of various malignancies are primarily attributed to their cells of origin; however, the degree of differentiation and location plays an important role in their ultimate radiosensitivity and radiocurability. The nutritional status of the patient and the condition of the supportive tissues surrounding the cancer are also of vital importance in the ultimate prognosis.

There are many different ways of treating cancer. Two methods are most effective for inducing remissions and eliminating the disease. These are surgery and radiation therapy. A third method, chemotherapy, is useful for palliation or supplementation of surgery and radiation therapy. Radiation therapy by means of either external radiation therapy or internal radioactive compounds is extremely effective in treating many forms of cancer. Radiation therapy may be used either pre- or postoperatively, before or after chemotherapy, or in combinations with both surgery and chemotherapy.

The use of radiation therapy to treat many forms of cancer has been covered in considerable detail in this chapter. Reduced to its most basic description, radiation therapy consists of the selective destruction of cancer while allowing the normal supportive tissues to repair and regenerate. If the radiation is successful in destroying all the cancer without causing irreparable damage to the patient, then a cure will result. If the cancer is able to withstand the complete course of radiation therapy and to regrow, then the radiation therapy has been unsuccessful. Surgery or chemotherapy, or both, may be utilized to treat radiation recurrences or residual tumor.

Chemotherapy is often used before and after radiation therapy with variable results. Chemotherapeutic agents are quite specific for the types of cancer against which they are effective. Most chemotherapeutic agents are not without their undesirable side effects.

Over the past 20 years an almost endless variety of approaches, countless studies and mathematical models, and untold millions of mice have been utilized in an attempt to make a quantitative assessment of the effects of ionizing radiations. The ultimate goal of all of these studies has been to attempt to discover a basic biologic rationale for the effects which we clinically observe when cancer is irradiated. We have yet to establish a solid bridge between theory and application. The knowledge gap between the experimental cancer researcher and the practicing clinical physician is narrowing. The time will eventually come when a biopsy of the patient's cancer may be grown, studied, and analyzed in a fashion yet to be discovered—in such a way that the ultimate formulation of the patient's successful treatment may be carried out in practically all cases of cancer.

We are a long way from realizing this final endpoint; yet, this end will be reached and theories will merge into facts which will eventually merge into "the ultimate cure for all cancer."

References

1. Andrews, J. R.: *The Radiobiology of Human Cancer Radiotherapy.* Philadelphia, W. B. Saunders, 1968.
2. Bogardus, C. T.: Radiation therapy for cancer of the bladder. *In* Maltry, E. (ed.): *Benign and Malignant Tumors of the Urinary Bladder.* Flushing, N.Y., Medical Examiner and Publishing Co., 1971.
3. Churchill-Davidson, I., Foster, C. A., Wiernik, G., Collins, C. D., Pizey, N. C. D., Skeggs, D. B. L., and Purser, P. R.: The place of oxygen in radiotherapy. Brit. J. Radiol., 39:321–331, 1966.
4. Churchill-Davidson, I., Sanger, C., and Thomlinson, R. H.: Oxygenation in radiotherapy. Brit. J. Radiol., 30:406–422, 1957.
5. Ellis, F.: The relationship of biological effect to dose-time-fractionation factors in radiotherapy. *In* Ebert, M., and Harold, A. (eds.): *Current Topics in Radiation Research*, ed. 4. New York, John Wiley, 1968.
6. Ellis, F.: Dose, time, and fractionation; A clinical hypothesis. Clin. Radiol., 20:1–7, 1969.
7. Ellis, F.: Fractionation in radiotherapy. *In* Deeley, T. J., and Woods, C. A. P. (eds.): *Modern Trends in Radiotherapy*, Vol. 1, London, Butterworth, 1967.
8. Fowler, J. F.: Experimental animal results relating to time-dose-relationships in radiotherapy and the "ret" concept. Brit. J. Radiol., 44:81–90, 1970.
9. Kroening, P. M., and Deiterman, L. H.: A table for the normalization of time-dose relationships. Amer. J. Roentgen., 112:803–805, 1971.
10. Moss, W. T., and Brand, W. N.: *Therapeutic Radiology Rationale, Technique, and Results*, ed. 3. St. Louis, C. V. Mosby, 1969.
11. Scanlon, P. W.: Radiotherapeutic problems best handled with split-dose therapy. Amer. J. Roentgen., 93:639–650, 1965.

8 CONCEPTS OF CLINICAL RADIATION PATHOLOGY

Philip Rubin, M.D., and George W. Casarett, Ph.D.

8.0 INTRODUCTION

The problems of radiation therapy are *in vivo* problems which involve the dynamic and interacting components of organized tissues and systems. Over many decades the histopathologic research on radiation effect *in vivo* in experimental animals and in humans has gradually contributed much information. However, one of the greatest obstacles to more rapid progress in the development of a biologic basis for radiation therapy has been the lack of due appreciation of the importance of this kind of information and the associated neglect of quantitative and mechanistic histopathologic research.

Essential to the development of a biologic basis of radiation therapy is the correlation of knowledge of cellular radiosensitivity and of the responses and interactions of parenchymal and supporting cells and tissues in relation to their proliferating and differentiating characteristics and their kinetics. To this end, radiobiologic research on cellular population kinetics and turnover rates, with the use of radioactive tracers, has been instrumental in more precisely quantitating certain cellular effects of irradiation. However, this work is still in its early phases. In addition, the functional dependencies and influences of organized tissues must be better known through meticulous study of physiologic alteration associated with morphologic change after irradiation. Due recognition must be given to the changes in microcirculation, vasculature, connective tissue, and other supporting tissues which are involved in histopathologic dynamics *in vivo*. Without such comprehension of the dynamic sequential events occurring in irradiated normal and neoplastic tissues, little progress will be made toward changing these events to advantage in radiation therapy.

The clinical manifestations of radiation lesions appear highly variable in different anatomic sites and include such diverse findings as a moist dermatitis, gastric ulceration, intestinal obstruction, nephritis, hypertension, cessation of bone growth, bone necrosis, decrease of salivation, liver failure, cardiomyopathies, demyelination of nerves, and cataracts. The list is hardly exhausted and could easily be expanded. The evidence is clear; the radiation lesions occur at different times and in highly varied clinical and pathologic forms.

However, the basic radiation lesions are essentially similar in the various organs. The clinical expressivity of the lesion will be determined by the nature and radiosensitivity of the cellular and tissue components of the organ and by the specific function of the organ. If the cellular and tissue organization of the irradiated organ is appreciated, our classifications of cellular, tissue, and organ radiosensitivity permit reasonable prediction of the course of development of the radiopathologic lesions and of the relative roles and predominance of parenchymal or vascular damage in the radiation reaction. The kinetics of the various cellular components in parenchymal, vascular, and connective tissues become a biologic time clock for the expression of such injury. It is within this context that seemingly different clinical manifestations of radiation injury are woven into a similar histopathologic fabric and explained.

8.1 CLASSIFICATION OF CELLS ACCORDING TO RELATIVE RADIOSENSITIVITY

Following is a working classification of the relative radiosensitivity of categories of cells according to the kinds of lives they lead (Figs. 8–1, 8–2). This classification is given in order of decreasing relative radiosensitivity and is based on the criterion of direct, acute cell death. This is defined as due to direct effects seemingly caused by mechanisms contained within the structure specified as being affected.

A. Vegetative Intermitotic (VIM) Cells (Class 1)

In general, this category contains the most radiation-sensitive of the cell types.

They are short-lived as individual cells, they are primitive, and they normally divide regularly to produce daughter cells, some of which will enter into a process of differentiation and others of which will not differentiate but remain vegetative intermitotic cells. This class includes cells such as the most primitive free stem cells of the hemopoietic tissues; the dividing cells in the intestinal crypts and gastric glands; the primitive Type A spermatogonia in the seminiferous epithelium; proliferating granulosa cells of developing ovarian follicles; and basal germinal cells of the epidermis and of epidermoid epithelia.

B. Differentiating Intermitotic (DIM) Cells (Class 2)

In general, this category contains relatively radiosensitive cell types which are, for the most part, somewhat less radiosensitive than vegetative intermitotic cells. There is some overlap between these two categories of cells, depending upon frequency of division of particular cell types. Cell types in this category are also relatively short-lived as individuals and are produced by divisions of vegetative intermitotic cells. They normally divide from time to time for a limited number of divisions, and they differentiate to some degree between divisions. The more differentiated they become, the less sensitive to radiation they become. This class includes cells such as the dividing differentiating cells of the various hemopoietic series in the inter-

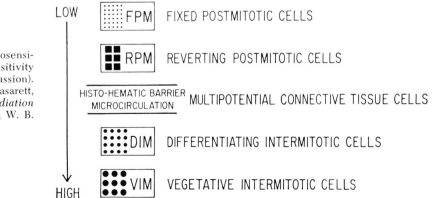

CELL RADIOSENSITIVITY

ORDER OF RADIOSENSITIVITY

LOW ── FPM   FIXED POSTMITOTIC CELLS

RPM   REVERTING POSTMITOTIC CELLS

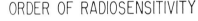
HISTO-HEMATIC BARRIER
MICROCIRCULATION   MULTIPOTENTIAL CONNECTIVE TISSUE CELLS

DIM   DIFFERENTIATING INTERMITOTIC CELLS

↓
HIGH   VIM   VEGETATIVE INTERMITOTIC CELLS

FIGURE 8–1 Cell radiosensitivity. Order of radiosensitivity (see text for further discussion). (From Rubin, P., and Casarett, G. W.: *Clinical Radiation Pathology.* Philadelphia, W. B. Saunders Co., 1968.)

CELL RADIOSENSITIVITY
POSSIBLE PATTERNS OF CELL FLOW

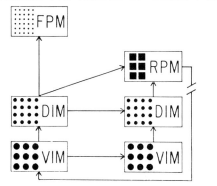

FIGURE 8–2 Cell radiosensitivity. Possible patterns of cell flow (see text for further discussion). (From Rubin, P., and Casarett, G. W.: *Clinical Radiation Pathology*. Philadelphia, W. B. Saunders Co., 1968.)

mediate stages of differentiation and the more differentiated spermatogonia (intermediate and Type B) and the spermatocytes in the seminiferous epithelium.

C. Multipotential Connective Tissue Cells (Class 3).

This category of cells is intermediate in position between the relatively radiosensitive cell types in Classes 1 and 2 and the relatively radioresistant cell types in Classes 4 and 5. These cells may divide irregularly or sporadically in time and in response to a variety of special stimuli. Their life span as individuals with respect to one form or function may be highly variable, but under normal conditions it is on the average longer than that of cells in Classes 1 and 2. This class includes such cells as endothelial cells, active fibroblasts, and mesenchymal cells.

D. Reverting Postmitotic (RPM) Cells (Class 4)

In general, this category of cells is relatively radioresistant. These cells have relatively long lives as individuals, do not normally undergo regular or periodic division in the adult, and generally do not divide except under abnormal conditions presenting special stimuli. Under an appropriate stimulus, usually involving damage, destruction, or loss of considerable numbers of cells of their kind or of cells which they are capable of producing, they can revert to a condition in which they divide to produce more cells of their kind or they undergo heterotypic transformations to produce cells of certain other kinds.

Some of the cell types of this class are highly specialized in function, while others are not. Some are epithelial and some are connective tissue elements. This class includes cells such as: the epithelial parenchymal cells and the duct cells in the salivary glands, liver, kidney, and pancreas; parenchymal cells of merocrine glands such as the sweat glands and of endocrine glands such as the adrenal, thyroid, parathyroid, and pituitary glands; cells of interstitial gland tissue of the gonads; cells of corpora lutea; sertoli cells; septal cells of the lung; fixed stem cells of various tissues, such as the reticulum cells in hemopoietic tissues; and perhaps some smooth muscle cells. The cells in this class may show considerable aging changes, but on division their daughter cells show a relative rejuvenation, and the disappearance of some of the aging changes.

E. Fixed Postmitotic (FPM) Cells (Class 5)

In general, the cells in this category are the most radioresistant of cells. Normally they do not divide, and have lost completely the ability to divide under any circumstances. They are highly differentiated morphologically and highly specialized in function. Some of them have very long lives and others have relatively short lives, but all undergo progressive aging changes until death (if they are not killed prematurely). The short-lived fixed postmitotic cells, when lost, are replaced by the action of vegetative or differentiating intermitotic precursor cells or both. If the loss of precursor cells is marked, the precursor cells may in some tissues be replaced by the action of reverting postmitotic primitive fixed stem cells. This class includes cells such as: the long-lived neurons and striated muscle cells, which are not replaceable; and the short-lived polymorphonuclear granulocytes, erythrocytes, spermatids, spermatozoa, superficial epithelial cells of the alimentary tract and epithelial cells of the sebaceous glands, all of which are replaceable.

8.2 CLASSIFICATION OF TISSUES ACCORDING TO RELATIVE RADIOSENSITIVITY

In keeping with the foregoing considerations of cellular radiosensitivity, various types of tissues are listed in Table 8–1 in the order of decreasing relative radiosensitivity on the basis of the relatively direct, acute, radiation-induced hypoplasia of the tissues; the chief mechanisms involved are indicated. Similarly, in Table 8–2 are listed various organs in their order of decreasing relative radiosensitivity on the basis of the relatively direct radiation effect on organs resulting in parenchymal hypoplasia by direct or indirect effect on the parenchyma. This would include effects due to intertissue mechanisms within the organs, such as effects on parenchymal tissues mediated through damage of the local fine vasculature and connective tissue reactions; here, too, the chief mechanisms involved in the organ effects are indicated.

Since it is difficult to establish the precise order of tissues of similar radiosensitivity,

the relative radiosensitivity is given in terms of high, fairly high, medium, fairly low, and low. There is much room for argument regarding the precise relative order of many of these tissues and organs, especially when different criteria are used. Furthermore, in the case of tissue or organ parenchymal hypoplasia secondary to damage of the vasculature and connective tissue reactions, it is recognized that, owing to the dose-dependent progressive nature of the damage and reactions in these supporting tissues, a moderate radiation dose may result in the development over a long period of time of a degree of parenchymal hypoplasia similar to that which may be caused by a large dose in a short period of time. Therefore, the order of relative radiosensitivity of the organs listed in Table 8–2 is based arbitrarily on the maximal degree of hypoplasia observed within two months; this is a period of time sufficient to observe most of the relatively direct destructive actions of radiation in tissues, the maximal degree of hypoplasia of parenchymal cells resulting from such actions,

TABLE 8–1 TISSUES IN DECREASING ORDER OF RELATIVE RADIOSENSITIVITY BASED ON RELATIVELY DIRECT TISSUE EFFECT (HYPOPLASIA)

Relative Radiosensitivity	Tissues	Chief Mechanisms of Hypoplasia
High	Lymphoid, hemopoietic (marrow), spermatogenic epithelium, ovarian follicular epithelium, intestinal epithelium	Destruction of vegetative or differentiating tissue cells of high mitotic frequency
Fairly high	Oropharyngeal stratified epithelium, epidermal epithelium, hair follicle epithelium, sebaceous gland epithelium, urinary bladder epithelium, esophageal epithelium, optic lens epithelium, gastric gland epithelium, ureteral epithelium	Destruction of vegetative or differentiating tissue cells of fairly high mitotic frequency
Medium	Ordinary interstitial connective tissue, neuroglial tissue (connective tissue of nervous system), fine vasculature, growing cartilage or bone tissue	Damage or destruction of connective tissue cells of moderate mitotic frequency, and damage of fine vasculature
Fairly low	Mature cartilage or bone tissue, mucus or serous gland epithelium, salivary gland epithelium, sweat gland epithelium, nasopharyngeal simple epithelium, pulmonary epithelium, renal epithelium, hepatic epithelium, pancreatic epithelium, pituitary epithelium, thyroid epithelium, adrenal epithelium	Hypoplasia secondary to damage of associated fine vasculature and connective tissue elements, with relatively less contribution by direct effects on parenchymal cells, which normally divide infrequently
Low	Muscle tissue, neuronal tissue	Hypoplasia secondary to damage of associated fine vasculature and connective tissue elements, with little contribution by direct effects on the parenchymal cells, which do not normally divide.

TABLE 8–2   ORGANS IN DECREASING ORDER OF RELATIVE RADIOSENSITIVITY BASED ON RELATIVELY DIRECT ORGAN EFFECT (PARENCHYMAL HYPOPLASIA)

Organ	Relative Radio-sensitivity	Chief Mechanisms of Parenchymal Hypoplasia
Lymphoid Organs Bone marrow (and blood) Testes Ovaries Intestines	High	Destruction of parenchymal cells, especially vegetative or differentiating intermitotic cells that are precursors to the mature parenchymal cells
Skin and other organs with epidermoid linings (cornea, oral cavity, esophagus, rectum, vagina, uterine cervix, urinary bladder, ureters, etc.)	Fairly high	Destruction of vegetative and differentiating intermitotic cells of stratified epithelium
Optic lens	Fairly high	Destruction of proliferating epithelial cells
Stomach	Fairly high	Destruction of proliferating epithelial cells
Fine vasculature	Medium	Damage of endothelium, plus some inflammatory reaction to destruction of associated, dependent, sensitive parenchymal cells
Growing cartilage	Medium	Destruction of proliferating chondroblasts, plus some damage of fine vasculature and connective tissue elements
Growing bone	Medium	Destruction of connective tissue cells and chondroblasts or osteoblasts, plus some damage of fine vasculature
Mature cartilage or bone, salivary glands, respiratory organs, kidneys, liver, pancreas, thyroid, adrenal, pituitary	Fairly low	Hypoplasia secondary to damage of fine vasculature and connective tissue elements with relatively less contribution by direct effects on parenchymal tissues
Muscles, brain, spinal cord	Low	Hypoplasia secondary to damage of fine vasculature and connective tissue elements, with little contribution by direct effects on parenchymal tissues.

and the regenerative capacity of parenchymal cells in relation to the damage to the fine vasculature and reactions of interstitial connective tissue.

8.3 KINETICS OF RADIATION PATHOLOGY OF ORGANS

The pathologic events in organs following exposure to radiation are determined in part by the radiosensitivity of parenchymal tissue relative to the radiosensitivity of the organ vasculature and stroma. Illustrated diagrammatically in Figure 8–3 are the radiopathologic events in an organ containing a rapid-renewal parenchyma consisting of VIM, DIM, and FPM cells in a stratified squamous epithelium, as found

in skin or epidermoid mucosae. Moderate doses of radiation can destroy many of the relatively radiosensitive (VIM and DIM) parenchymal cells by relatively direct mechanisms. It can also reduce production of cells which normally flow into the postmitotic (FPM) compartment, resulting in hypoplasia of the parenchyma, with relatively little mediation of this acute effect through vascular damage, circulatory impairment, and connective tissue reaction. With large doses the parenchymal compartment may be lifted or sloughed as a result of acute edema secondary to acute vascular damage. The ability of the parenchymal tissue to regenerate depends not only upon the survival of VIM parenchymal cells and their ability to proliferate but also upon the integrity of the supporting stroma

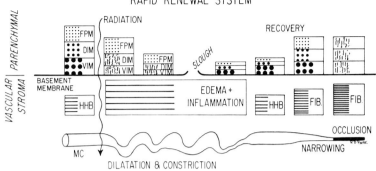

FIGURE 8–3 Kinetics of radiation pathology. Rapid renewal system (see text for further discussion). (From Rubin, P., and Casarett, G. W.: *Clinical Radiation Pathology.* Philadelphia, W. B. Saunders Co., 1968.)

and circulation. These factors permitting, the parenchyma may regenerate and the acute edema may subside, but there may be delayed parenchymal hypoplasia or even delayed frank necrosis owing to progressive vascular and interstitial fibrosis (increased histohematic connective tissue barrier (HHB) and circulatory impairment which are dose-dependent in rate of progression. Large doses may lead to rapid vascular occlusion and delayed frank necrosis. With lesser doses and rates of progression of vasculoconnective tissue changes and circulatory impairment, the parenchyma may atrophy more gradually and, when stressed, may show its limited reserve capacity to respond.

In organs with slowly renewing or non-renewing parenchyma, the parenchyma consists of reverting postmitotic (RPM) cells or fixed postmitotic (FPM) cells (Fig. 8–4). There is little or no direct acute destruction of these relatively radioresistant parenchymal cells, even with the substantial dose schemes utilized clinically. The changes in the vascular stromal compartment chiefly determine the course of radiopathologic events, both acute and delayed.

If the dose is not large enough to destroy parenchyma acutely through severe acute damage of circulation, the parenchyma is affected as a consequence of more slowly progressive vascular and interstitial fibrosis (HHB) and compromise of the microcirculation.

8.4 CLINICAL EVENTS

The sequence of clinical events after the initiation of radiation therapy will be considered in terms of four successive periods of time of arbitrary length, as follows: acute clinical period (first six months); subacute clinical period (second six months); chronic clinical period (second through fifth years); and late clinical period (after five years).

The diagrams in Figures 8–5 and 8–6 illustrate generally, with respect to these clinical periods, the waxing and waning (vertically) of organ damage with time

FIGURE 8–4 Kinetics of radiation pathology. Slow renewal system (see text for further discussion). (From Rubin, P., and Casarett, G. W.: *Clinical Radiation Pathology.* Philadelphia, W. B. Saunders Co., 1968.)

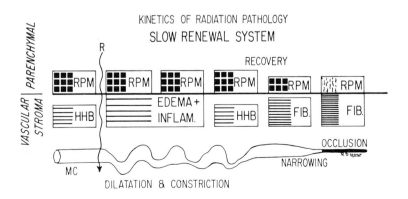

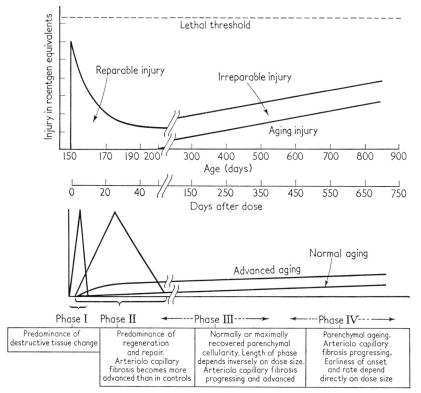

FIGURE 8–5 Diagram of the course of radiation injury and recovery and the progression of residual damage and nonradiation damage (aging and pathology). Time scale for the rat. (From Casarett, G. W.: Concept and Criteria of Radiologic Aging. *In* Harris, R. J. C. (ed.): *Cellular Basis Aetiology of Late Somatic Effects of Ionizing Radiation.* New York, Academic Press, 1963.)

(horizontally) in the sequence of acute damage, recovery from acute damage, and persistence or progression of residual damage. The upper lines depict radiation damage of different degrees. The bottom line indicates the accumulation of organ damage with time or "aging," as a result of causes other than the radiation in question, that may be additive to radiation damage in effect or consequence. The rising arrows (Fig. 8–6) indicate the precipitation of damage from subclinical or clinical levels to clinically significant or even lethal levels, as a result of complications such as trauma or infection or as a result of deterioration of the vasculature and failure of the blood circulation. No precise values or relationships are intended for the slopes or shapes of the graph lines.

A. Acute Clinical Period
(Fig. 8–6)

The accumulation of acute organ damage (histopathologic Phase I) during the first

part of this period, i.e., during the course of the fractionated radiation treatment, is depicted on the graph by the sharp initial rise in the radiation damage. Although recovery processes are operating between radiation exposures, the destructive processes predominate during the course of radiotherapy. The steepness of the radiation damage curve depends upon the relative radiosensitivity of the organ, the dose, and the schedule of fractionation. The recovery from acute organ damage (histopathologic Phase II) after the cessation of the course of radiotherapy is depicted by the gradual decline in the radiation damage after the peak of acute damage. The steepness of the recovery curve is usually greater with lesser degrees of acute radiation damage and complicating factors.

Whether or not the radiation damage of an organ is sufficient to reach levels of clinical significance or to exceed tolerance limits and cause death in the acute clinical period depends upon the particular func-

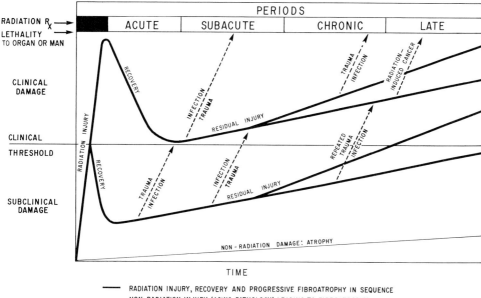

FIGURE 8–6 This diagram illustrates generally, with respect to clinical periods, the waxing and waning (vertically) of organ damage with time (horizontally) in the sequence of acute damage, recovery from acute damage, and persistence or progression of residual damage. The heavy continuous lines depict radiation damage of different degrees or after radiation doses of different size. The lighter continuous line indicates the accumulation of organ damage with time or "aging," as a result of causes other than the radiation in question, that may be additive to radiation damage in its effect or consequence. The rising broken arrows indicate precipitation of damage from subclinical or clinical levels to clinically significant or even lethal levels, as a result of complications such as trauma or infection or of deterioration of the vasculature and failure of blood circulation. No precise values or relationships are intended for the slopes or shapes of the graph lines. (From Rubin, P., and Casarett, G. W.: *Clinical Radiation Pathology.* Philadelphia, W. B. Saunders Co., 1968.)

tion of the organ, the relative radiosensitivity of the organ, the volume irradiated, the dose, the schedule of fractionation, and the occurrence or absence of complicating factors. In the case of some organs, with certain schedules of radiotherapy, the first part of the acute clinical period or even the whole of this period may be clinically silent, with clinically significant changes appearing for the first time, if at all, in later clinical periods as a result of deterioration of the vasculature and occurrence of complications.

B. Subacute Clinical Period

In the radiation damage graphs in Figure 8–6, the leveling of the slope or the plateau of the recovery portions of the curves above the threshold or "aging" damage levels during the subacute clinical period depicts the end of recovery from acute damage (end of histopathologic Phase II) or the per-

sistence or early progression of permanent residual damage (histopathologic Phase III). The histopathologic radiation damage underlying clinically significant problems that arise during the subacute clinical period, with or without added complications, are therefore subacute or chronic in character, with deterioration of the vasculature and impaired circulation playing an important role.

C. Chronic Clinical Period

In the radiation damage graphs in Figure 8–6, the gradually rising lines depict an increase in degree of chronic organ damage. This occurs by means of the progression of permanent residual radiation damage, the addition of aging damage (histopathologic Phases III and IV), or both. The clinically significant problems arising during this clinical period are usually the result of the chronic deterioration of the organ's vasculature and circulation, substantial increase in the histohematic connective tissue barrier, secondary degeneration of dependent parenchyma, and a reduction in resistance to complicating factors such as infection, trauma, or functional stress.

D. Late Clinical Period

The histopathologic and clinical developments during this clinical period are essentially similar to those described for the chronic clinical period, except for the slower progression of permanent residual radiation damage and a greater dependence upon the addition of the damage of aging. Radiation carcinogenesis can be manifested during this period and is usually preceded by some manifestation of chronic radiation damage.

8.5 CLINICAL-PATHOLOGIC COURSES IN SPECIFIC ORGANS

A. Skin

In Figure 8–7, the epidermis covering the dermis, and the proliferating epithelium of hair follicles and sebaceous glands within the dermis, are rapidly renewing cell systems.

To many patients and physicians, skin reactions following irradiation are synonymous with radiation therapy since they are the visible part of the reaction. There is no sensation as a course of irradiation proceeds, but when a critical dose level is reached, after a latent period of two to three weeks, there is a sequence of alterations: erythema; dry or moist desquamation; alteration of skin adnexae, such as epilation, decrease in secretions of sebaceous glands, and decrease in sweating; fol-

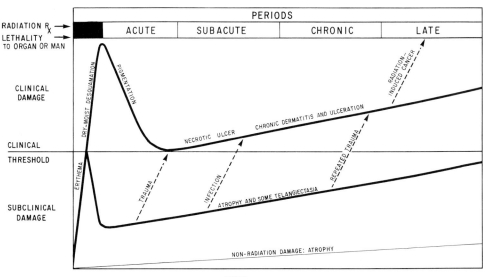

FIGURE 8–7 Clinicopathologic course: irradiated skin. When radiation damage is viewed against a background of normal aging in which atrophy occurs, two possible courses out of many are illustrated. The lower line illustrates the effect of an erythematous dose level with rapid recovery and minimal changes, an effect which rarely reaches clinical significance. Trauma or infection may unmask latent radiation change, since irradiated skin has less resistance and heals more slowly than normal skin. The top line shows the probable damage from a large dose of irradiation in which a moist desquamation occurs and in which atrophy and pigmentation are immediately evident. A necrotic ulcer may occur as a result of minimal trauma. Chronic dermatitis, telangiectasia, ulceration and, in some instances, radiation-induced cancer may follow in time. The most typical course in patients receiving therapeutic radiation lies in the zone between the two heavy lines; with supervoltage irradiation the typical course lies closer to the lower line. (From Rubin, P., and Casarett, G. W.: *Clinical Radiation Pathology.* Philadelphia W. B. Saunders Co., 1968.)

lowed by eventual recovery. The new skin is often thinner, there may be atrophy and depigmentation or increased pigmentation and telangiectasia. These changes, their severity, and the recovery from them are dose-dependent and in modern radiation therapy may be avoided by supervoltage techniques which lead to skin sparing. Severe necrosis is usually accidental and is rarely produced deliberately in practice. However, due to secondary factors such as trauma, infection, or severe cold, an ulcer may appear in an irradiated site months or years later. This is due to loss of vascular integrity, which renders the skin more vulnerable. Likewise, a fibrosing reaction may produce a heavy cicatrix under the treatment field on some occasions.

If a chronic radiodermatitis is produced, a radiation-induced skin cancer may result. This event, however, is extremely rare with current practice techniques and relates more to populations receiving repeated small doses, such as physicians doing fluoroscopy in an unprotected fashion.

The relationships between degree of skin reactions and dose, particularly when the dose is given fractionally, are as follows:

a) The biologic effect is directly proportional to the total dose delivered.

b) The biologic effect is inversely related to the time in which a given dose is delivered.

c) A fractionated dose is less effective than a single dose in producing skin erythema. The relative effectiveness of a fractionated dose is dependent on the intervals between fractions, or a greater total dose is required to produce the same end effect.

d) As the intervals between the fractions are extended, greater recovery occurs, and therefore larger dose fractions or a greater total dose is required to produce the same end effect.

e) If the fractions are delivered daily, the effects on skin are similar to those caused by continuous irradiation, within certain limits.

f) Recovery between large dose increments is slower than between smaller increments, and the damaging effect builds up more rapidly than would be predicted by some time-dose plots in current use.

Much of the dose-time data has been embodied in an isoeffect (similar effect) plot which is referred to as a Strandqvist line (Fig. 8–8). By plotting a series of observations on skin reactions of different degrees

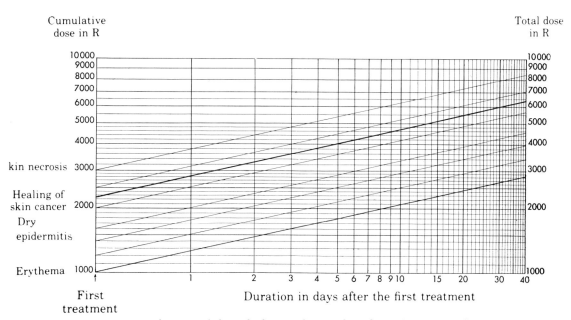

FIGURE 8–8 Fractionation diagram of the calculation of equivalent doses. (From Strandqvist, M.: Studien über die kumulative Wirkung der Röntgenstrahlen bei Fraktionierund. Acta Radiol. (suppl.). 55:1–300, 1944.)

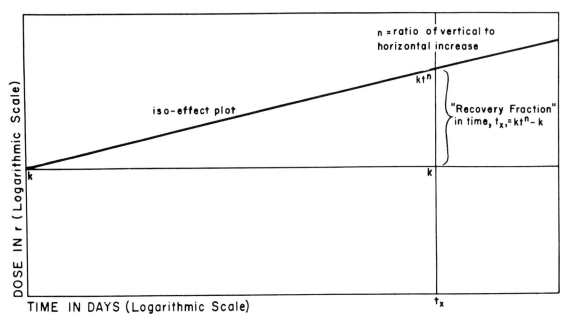

FIGURE 8–9 Recovery plot. Derivation of "recovery fraction," $kt^n - k$. Radiosensitivity connotes not only susceptibility to injury, but also the capacity to recover from injury. Symbols: k is the dose required to produce a given response when administered in a single sitting and thus is an index of susceptibility to injury; kt^n is the dose required to produce the same response when administered in t_x days. The difference between the two, $kt^n - k$ is an index of the capacity to recover from injury. (From Andrews, J. R., and Moody, J. M.: The dose-time relationship in radiotherapy. Am. J. Roentgenol., 75:590–596, 1956.)

of severity against a log-log scale relating dose and time, best fit isoeffect lines are constructed.

Mathematical analysis of time-dose plots permits formulation of a recovery factor (Fig. 8–9) from a general equation:

$$Y = kX^n \quad \text{or} \quad D = kt^n$$

where D is the total dose, t is the time in days for a specific effect to take place, k is the single dose for a specific effect, and n is the value of an exponent derived from the slope of the line. For moist desquamation reactions of skin, the following has been suggested:

$$D = 1500 \ rt^{0.32}$$

For probability of three per cent necrosis for smaller fields,

$$D = 2700 \ rt^{0.27}$$

has been proposed. In actuality, both equations are hypothetical. The variation in k, believed to parallel the radiosensitivity of the tissue, is well recognized to vary with the end point and field size, and recovery rates are not constant. Nevertheless, this type of concept is important in quantification of radiation effects and is applicable in clinical therapeutics.

Recently (1970) a new tolerance nomogram,

$$D = k \sqrt[3]{\frac{T}{L}}$$

has been offered, where D is the cumulative dose of daily treatments in rads to produce a given reaction, T is the overall time in days (including the first treatment), L is the equivalent diameter in centimeters of the radiation field, and k is the proportionality factor referring to the dose to produce a specific reaction when administered to a field of one centimeter diameter. The k factor for three per cent necrosis for late damage appears to be 3100 rads. Applying a similar formulation suggests a k factor of 3300 rads for oral mucosa and upper respiratory tract.

B. Oral Mucosa

The sequence of radiation-induced changes in the mucosa of the upper diges-

FIGURES ILLUSTRATING THE EVOLUTION OF MUCOUS MEMBRANE AND CUTANEOUS LESIONS OF THE
NORMAL EPITHELIUM IN ROENTGEN THERAPY OF SQUAMOUS EPITHELIOMAS
OF THE HYPOPHARYNX AND LARYNX.

The Whole is Composed of Three Equal Periods of Two Weeks Each or Six Weeks.

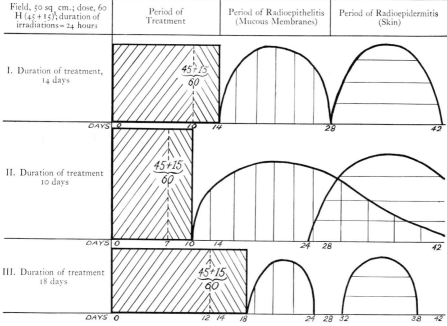

FIGURE 8-10   Physical factors. The evolution of mucous membrane and cutaneous lesions of the normal epithelium in roentgen therapy of squamous epitheliomas of the hypopharynx and larynx. The three periods are
equal—two weeks each, or a total of six weeks. (From Coutard, H.: Roentgen therapy of epitheliomas of tonsilar
regions, hypopharynx, and larynx from 1920–1926. Am. J. Roentgenol., 28:313–331, 1932.)

tive and respiratory tract is similar to that
in skin, but the radiation mucositis appears
earlier than the dermatitis.

A cyclic mucositis pattern initially identified in 1932 is the basis of the clinical
development of fractionation schedules
which would reduce the intensity of
normal mucosal reactions without sparing
the regional tumor (Fig. 8–10).

The information gathered in quantification of radiation-induced mucositis is one
of the cornerstones in modern radiotherapy.
The combined effects of irradiation and
chemotherapy are well studied in this
accessible site. The tenets of differential
effects in tumors and normal tissues have
made cancers of upper passageways an
excellent target group for such study. One
of the techniques for assessment of radiopathologic effects—exfoliative cytology—
has been applied to gain prognostication of
tumor response. The pattern of cytologic
vacuolization, enlargement of cell and

nucleus, and occurrence of double nuclei
appears within two weeks of irradiation at
the 1000- to 2000-rad level. The value of
cytologic changes has not proven itself in
field testing in selecting the favorable
responders from the unfavorable tumor
responders.

C. Alimentary Tract (Figs. 8–11, 8–12, 8–13)

The onset of acute esophagitis, gastritis,
enteritis, colitis, and proctitis occurs between one and three weeks following irradiation, depending on a variety of factors
of which organ volume and depth dose are
most critical. The initial manifestations
are those of an acute dysfunction similar to
that from other inflammatory causes.

In clinical dose prescriptions, although
substantial histologic recovery from acute
effects may occur, some measurable physiologic parameters can be seen to remain

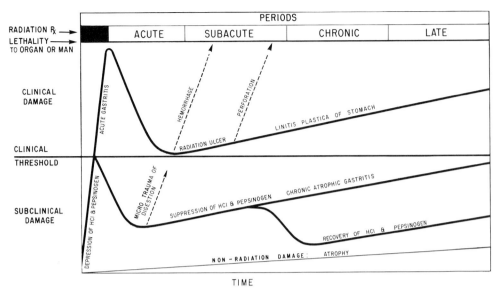

RADIATION INJURY, RECOVERY AND PROGRESSIVE FIBROATROPHY IN SEQUENCE
NON-RADIATION INJURY (AGING, PATHOLOGY) LEADING TO FIBROATROPHY
COMPLICATIONS (INFECTION, TRAUMA, STRESS) LEADING TO CLINICAL SYMPTOMS AND SIGNS

FIGURE 8–11 The initial damage produced by irradiation of the esophageal mucosa occurs rapidly and is similar to that in the oral mucosa. At lower dose levels (lower line) of 1000 to 2000 R, the mucosal damage, from which there is rapid recovery, may result in subtle changes which rarely prove to be clinically significant. In some cases, the addition of the microtrauma of swallowing, particularly of irritating foods or of foods at the extremes of temperatures, may alter the direction and slope of the lower heavy line, but rarely does it reach the clinical threshold. The upper heavy line illustrates the more dramatic sequence of events which can occur in an irradiated cancerous esophagus. The complications of hemorrhage and perforation and fistula do not occur in normal esophagi even at high doses, i.e., 6000 to 7000 R. In the chronic clinical period, stricture formation does occur as a result of large doses and represents muscle as well as mucosal damage. The zone between the two lines covers the range of possible courses most often encountered in clinical radiotherapy. (From Rubin, P., and Casarett, G. W.: *Clinical Radiation Pathology.* Philadelphia, W. B. Saunders Co., 1968, p. 173.)

	2500 r to 3400 r	3500 r to 4400 r	4500 r to 5400 r	5500 r to 6400 r
NUMBER OF CASES	15	32	61	22
PERCENT NO INJURY	80%	75%	50%	37%
TOTAL PERCENT INJURED	20%	25%	50%	63%
ULCER, WITH PERFORATION OR OBSTRUCTION			11%	18%
RADIATION ULCER	7%		15%	14%
RADIATION GASTRITIS		21%	21%	32%
RADIATION DYSPEPSIA	13%	3%	2%	

FIGURE 8–12 Physical factors: severity of stomach injury. Types of stomach injuries and their incidence in relation to tissue dose. (From Friedman, M.: Calculated risks of radiation injury of normal tissue in the treatment of cancer of the testes. Proc. 2nd Nat. Cancer Conf., *1*:390, 1952.)

NUMBER OF CASES	11	9	20	23	57
PERCENT NO INJURY	82%	89%	90%	83%	63%
TOTAL PERCENT INJURED	18%	11%	10%	17%	37%
PERFORATION					5%
PARTIAL OBSTRUCTION	9%	11%	5%	13%	25%
ASYMPTOMATIC CONSTRICTION	9%		5%	4%	7%

4000 r to 4400 r 4500 r to 4900 r 5000 r to 5400 r 5500 r to 5900 r 6000 r to 6400 r

FIGURE 8–13 Variable factors: type and incidence of colon injury in relation to dose. (From Friedman, M.: Calculated risks of radiation injury of normal tissue in the treatment of cancer of the testes. Proc. 2nd Nat. Cancer Conf., *1*:390, 1952.)

definite associated morphologic changes in the intestine were documented.

The later radiopathologic sequelae may include ulcer and stricture as clinical expressions of injury in the alimentary tract. Perforation, hemorrhage, and obstruction are serious problems. Such late injury is due to vascular damage primarily, and the obliteration of fine vessels leads to the pattern of infarctive necrosis. These lesions may be fatal and require meticulous handling of bowel at surgery to avoid introduction of new injury and further impairment of blood supply. In the stomach, ulcer is often associated with hemorrhage and perforation. In the rectum and colon it can appear clinically as a pseudocarcinoma.

The quantitative dose-time data are derived largely from the Walter Reed experience in treating testicular tumors. Dose-response data indicate that at the 5000-rad to 6000-rad level injurious effects increase in different parts of the gastrointestinal tract (Figs. 8–12, 8–13). The esophagus and rectum have been relatively more tolerant of larger doses as compared with the stomach and small intestine.

D. Major Digestive Glands

Salivary Glands. Interest in the major digestive glands has increased because of changing concepts of their vulnerability to irradiation. The salivary glands are

depressed for relatively long times. For example, the gastric mucosa in serial biopsies returns to a normal cellular appearance within one or two years after 2000 rads, while pepsin and free hydrochloric acid remain depressed. In 1965, a correlation was found between altered fat absorption and dosage level in the small bowel. In 1966, the dose-effect relationship for leakage of plasma protein in intestine as measured by PVP ^{131}I was found, and

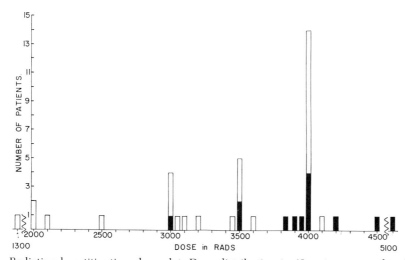

FIGURE 8–14 Radiation hepatitis: time-dose plot. Dose distribution in 40 patients treated with irradiation of the entire liver at 1300 to 5100 rads. The incidence of radiation hepatitis appears to be related to the dose of hepatic radiation given. □ = Total number of patients; ■ = radiation hepatitis. (From Ingold, J. A., et al.: Radiation hepatitis. Am. J. Roentgenol., *93*:200–208, 1965.)

known to be altered, and xerostomia is frequently a complication after fractional irradiation. Studies in 1965 identified the acute changes in elevated serum amylase and sialography due to high intense exposure. This is associated clinically with intense glandular swelling which can be attributed partly to changes in the endothelium of the fine vasculature, congestion and increased permeability, interstitial edema and partly to narrowing of excretory ducts due to the presence of such edema.

Liver. The liver, long regarded as radioresistant, has been shown to manifest acute and chronic injury with clinical dose ranges. Observations have established radiation hepatitis as a distinct clinical syndrome resulting in ascites and liver failure. The majority of specimens studied showed a typical change in the centrolobular region consisting of severe sinus congestion, hyperemia, and hemorrhage due to occlusion of small hepatic veins. Quantitative data indicate that this injurious effect begins at

between 3500 and 4500 rads, and the volume involved determines its clinical severity (Figure 8–14).

E. Urinary Structures (Fig. 8–15)

Kidney. The clinical syndromes of *radiation nephritis* have a common basis in radiation pathology. The misconception about the general radioresistance of the kidney had been perpetuated largely by omission and neglect in the radiologic literature. A series of reports in the fifties laid the foundation for present concepts of tolerance. The basic histopathogenesis involves primarily the damage of arterioles and capillaries, with subsequent important contribution by the induced hypertension, leading to arteriolonephrosclerosis. Acute radiation nephritis may be pictured as a syndrome in which the arteriolonephrosclerotic process progresses at such a rapid rate to such a marked degree that the clinical signs and symptoms of hypertension

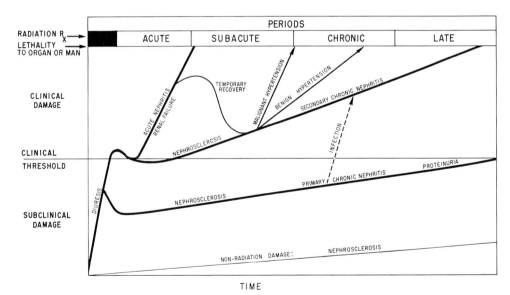

FIGURE 8–15 Clinicopathologic course in the kidney. The immediate acute period following fractionated therapeutic irradiation is silent clinically. The pathologic changes are subtle and spotty initially and are seen mainly in the vascular bed. The essential lesion is an arteriolar nephrosclerotic process which is progressive. Its rate of progression is usually determined by volume, dose, and time factors. These manifestations, depending on the rate and degree of the arteriolar nephrosclerotic process, lead to the insidious clinical onset of one or any combination of the following: acute renal failure, malignant hypertension, primary or secondary chronic nephritis, benign hypertension, proteinuria or anemia. Recovery from the acute renal failure does not alter the underlying pathologic picture, and the prognosis remains poor. (From Rubin, P., and Casarett, G. W.: *Clinical Radiation Pathology.* Philadelphia, W. B. Saunders Co., 1968.)

and cardiorenal and hemopoietic failure develop six to 12 months, sometimes earlier or later, after irradiation.

The clinical renal syndromes are manifested more specifically as acute renal shutdown, proteinuria, benign hypertension, and malignant hypertension. The course is varied, and reversibility of the acute manifestations into a more chronic course is possible. Complete recovery is only possible if the damage is unilateral and if the diseased kidney is surgically resected. The quantitative dose-response data upon which tolerance levels have been based are as follows:

a) A homogeneous dose of 2300 rads delivered to the *whole* of both kidneys may cause hypertension and renal failure.

b) The risk of renal failure may be minimized by ensuring that one-third of the volume of the kidney is outside the field or is at least irradiated with as low a dose as possible.

c) In adults treated six days each week, a dose of 2800 rads in five weeks to the *whole* of both kidneys is associated with a high risk of fatal radiation nephritis.

d) The quality of irradiation is important in that supervoltage (^{60}Co gamma) irradiation is less damaging than orthovoltage (280 kV).

Bladder. The bladder has a rapid-renewal mucosal epithelium; the effects of irradiation on this mucosa are similar to those on skin. The clinical manifestations are related to acute or chronic cystitis, ulceration, and contracture, depending on the dose and volume of tissue irradiated. Associated infection and cancer, however, account for many of the later effects and complicate the establishment of meaningful dose-response curves on clinical data. Of particular interest is the variety of irradiations utilized in bladder cancers and their late effects.

F. Gonads

Of more recent development are studies on the effect of fractionation of dose, as compared to single doses, on testes. Certain modes of fractionation of radiation doses may be much more effective in permanently damaging the spermatogenic epithelium than single doses or other modes of fractionation; i.e., complete and permanent sterility may result with lower total doses with such critical, highly efficient fractionation modes than with a single exposure or other modes of fractionation. The basis for this seems to be that the relatively radiosensitive proliferating spermatogonia are destroyed most efficiently (with a minimum of "wasted" radiation) in mitosis-linked necrosis by such critical modes of fractionation; and they draw the less radiosensitive, less frequently dividing, spermatogonial stem cells into the proliferating, more radiosensitive state to be killed efficiently in the same way by repeated dose fractions.

In the ovary, as contrasted to the testes, radiation destruction of the relatively sensitive gametogenic epithelium of developing follicles and inhibition of successful development (or delayed destruction) of primitive follicles reduce not only gamete production but also much of the production of sex hormones. Consequently, in the female, the process of radiation sterilization of the gonads may cause the production of an artificial menopause with marked secondary effects on secondary genitalia and sexual characteristics. In contrast, in the male, the separate and more dependent radioresistant interstitial cells of Leydig are spared and there is little or no secondary effect on secondary sexual apparatus and characteristics.

The tolerance doses for permanent testicular sterility are given as between 450 and 600 rads. The fact that certain critical modes of fractionation may lower this dose has been noted. The doses for ovarian sterilization depend upon the surviving number of primordial ovocytes, because there is no repopulation of stem cells as in the testes. One investigator believes that the ovarian sterilization dose is at the level of 2000 to 3000 rads, but others present convincing data for levels between 600 and 700 rads in humans.

G. Respiratory System (Fig. 8–16)

The past decade has seen a resurgence of interest in radiation reactions involving the lung. A wide variety of terms has been used to describe the effects of irradiation of pulmonary tissues, termed by various workers as radiation pulmonitis, radiation

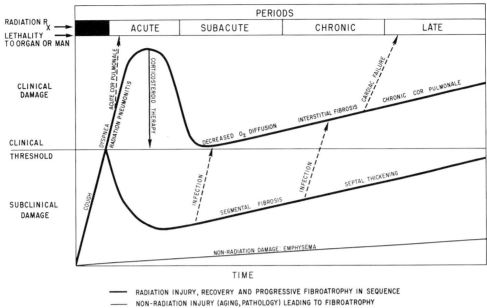

FIGURE 8-16   Clinicopathologic course: the lung. Pulmonary radiation reaction is usually manifested clinically after a course of irradiation is completed. With low doses, as depicted by the lower heavy line, pathologic changes are subtle and consist of some segmental fibrosis or septal thickening. Large doses given to more than half of the total lung volume can lead to dyspnea and in severe cases to acute cor pulmonale. Corticosteroid therapy can reverse this acute phase, but interstitial fibrosis continues, leading to altered pulmonary physiology. In the chronic period, chronic cor pulmonale and cardiac failure may occur eventually. (From Rubin, P., and Casarett, G. W.: *Clinical Radiation Pathology.* Philadelphia, W. B. Saunders Co., 1968.)

pleuropneumonitis, radiation reaction in the lung, radiation pulmonary changes, radiation lung fibrosis, or scarring. For simplicity, the term radiation pneumonitis is advocated, and this should be distinguished in a pathologic sense from the inflammatory pneumonitis characterized by acute inflammatory cell infiltration of the septa or alveoli. In a radiation pneumonitis, the first phase of the reaction is predominantly one of plasmatic exudation into alveolar walls and alveoli due to the changes in the endothelium of fine vasculature. Associated and subsequent histopathologic changes in the lung include hyperemia and vascular congestion; lymphangiectasis; leakage of red cells and diapedesis of some hemogenous polymorphonuclear leukocytes in alveolar spaces; increases in phagocytic cells; increases in mucous secretion by bronchial epithelium and small degrees of degenerative changes in small numbers of alveolar and bronchial epithelial cells; and eventually the development of chronic inflammation, fibroblastic activity, and progressive fibrosis. On a pathologic basis,

radiation pneumonitis cannot be arbitrarily and sharply divided into an acute or exudative and a chronic or fibrotic period, since one may merge subtly into or with the other or partial or complete resolution may occur, depending upon the radiologic and clinical factors involved.

The same is true of the clinical syndromes, which are not clear-cut and cover the entire spectrum, reflecting the pathologic changes. If the volume of lung included in the treatment fields is small, the acute phase can be asymptomatic, and only in the later stages will fibrosis be detected on chest films.

If the whole of both lungs is included in the treatment field, however, an acute decompensation with pulmonary edema can produce a fatal, acute cor pulmonale. The basic lesion is a capillary-alveolar block. This has been studied in the laboratory as well as clinically. Several workers present correlative laboratory and clinical experiences in which an attempt has been made to study serially the pathophysiologic changes. The most sensitive parameters are the oxygen content and oxygen tension of arterial blood, particularly after exercise, and the diffusing capacity for carbon monoxide. Lung volume is measured by total lung capacity, vital capacity, and reduced residual volume; the ventilation parameters, such as respiratory volume, frequency, and total ventilation per minute, likewise are altered once the process is manifest.

Quantitative dose response data are being developed, and the importance of volume has been emphasized in a number of studies. When the whole of both lungs is included in the treatment field, even at daily dose rates of 150 rads, decompensation is expected after doses between 2500 and 3000 rads. When a portion of the lung is included in the treatment field and the end point is the production of lung fibrosis, varying degrees of injury are recorded at the 4000-rad level. Using similar techniques in breast carcinoma patients, the degree of pleuropneumonitis in the supraclavicular axillary field has been determined. With 250-kV X-rays there was a 44 per cent incidence of pleural pulmonary reactions in contrast to 20 per cent with Cobalt-60 gamma irradiation. The reasons for this difference in effect need further clarification. There is an increase in transmission through the lung tissue with supervoltage irradiation which, unless accounted for, can give false lower dose values.

Recent work using human and experimental mouse data, has shown correlations for single dose and fractional dose mouse data which corroborate the slope of clinical dose-response curves (Fig. 8–17). The corroboration which was developed for lung deserves similar exploration in other organs and sites. The tolerance doses that were developed for exposure of both lobes of lungs are 2650 rads for a five per cent injurious effect and 3050 rads for a 50 per cent injurious effect. This confirms other studies in terms of tolerance dose levels.

H. Cardiovascular System

A reappraisal of the problem of heart tolerance to irradiation has been undertaken by a number of investigators in the past decade. The observation that the heart was extremely resistant to irradiation, which was developed in human and animal studies in the twenties, thirties, and forties is open to re-examination. Early experiments (1941), using rats, set the clinician to believe that the heart can withstand large doses. At the level of 7500 rads for one month, minimal histopathologic changes were noted. Even larger doses, up to 10,000 rads, produced no myocardial changes, and at 20,000 rads there were no pericardial changes. Clinical studies in humans demonstrated that EKG changes in T waves were due to locational organizational factors of heart, lung, diaphragm, and chest wall. More recent studies have indicated that in patients receiving chest irradiation, such as for Hodgkin's disease and breast cancer, transient EKG changes are noted, but most of these are reversible and of no later significance.

Later reports (1967) have challenged the view that the heart is radioresistant. Radiation-induced heart disease appeared more than a year after irradiation in 3.4 per cent of patients irradiated prophylactically following mastectomy for breast carcinoma

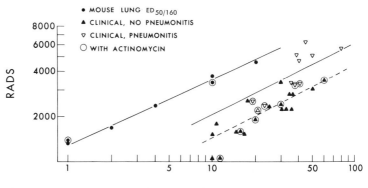

FIGURE 8–17 Parallel slope of line with single doses and fractionated doses in the development of radiation pneumonitis. (From Philips, T. [presented at the Symposium on Clinical Radiation Pathology]. In *Frontiers of Radiation Therapy and Oncology*, vol. 7. White Plains, N.Y., Albert J. Phiebig, in press.)

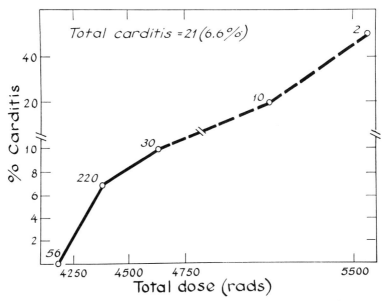

FIGURE 8–18 Graphic representation of the number of radiation-induced heart disease in patients treated after a year. The most common syndrome was radiation pericarditis; also noted were myocardial lesions and pancarditis. (From Stewart, J. R., and Fajardo, L. F.: Dose response in human and experimental radiation induced heart disease. Application of the nominal standard dose (NSD) concept. Radiology, 99:403–408, 1971.)

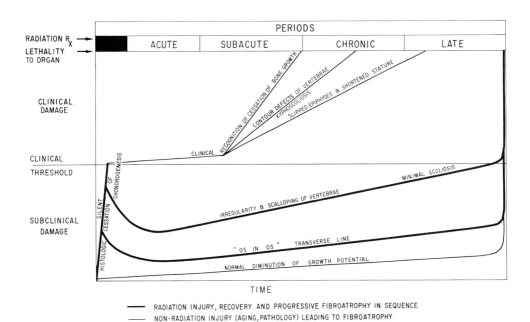

FIGURE 8–19 Clinicopathologic course: growing bone and cartilage. The cessation of chondrogenesis can occur with moderate doses. Although the acute clinical period is silent and clinical manifestations are delayed, there is *no* silent period in a histopathologic sense. The roentgenographic changes can be detected in the latter part of the acute period or early in the subacute period. Depending upon the dose delivered and the age of the patient, changes can range from transverse lines indicative of temporary cessation of bone growth to contour abnormalities suggestive of achondroplasia. The vertebral effects are well appreciated, since axilla irradiation is common for childhood abdominal tumors such as Wilms' tumor and neuroblastoma. Since bone formation is secondary to chondrogenesis in endochondral bone production, the effect is magnified in time in comparison with normal growth parameters. (From Rubin, P., and Casarett, G. W.: *Clinical Radiation Pathology.* Philadelphia, W. B. Saunders Co., 1968.)

and in 5.8 per cent of patients irradiated for malignant lymphoma. The most common syndrome was that of radiation pericarditis; also noted were myocardial lesions and pancarditis. The new data set tolerance doses for fractionated irradiation at 4300 rads for the five per cent injurious level and approximately 6000 rads for the 50 per cent injurious level when the entire heart is included in the treatment field (Fig. 8–18).

I. Growing Cartilage and Bone

The relative radiosensitivity of growing cartilage (Fig. 8–19) was appreciated by investigators shortly after pathologic effects of irradiation on tissues were first noted. This organ system has been selected for studying various effects of irradiation because of the ease of measurement. A number of laboratory investigations were done in the forties and fifties and correlated with the clinical findings. The important clinical site which has been studied has been that of the axial skeleton because of the relative

frequency of irradiation for abdominal tumors in childhood.

The quantitative dose-time data that are available, therefore, related to the changes in the skeletal vertebral system. Certain types of vertebral changes were dose-dependent (Fig. 8–20) and were of three varieties:

a) Horizontal transverse lines or an os-in-os configuration within vertebrae.
b) An irregularity or scalloping of the vertebral plates associated with the loss of axial height, through more pronounced trabeculation, and severe changes in groove pattern.
c) Gross contour abnormalities as seen in contour dysplasias.

The major clinical problem was the development of scoliosis which, in most instances as the child grew, was not of a progressive nature.

There are no clinical manifestations during the acute period despite the severe histopathologic alterations that are taking place. Changes induced in growing car-

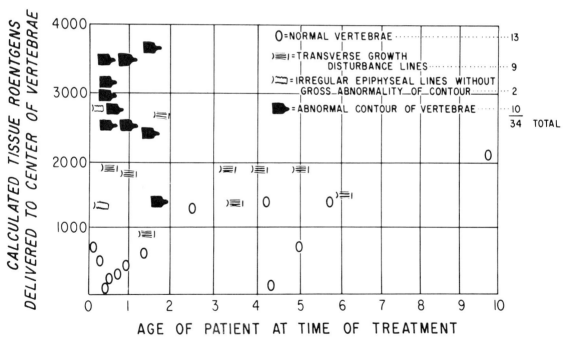

FIGURE 8–20 Variable factors: age-dose relationship. Graphic presentation of the status of 34 patients still living. Each point represents a patient and is placed according to his age at the time of treatment (abscissa) and the tissue roentgens delivered to the center of the vertebra (ordinate). The roentgenographic findings on follow-up examination, two years and seven months to 13 years after irradiation, are shown by schematic drawings. Note that the 12 patients showing no detectable abnormality on follow-up (if we allow for some change with advancing age) lie predominantly in the lower dosage range. The 10 patients showing the severest change lie in the high dosage area and in the lower age level at the time of treatment. (From Neuhauser, E. B., Wittenborg, M. H., Bergman, C. Z., and Cohen, J.: Irradiation effects of roentgen therapy on growing spine. Radiology, 59:637–650, 1952.)

tilage are eventually reflected, however, in disordered bone growth. The selective irradiation of the various sites in long bones results in a variety of abnormalities in bone modeling. Selective effects also can be produced by the administration of bone-seeking radioisotopes which concentrate in different segments of the bone, resulting again in various types of abnormalities in growth and development.

J. Mature Cartilage and Bone

Radionecrosis of mature bone and hyaline cartilage is due to a combination of factors: irradiation, infection, and trauma. That is, radiation effects act to render these tissues more susceptible to damage by other noxious agents and conditions. A number of sites are particularly notable in this respect because of the inclusion of these sites in treatment. Thus, osteonecrosis of the mandible, dental caries, contour necrosis of laryngeal cartilage, osteonecrosis of the femoral head, fractures of ribs, and skull changes have not been uncommon complications of radiation therapy.

The bulk of the evidence indicates that the principal factor in radiation damage to mature bone and cartilage is the damage of the fine vasculature supplying the structures, with degeneration and loss of dependent parenchymal cells being secondary to interference with blood supply and with changes in matrix being secondary to either or both of these changes. In the case of mature bone, the damage to the intraosseous vasculature, with occlusion of the fine vasculature and canaliculae and secondary loss of osteocytes, and the damage to periosteal vasculature and endosteal vasculature are of prime importance in the pathogenesis of radiation-induced damage. In the case of mature cartilage, which does not contain fine vasculature within it and which is regenerated by connective tissue cells from the surrounding perichondrium, the radiation damage to the surrounding fine vasculature and connective tissue (perichondritis) is of prime importance in the development of radiation damage.

Quantitative time-dose information is based upon a blend of clinical experience and laboratory investigation. Results from these efforts indicate that dose levels above 6000 rads are required before such compli-

cations are seen. Pertinent to the subject of bone and cartilage observation, fractures do not heal following moderate courses of irradiation to the 2000-rad level. The reason for the interference with callus formation is that the anchoring callus forms through an endochondral pathway which is particularly susceptible to radiation. Pinning of long bones is essential, therefore, to insure healing of pathologic fractures where irradiation is involved.

K. Central Nervous System

The assumption that the central nervous system is resistant to radiation has never been established. As reports of late necrosis of the central nervous system appear in the clinical literature, experimental investigations of this problem have increased. Most experimental studies have employed single radiation exposures in animals, but direct extrapolation in human radiotherapeutic situations remains limited. To define brain tolerance is vital, and efforts to construct time-dose isoeffect plots have been exerted by some critical observers. The information remains sparse because a number of criteria must be met before such information can be accurately recorded. These include precise dosimetry, irradiation of normal brain to a variety of dose levels, and pathologic proof that the complication is indeed a radiation complication. Since most patients irradiated to the brain region are those with brain tumors, many of whom have been operated upon, the required information is very difficult to obtain.

The clinical course of an irradiated patient is likewise difficult to evaluate because of the circumstances—namely, brain tumor. Although radiation edema has been postulated to occur when symptoms worsen during the early part of the course of treatment, there is no unequivocal evidence to substantiate this. Single doses from 2000 to 5000 rads have produced no significant change in the water content of brain tissue at four to 10 days after irradiation. The later changes which occur in the subacute and chronic clinical periods often present as a recapitulation of the initial symptoms related to the brain tumor. Since the radiation dose is concentrated on this region, there is a differential diagnostic problem as to whether the tumor is recurring or the symptoms and signs are due to irradiation complications. The information with regard to radiation myelitis is usually more meaningful because the normal spinal cord has been included in treatment fields about lesions in the head, neck, and thoracic area. Radiation myelitis should be suspected if motor and sensory signs and symptoms occur which are referable to a segment of the spinal cord which has been included in treatment fields. In addition, the diagnosis is substantiated if the cerebrospinal fluid is normal (in all respects, save for the possible presence of excess protein) and radiographs of the spine are normal.

Although there is considerable contradiction and disagreement in the results and interpretation in studies of the response of the nervous system to irradiation, especially in respect to sequence of events and primary and secondary roles of various changes in the pathogenesis of radionecrosis of tissue, certain conclusions are warranted. Semantic imprecision also serves to perpetuate such disagreements. For example, the disagreement concerning relative roles of vascular damage and direct nerve cell damage in the radionecrosis of nerve tissue is usually stated in very general terms but actually is often based upon limited concepts of vascular damage and its significance. Arguments against primary involve-

ment of vascular damage usually take into account the histologic relationship of only the obvious occlusive changes in the larger vessels to the distribution of radionecrosis, with little significance being given to other and earlier more subtle and widespread vascular changes and their prominent consequences in the form of impaired circulation, edema, and inflammation. In brief, the radiopathologic observations and experiments strongly support the contention that radiation-induced vascular damage is primary to parenchymal damage and may cause most of the parenchymal damage involved in the development of radionecrosis of nervous tissue.

The quantitative dose-response information, however limited, is mentioned in the literature; the details of mechanisms by which vascular damage may cause such lesions at different times at different dose levels vary and add to the confusion. The early and persistent changes in the capillaries and the blood-brain barrier, with associated increase in resistance to blood flow, erythrocyte aggregation, stasis, edema, inflammation, microthrombi, and ischemia, may lead to parenchymal cell damage; they may eventually lead to frank necrotic lesions, as well as to the more slowly developing occlusive lesions in larger blood vessels, but with different time intervals. The similarity of slope of the time-dose relation-

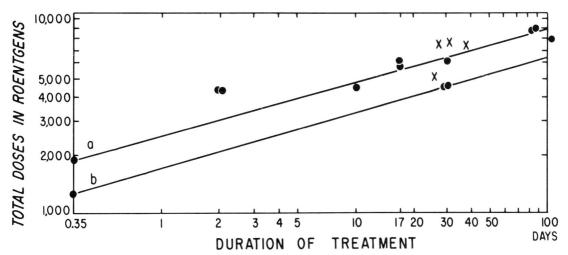

FIGURE 8-21 Physical factors. Time-dose: brain. In this modified Strandqvist diagram, the dots denote 13 cases from the literature; the crosses, four cases reported by Lindgren. The slope of the two lines is 0.26. The dosage level at line *a* involves a great risk of cerebral necrosis. Line *b* shows the lowest dosage level producing necrosis in brain tissue. (From Lindgren, M.: On tolerance of brain tissue and sensitivity of brain tumors to irradiation. Acta Radiol. (suppl.), *170*:1–73, 1958.)

ship (Fig. 8–21) for delayed radiolesions in brain and skin of rabbits led to the conclusion that a common substrate for these types of injuries exists. Judging from morphologic changes, the conclusion was that the vascular elements were the ones at risk for the development of this lesion. Furthermore, the slopes of the time-dose curves should be the same for tolerance of the skin and brain of other mammals, including man.

L. Eye

The organs of special sense, particularly the eye, have been intensively studied since the advent of medical radiation at the turn of the century. There has been much concern with radiation cataractogenesis, and this is one of the most thoroughly explored phenomena with regard to radio-

pathologic mechanisms and dose-response information. Biochemical studies, with attention to enzyme systems and protection, have also been done.

The lens is an interesting system in that there is no cell removal and therefore the injured cells form the cataract. The most vulnerable cells are the proliferating anterior epithelial cells located near the equator of the lens. Normally, the cells migrate posteriorly and become translucent, forming the posterior surface of the lens. The production of a radiation cataract by defective cells and fibers occurs first, therefore, at the posterior surface of the lens as a donut-shaped lesion.

When duration of treatment is between three weeks and three months, the minimal dose to induce cataract formation is 400 rads, and at levels beyond 1200 rads lenticu-

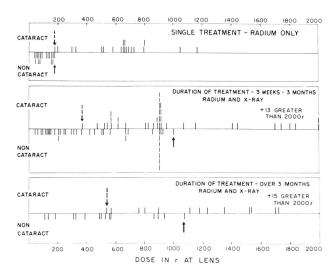

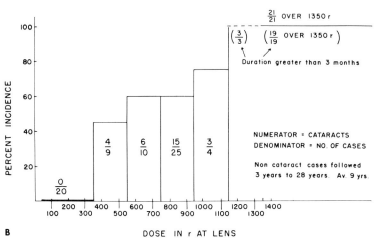

FIGURE 8–22 Dose in r at lens of the eye. Variable factors: time-dose. Incidence of cataracts following x- and gamma irradiation. A, Doses of x- or gamma radiation to the lens in 97 cases of radiation cataract and 70 cases without lens opacities. B, Incidence of cataracts. The treatment period was three weeks to three months. (From Merriam, G. R., Jr., and Focht, E. F.: Radiation dose to the lens in treatment of tumors of the eye and adjacent structures. Possibilities of cataract formation. Radiology, *71*:357, 1958.)

lar opacities are almost certain to occur (Fig. 8–22). Cataracts do not as a rule become progressive until the dose exceeds a level of 1350 rads. From the clinical data recorded to date, the child at the age of one year has the same radioresponsiveness as the adult.

In contrast to the eye, the ear has not been as intensively studied.

M. The Endocrine Glands

In general, because of the relative resistance of the parenchymal cells of the mature pituitary, thyroid, parathyroid, and adrenal glands to the direct cytocidal actions of radiation, the early and late lesions caused by radiation in these glands are largely the result of damage to the fine vasculature, with impairment of circulation and secondary degeneration of dependent parenchymal cells. In this respect, the sinusoidal vasculature of some of the endocrine glands (pituitary and adrenal) might conceivably offer some protection. The interpretation of the direct effects of radiation on endocrine glands is made difficult by the complex functional interrelationships of these glands among themselves and with other organs and tissues. Careful distinction must be made between the changes in the gland cells that reflect functional responses to other glands and tissues and those changes in cells that are the results of radiation damage to cells. Therefore, the radiation effects in endocrine glands are best observed—although they are not completely uncomplicated by interglandular influences—under conditions of radiation localized to the individual glands. This requirement for selective endocrine gland irradiation has been met with proton beam irradiation or Yttrium-90 implantation of the pituitary gland and radioiodine treatment of the thyroid gland. Considerable literature has developed describing the radiation pathophysiology involved in these organ systems. The thyroid gland in particular is of interest because of the possible role of auto-immune mechanisms, i.e., secondary antigen and antibody formation producing late radiopathologic changes. The adrenal gland has not been studied in this fashion; such studies are further complicated by the fact that radiation itself is a "stress" causing indirect effects.

N. Hemopoietic Tissues and Blood

The sequence of changes in the number of circulating blood cells of various kinds after irradiation is largely a reflection of the effects of irradiation on the radiosensitive precursor cells in the hemopoietic tissues, the kinetics of hemopoietic cell maturation, and the survival times of blood cells in the circulation. Although much of the literature deals with whole-body irradiation, of particular concern in clinical radiation therapy are the effects of segmental irradiation upon bone marrow regeneration. After whole-body exposure, a depression in leukocytes, particularly the lymphocytic fraction, occurs first. This is followed by a reduction in granulocytes, then thrombocytes, and lastly erythrocytes (Fig. 8–23A). In contrast to the changes noted in the circulating blood cells, the effects on stem cells in the marrow population differ. The initial reduction is in the erythroid followed by a reduction in cells of the granulocytic series.

Four general categories of clinical course and prognosis after single whole-body doses or irradiation are: more than 600 rads, survival virtually impossible; 200 to 600 rads, survival possible; under 200 rads, survival probable; less than 100 rads, survival virtually certain.

With single doses in the range of 600 or more rads to the whole body, survival is virtually impossible even with excellent medical care and application of known therapeutic measures. After doses of 200 to 600 rads, severe hemopoietic syndromes may develop, but recovery may occur and survival is possible if appropriate medical care is provided for developing signs and symptoms.

Segmental irradiation of the bone marrow with relatively large doses does not cause bone marrow degeneration. As an example, with doses beyond 3000 rads, patients with breast cancer seem to show little to no evidence of bone marrow degeneration from periods of two to three months up to 18 months.

There is renewed interest in irradiation of lymph nodes and lymphoid tissue, particularly with the introduction of total lymph nodal irradiation; whole-body doses of 600 rads in rats lead to lymphocytic depletion in lymph nodes. By contrast, localized irradiation of lymphoid tissue up

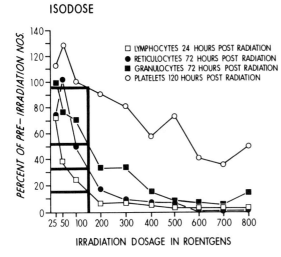

ISODOSE

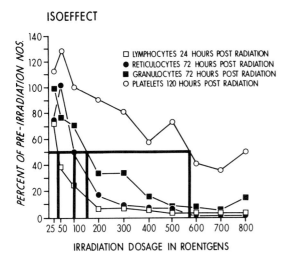

ISOEFFECT

FIGURE 8-23 Radiation sensitivity is best defined as a dose response curve in which a range of effects and doses are documented, as in this response of different elements of blood to increasing doses of total body irradiation. Radiosensitivity of different tissues or cells can be expressed in either of two ways: *A*, For a similar dose, a range of response, often cell death, is recorded. For 150 rads, the per cent of depression of the pre-irradiation level of the blood element provides an ordering of radiosensitivity: lymphocytes, reticulocytes, granulocytes, and platelets. *B*, For a similar effect, a range of doses is recorded, and these in turn express an order of radiosensitivity. For a 50 per cent reduction to pre-treatment level counts, the blood elements in this order require greater doses: lymphocytes (40 R), reticulocytes (100 R), granulocytes (150 R), and platelets (575 R). (From Rubin, P., and Casarett, G. W.: *Clinical Radiation Pathology.* Philadelphia, W. B. Saunders Co., 1968.)

to doses of 3000 rads leads to temporary depletion and rapid recovery of the lymphocytic population after a week. The awareness of the regional lymph nodal role in providing immunity is serving as a stimulus to investigators to determine the effects of modest doses on lymph node barrier function and cellular immune functions.

8.6 THE TOLERANCE DOSE

After seven decades of radiotherapeutic practice, precise knowledge of tumoricidal doses and of tolerance of normal tissues in various radiation regimens is lacking. More accurate laboratory as well as clinical definition in reporting radiation-induced physiologic and pathologic changes is imperative. Among clinicians, there is still an all too prevalent black and white concept of radiation injury. The attitude of many physicians and pathologists seems to be that irradiation causes all the complications in cancer patients receiving radiation therapy. At the other extreme, many therapeutic radiologists assume that most organs are safely within the tolerance levels of their dose schedules. The importance of time-dose-volume factors in radiation therapy is well recognized but has been inadequately documented. As supervoltage irradiation now allows the delivery of greater depth doses, the so-called radioresistant structures are recognized as vulnerable. With longer follow-up studies of irradiated patients cured of cancer, the importance of time in the development of radiation-induced lesions has become more apparent.

The radiation therapist is admittedly treating to "tolerance" doses rather than to specific "tumoricidal" doses. The risks are poorly defined, and therapeutic ratios remain largely abstractions rather than concrete estimates. The amount of radiation damage that is acceptable for the purpose of curing a cancer remains one of personal philosophy as long as the overlapping zones of normal tissue tolerance and tumor curability are inadequately defined.

To define radiation sensitivity and radiation resistance, the investigator needs to follow clear lines of study and expression. The term "radiation sensitivity" can best be expressed as a dose response curve. Either a range of doses is utilized to study an isoeffect or an isodose is used to elicit a range of effects in a tissue (Fig. 8–23). A dilemma is presented by the need to utilize appropriate indices in coping with the spectrum of biologic systems, the variety of physiologic and pathologic processes in different organs, the differences in cell kinetics of parenchymal cell populations, and the recovery (repair and regeneration) capacities of systems in vivo.

Before approaching the problem in the laboratory, all of the factors involved in a radiation response must be defined. There is an assortment of biologic and physical variables. Precise statement of the biologic endpoint in the study is critical to the definition of radiation sensitivity. Although lethality is frequently used, the end point is often a point in the course of a process, such as alterations in physiologic function, enzyme production, or cell proliferation. The extent to which the parameters are quantifiable and relevant to clinical problems influences the usefulness of experimental studies in radiation pathology as related to therapeutics.

The clearness and convenience of single dose studies in animals is obvious. However, the practical yield of such studies alone is limited in its application to clinical work. Most radiation pathology studies are unfortunately of this genre and are short-term as well. To move beyond single dose study means juggling total dose, total time, fractional dose, fractional numbers, fractional interval, and interrupted versus continuous administration into a potpourri of time-dose data in which it is impossible to keep all factors but one fixed. Usually, only a few factors are kept constant while more than one are varied, and some factors are ignored for reasons of expedience or relative unimportance.

Borrowing such terms as the D_0 or D_Q of mammalian cell biology and grafting them onto clinical settings have resulted in few takes. Such information is not known for most normal tissue studied in laboratory animals and is lacking for the more complex human situation. Its application to tumors is likewise debatable unless one can devise systems correlating the in vitro quantitative work with the in vivo studies. The applications of such information to normal tissue tolerance in vivo remains unclear and uncharted.

Few clinical definitions of radiation sensitivity cannot be challenged. An understanding of a biologic index and its translation into clinical terms is at issue. Radiation sensitivity, to the clinician, means the difference in the same radiation response to a given dose or range of doses in different tissues and organs. The response referred to is usually a severe complication, such as marked impairment or necrosis, producing objective and subjective symptoms and signs. If the organ is vital, lethality can result. The minimal reaction can also be scored. The difficulty resides in the incongruity of the responses of specific cell types, specific tissues, and various organs with different tissues. The response must also be scored in time after irradiation. Thus, a rapid-renewal system, such as the urinary bladder epithelium, may be severely damaged after 4000 to 6000 rads in six weeks at the completion of this course of irradiation, whereas the kidney epithelium irradiated to the same dose level may show few measurable alterations at that time. However, six to 12 months later the bladder may be functioning normally, but the renal tissue may be completely and irreversibly atrophied if its entire volume was irradiated.

A number of expressions of tolerance have evolved, but new definitions are required. The quantitative aspects of the radiation pathologic dose-effect relationships have recently been expressed in the Nominal Standard Dose (NSD), a System of Quantitative Correlation of Treatment Schedules (SQCTS), and equivalent dose nomograms.

The concept herein advocated is that of the tolerance dose. This concept involves a modification of the historical expression used for describing the lethality of animals exposed to irradiation, the mean lethal dose or $LD_{50/30}$. The tolerance dose is an attempt to express the minimal and maximal injurious dose *acceptable* to the clinician in the different clinical settings described previously. This requires the assignment of an arbitrary but useful percentage of complications. A five per cent severe complication rate up to five years after therapy could be assigned as the minimal level and a 50 per cent severe complication rate as the maximal level. In favorable circumstances the radiation therapist would not be willing to exceed the minimal rate, and in unfavorable conditions he would be unwilling to exceed the maximal.

The minimal tolerance dose is defined as the $TD_{5/5}$—the dose which, when applied to a given population of patients under a standard set of treatment condi-

TABLE 8–3   RADIATION TOLERANCE DOSES

Organ*	Injury at 5 Years	1–5% (TD$_{5/5}$)	25–50% (TD$_{50/5}$)	Volume or Length
Skin	Ulcer, severe fibrosis	5500	7000	100 cm³
Oral Mucosa	Ulcer, severe fibrosis	6000	7500	50 cm³
Esophagus	Ulcer, stricture	6000	7500	75 cm³
Stomach	Ulcer, perforation	4500	5000	100 cm³
Intestine	Ulcer, stricture	4500	6500	100 cm³
Colon	Ulcer, stricture	4500	6500	100 cm³
Rectum	Ulcer, stricture	5500	8000	100 cm³
Salivary	Xerostomia	5000	7000	50 cm³
Liver	Liver failure, ascites	3500	4500	Whole
Kidney	Nephrosclerosis	2300	2800	Whole
Bladder	Ulcer, contracture	6000	8000	Whole
Ureters	Stricture, obstruction	7500	10,000	5–10 cm
Testes	Permanent sterilization	500–1500	2000	Whole
Ovary	Permanent sterilization	200–300	625–1200	Whole
Uterus	Necrosis, perforation	>10,000	>20,000	Whole
Vagina	Ulcer, fistula	9000	>10,000	5 cm
Breast (child)	No development	1000	1500	5 cm³
Breast (adult)	Atrophy and necrosis	>5000	>10,000	Whole
Lung	Pneumonitis, fibrosis	4000	6000	Lobe
			2500	Whole
Capillaries	Telangiectasia, sclerosis	5000–6000	7000–10,000	–
Heart	Pericarditis, pancarditis	4000	>10,000	Whole
Bone (child)	Arrested growth	2000	3000	10 cm³
Bone (adult)	Necrosis, fracture	6000	15,000	10 cm³
Cartilage (child)	Arrested growth	1000	3000	Whole
Cartilage (adult)	Necrosis	6000	10,000	Whole
			absorbed dose	
CNS	Necrosis	5000	>6000	Whole
Spinal Cord	Necrosis, transection	5000	>6000	5 cm³
Eye	Panophthalmitis, hemorrhage	5500	10,000	Whole
Cornea (L.b.)	Keratitis	5000	>6000	Whole
Lens	Cataract	500	1200	Whole
Ear (inner)	Deafness	>6000	–	Whole
Vestibular	Meniere's syndrome	6000	10,000	Whole
Thyroid	Hypothyroidism	4500	15,000	Whole
Adrenal	Hypoadrenalism	>6000	–	Whole
Pituitary	Hypopituitarism	4500	20,000–30,000	Whole
Muscle (child)	No development	2000–3000	4000–5000	Whole
Muscle (adult)	Atrophy	>10,000	–	Whole
Bone marrow	Hypoplastic	200	550	Whole
		2000	4000–5000	Localized
Lymph nodes	Atrophy	4500	>7000	–
Lymphatics	Sclerosis	5000	>8000	–
Fetus	Death	200	400	–

*There is no dose-data available for the pancreas, gallbladder, or aorta.

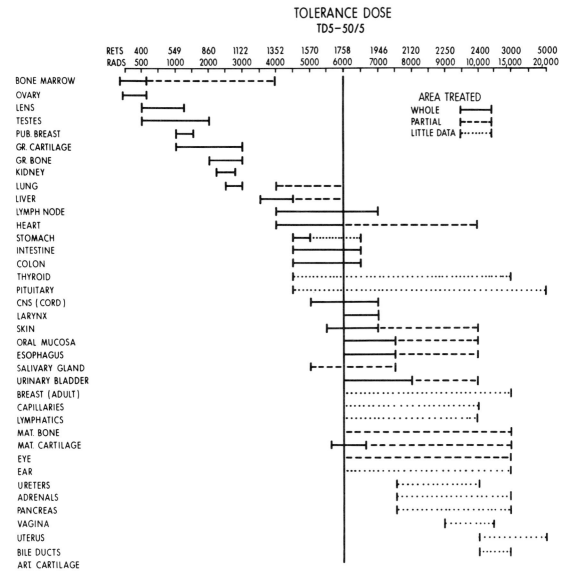

FIGURE 8–24 Tolerance doses for different organs. $TD_{5-50/5}$. These estimates for tolerance doses or injurious doses resulting in severe complications at each organ site are based in part on personal experience and in part upon the time-dose data recorded in individual organ sections by Rubin and Casarett (1968). It represents the authors' personal value system in decision making. When the dose to the whole or a large segment of an organ in the treatment field approaches the $TD_{5/5}$ level, we attempt to shield or exclude the structure if it is vital. Depending upon the risks and gains involved, we will vary the dose beyond the $TD_{5/5}$ level, but only in rare circumstances are we willing to approach the $TD_{50/5}$ level for a vital structure because of the risk of severe complication. RET dose is calculated for each rad dose shown and is not a sample linear relationship. (From Rubin, P., and Casarett, G. W.: A direction for clinical radiation pathology: the tolerance dose. *In* Vaeth, J. (ed.): *Frontiers of Radiation Therapy and Oncology.* Baltimore, Karger, Basel, and University Park Press, 1972, vol. 6, p. 13.)

tions, results in no more than a five per cent severe complication rate within five years after treatment.

The maximal tolerance dose is defined as the $TD_{50/5}$ dose; this, when applied to a given population of patients under a standard set of treatment conditions, results in a 50 per cent severe complication rate within five years after treatment.

The limit of tolerance is a clinical concept and is dependent on the importance of the tissue or organ to the organism's survival. The accessibility of the structure to observation and the detectability of injury help to determine the so-called "latent period" or "subclinical" level of injury. If serial histopathologic analysis were possible or sensitive functional tests were available for each organ system, our view of an acceptable reaction would be altered. It is important to the clinician to be able to predict with reasonable certainty the risk of injury (five to 50 per cent in five years) which is associated with the treatment dose (Fig. 8–23B).

In Table 8–3 are tabulated estimated minimal injurious doses ($TD_{5/5}$) and maximal injurious doses ($TD_{50/5}$) on the basis of personal experience and time-dose plots in the literature. However, in the table, broader ranges of incidence (one to five per cent and 25 to 50 per cent) are used because of limitations in clinical data interpretation. The standard set of conditions referred to are supervoltage therapy (one to six MeV), fractionation of 1000 rads per week, five daily fractions and a two-day rest, and treatment completed in two to eight weeks, depending on the total dose. Volumes or lengths irradiated are shown in a separate column. These dose ranges (Fig. 8–24) are hypothetical but represent our concept of tolerance doses in current practice, with the common fractionation regimen noted.

8.7   SUMMARY

In summary, if tolerance doses are arranged by dose level, the following observations are apparent:

A. *At the 1000- to 2000-rad level* there are some tissues which are markedly damaged. For example, the gonads, ovaries, and testes, are sterilized; the developing breast, growing bone, and growing cartilage would be severely damaged; bone marrow, if totally exposed to 1000 rads, would be rendered markedly hypoplastic; the optic lens would develop progressive cataract; and the fetus or the adult, if exposed to a dose of 1000 rads, would die. Doses greater than 2000 rads might be required to completely arrest growing bone and cartilage and to prevent localized segments of damaged bone marrow from regenerating.

B. *At the 2000- to 4500-rad level* the moderate dose range, minimal incidence levels of severe complications would result if the whole (or large portions) of the stomach, intestine, and colon were exposed. Liver and kidney, previously thought to be radioresistant, are vulnerable in this range if whole organs are irradiated. Lung is affected at dose levels similar to those affecting the kidney if all of both lungs is treated beyond 2500 rads. The heart has been demonstrated to be vulnerable when its entire volume is treated beyond 4500 rads. The thyroid and pituitary have been affected in certain situations. Developing muscle, unlike adult muscle, can be rendered atrophic. Lymph nodes will atrophy at this dose level.

C. *At the 5000- to 7000-rad level* a small incidence (one to five per cent) of severe complications will occur in a variety of epithelial structures, including skin, oral mucosa, esophagus, rectum, salivary glands, pancreas, urinary bladder, mature bone and cartilage, central nervous system, spinal cord, eye, ear, and adrenal glands. These organs, if exposed to higher doses (7500 rads), would develop severe complications in an incidence in the steep part of a dose-responsive curve (25 to 50 per cent injury).

D. *At the highest levels* of dose in clinical radiation therapy (7500 rads), there are some structures which are tolerant in terms of severe complications: the ureters, the uterus, the vagina, breast (adult), muscle (adult), blood, bile ducts, and articular cartilage. The latter, from the results of our experimental studies, is perhaps among the most radioresistant of tissues.

In conclusion, the design of this chapter is to present basic concepts in radiation pathology in a concise fashion. The correlation of clinical syndromes and their basis in the physiopathologic alterations of parenchymal cellular compartment and the microcirculation has been discussed. Available quantitative dose-time data has been emphasized at specific tissue and organ sites. It is the hope of the authors that by defining the limits of tolerance of normal tissues and organs, a sound basis will be provided for optimum radiation therapy.

References

1. Andrews, J. R., and Moody, J. M.: The dose-time relationship in radiotherapy. Amer. J. Roentgen., 75:590–596, 1956.
2. Barendsen, G. W.: In *Time and Dose Relationships in Radiation Biology as Applied to Radiotherapy.* National Cancer Institute – AEC Monograph. Upton, N.Y., Brookhaven National Laboratory, Aug., 1970.
3. Casarett, G. W.: Concept and criteria of radiologic aging. *In* Harris, R. J. C. (ed.): *Cellular Basis and Aetiology of Late Somatic Effects of Ionizing Radiation.* London, Academic Press, 1963.
4. Ellis, F.: The relationship of biological effect to dose-time fractionation factors in radiotherapy. *In* Eberhard, M., and Howard, A. (eds.): *Current Topics in Radiation Research,* Vol. IV. London, North-Holland Publishing Co., 1968.
5. Lindgren, M.: On tolerance of brain tissue and sensitivity of brain tumors to irradiation. Acta Radiol. (Stockholm) (Supp.), 170:1–73, 1958.
6. Luxton, R. W.: The clinical and pathological effects of renal irradiation. *In* Buschke, F. (ed.): *Progression in Radiation Therapy,* Vol. II. New York, Grune and Stratton, 1962.
7. Merrian, G. R., Jr., and Focht, E. F.: Radiation dose to the lens in treatment of tumors of the eye and adjacent structures; possibilities of cataract formation. Radiology, 71:357, 1958.
8. Rubin, P., and Casarett, G. W.: *Clinical Radiation Pathology.* Philadelphia, W. B. Saunders, 1968.
9. Stewart, J. R., and Fajardo, L. F.: Dose response in human and experimental radiation induced heart disease; application of the nominal standard dose (NSD) concept. Radiology, 99:403–408, 1971.
10. Von Essen, F. F.: Clinical radiation tolerance of the skin and upper aerodigestive tract. *In* Vaeth, J. (ed.): *Frontiers in Radiation Therapy and Oncology.* New York, S. Karger, in press.

9 ACUTE EFFECTS

Acute Radiation Syndrome

William S. Maxfield, M.D., Gerald E. Hanks, M.D.,
Donald J. Pizzarello, Ph.D., and Leo H. Blackwell, Ph.D.

9.0 INTRODUCTION

Whole body radiation delivered in a period of seconds to minutes produces a clinical pattern termed the acute radiation syndrome. The pattern response to whole body radiation is dependent upon the total dose of radiation received. In many ways, the acute radiation syndrome follows the well known pattern of response of viral infections. The exposure to whole body radiation is similar to inoculation of a virus into the body. After the exposure to radiation, there is a delay until the prodromal reaction to the radiation, or to a viral infection, is clinically evident. Following this mild initial reaction, there is a latent period, lasting until the specific pattern of damage from the acute whole body radiation is evident as the specific disease pattern. This phase corresponds to the specific disease patterns of a viral disease.

Data concerning the acute radiation syndrome have been drawn from many sources. Animal experiments have provided significant understanding of the various phases of the acute radiation syndrome. On the human level, data have been drawn from experience with local radiation therapy, whole body radiation therapy, the Japanese atomic bomb casualties, and nuclear accidents. The various patterns shown in the phases in the acute radiation syndrome have been well documented from these sources.

9.1 THE LD$_{50}$ CONCEPT

The pathogenesis of radiation injury at the cellular and organ level has been outlined in Chapter 8. The measuring of radiation effect is a problem because of the delay between the time the radiation is received and the time that the full clinical effects of the radiation dose are manifest. In measuring radiation effect, a concept of the lethal dose 50 (LD$_{50}$), the end point for measuring the effect of acute radiation exposure, has been borrowed from the field of pharmacology (see Figure 9–1). The lethal dose 50 is defined as the dose of any agent or material that causes a mortality of 50 per cent in the experimental group. The lethal dose 100 is defined as the dose of an agent or material that produces a 100 per cent mortality in an experimental group. For radiation exposure, an additional expression of mortality within a specific period of time is employed, LD$_{50/30}$, which is defined as a 50 per cent mortality occurring within 30 days. This is the term applied to most animal studies. For severe acute radiation exposures, the term LD$_{100/88}$ has been employed referring to 100 per cent mortality within 88 hours. Of these, the LD$_{50/30}$

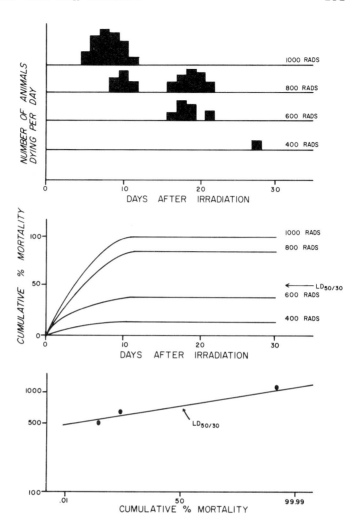

FIGURE 9-1 Mortality patterns after irradiation. The top panel shows the number of irradiated animals dying on a given day as a function of dose. The center panel shows the cumulative per cent mortality after exposure. The lower panel shows a plot of the log of the cumulative per cent mortality against dose. This is a "probability" (or probit) plot which aids in the estimation of the LD$_{50/30}$.

is the more common term. For human radiation exposure, the LD$_{50/60}$ has been established at approximately 400 to 450 R whole body radiation exposure from electromagnetic or neutron exposure, or both, as measured in air. In terms of absorbed dose this would be in the range of 300 to 350 rads (see Chapter 8).

Within a given population of human beings or experimental animals there are many factors which influence the response of the individual to whole body radiation. Briefly stated, the young and the old appear to be more radiosensitive than the middle-aged individual. The female appears to have a greater degree of tolerance to radiation than does the male. In addition, environmental factors may affect the response to radiation exposure. If the environment is kindly, the radiation effect is lowered, while a hostile environment, one requiring exercise, tends to enhance the damage from a given dose of radiation. If an area of the body is shielded (e.g., the spleen or bone marrow), then the effect of a given dose of radiation is decreased. The presence of infection markedly increases the mortality from radiation exposure. The effect of pharmaceutical agents administered prior to irradiation and methods of treatment after radiation exposure will be discussed later in this chapter. In addition to general factors which modify the response to radiation for a given population, there are also individual sensitivities to radiation.

An individual may show a normal response to radiation exposure or may be either hypo- or hypersensitive to radiation. Approximately 50 per cent of the population falls into the normally sensitive group, with 25 per cent being hypersensitive and 25 per cent being hyposensitive.

9.2 THE ACUTE RADIATION SYNDROMES

The major patterns of the acute whole body radiation syndrome in man can be divided into four forms, with a further division into two sub-groups under the hemopoietic form (Table 9–1). Experimental animals show a similar pattern, but the radiation dose required to produce the syndrome varies with the species, as does the time sequence of the response. The major patterns include a subclinical form and three clinical forms known as the hemopoietic, the gastrointestinal, and the central nervous system (cerebrovascular). Organ systems are named because the predominant effects of the radiation dose at the various levels are clinical symptoms due to damage of these organs. The form that is manifest is directly dose-dependent, but the factors modifying response to radiation may vary the clinical pattern of damage for a given individual. The response to a dose of whole body radiation, therefore, is not as specific as outlined below; however, this outline may serve as a guide for

evaluation of acute whole body radiation exposure.

A. Subclinical Form

Radiation exposures up to 200 R* whole body acute dose usually produce the subclinical form of radiation exposure. This form consists of predominantly psychic anxiety with tachycardia, vasomotor symptoms frequently with nausea and vomiting, but usually a normal peripheral blood count. The psychic anxiety with associated symptoms persists until the radiation dose is known or until the individual can be assured that on the basis of clinical evaluation his radiation exposure was of minimal degree.

B. Hemopoietic Syndrome

The hemopoietic form occurs with radiation exposure from 200 to 600 R. The hemopoietic form is divided into two sub-groups: a mild form, which occurs at doses between 200 and 400 R, and the severe form, occur-

*In this section the irradiations are quantitated in units of exposure (roentgens in air). Because of problems of estimation of absorbed doses in many studies, the earlier convention of R in air will be used.

TABLE 9–1   THE ACUTE RADIATION SYNDROME

Form	Dose in Air (R)	Clinical Manifestation	Result
Subclinical (1)	200 or less	Usually asymptomatic to minimal prodromal symptoms	No evidence of damage in most individuals, except at higher part of dose range
Hemopoietic Mild Form (II)	200–400	Transient prodromal symptoms of nausea and vomiting, mild to moderate laboratory and clinical evidence of hemopoietic derangement.	Maximum depression at 3 weeks, recovery in 5–6 weeks. Complete in 4–6 months.
Severe Form (III)	400–600	Severe hemopoietic complications and some evidence of gastroenteric damage in upper dose range.	$LD_{50/60}$ is 400–450 R. Requires bone marrow transplants and other supportive measures
Gastrointestinal (IV)	600–1000	Severe prodromal symptoms of nausea, vomiting, and diarrhea. Some recovery then return of severe diarrhea with blood and electrolyte loss.	Progress to shock and death 10–14 days
Cerebral (V)	1000 and above	Burning sensation at exposure, confusion. Partial recovery then progressive confusion and shock.	Death in 14–36 hours

ring at doses between 400 and 600 R. It should be remembered that the $LD_{50/60}$ for human radiation exposure is approximately 400 to 450 R; therefore, at the 400 to 500 R level without treatment there is a 50 per cent chance of mortality. The hemopoietic form consists of a prodromal phase starting a few hours after the exposure and lasting for usually 24 hours with mild to moderate nausea and vomiting. During the first day, the leucocyte count will usually increase,* although the lymphocyte count in differential study will start to drop. After the prodromal phase there is a latent period lasting from a few days to three weeks during which there may be mild weakness and fatigue. At the end of the latent period, the clinical symptoms secondary to depression of the hemopoietic system will begin to be evident. In the mild phase of the hemopoietic form of the acute radiation syndrome, effect on the hemopoietic system is usually evident by sore throat, fever, malaise, and fatigue, with possible development of purpura as the platelet count drops. The hemoglobin and the white count will show progressive decrease. This period of pancytopenia will last from three to four weeks. Epilation occurs at about three weeks after the radiation exposure. There is usually moderate weight loss with recovery of the hemopoietic system starting in the fifth week with virtually complete recovery by three to six months. As a long-term sequela, there is usually an elevated sedimentation rate and fatigue which may persist for months. For the severe phase of the hemopoietic form, the onset of the specific disease is usually earlier, with depression of the hemopoietic system being more severe. Without treatment, the majority of the individuals in this dosage range will die from infection or bleeding secondary to the severe bone marrow depression. With therapy, as will be discussed later, there is a chance of improving survival.

C. Gastrointestinal Syndrome

The gastrointestinal form of the acute radiation syndrome occurs between 600 and 1000 R or greater whole body radiation ex-

*The reason for the transitory leucocytosis is not the result of increased production of cells. More likely it follows from the release of cells from "storage" areas, such as the spleen or bone marrow.

posure. The onset of the prodromal symptoms usually occurs within a few hours after the exposure. There is often severe nausea and vomiting, occasionally accompanied by diarrhea, producing watery stools and severe cramps. The total leucocyte count shows a significant increase, but there is rapid fall in the lymphocyte count to zero. After the first 24 to 48 hours, the patient may feel better as he enters the latent phase, which may last from the second day to approximately one week. At the end of this latent phase, there is return of severe nausea, vomiting, and diarrhea with fever. The cellular elements of the hemopoietic system start to fall at about one week, and at this time there is return of nausea and vomiting, which progresses to bloody diarrhea, shock, and death, occurring from 10 to 14 days after the acute radiation exposure.

D. Central Nervous System Syndrome

The central nervous system form of the acute radiation syndrome occurs at radiation doses above 1000 R. The exposure to radiation at this level produces a sensation of burning within a few minutes. There is the development of severe nausea and vomiting usually within ten minutes; loss of consciousness sometimes occurs. Within the first hour, ataxia and confusion with prostration develop. There is a tremendous increase in the white count initially reaching levels of 40,000 or more, but the differential will show essentially no lymphocytes. The patient may go into a latent period with apparent improvement for several hours; however, in five to six hours there is onset of watery diarrhea, cyanosis with respiratory distress, which progresses to shock and decrease in urine production at 10 to 14 hours. These processes continue, and death occurs at 20 to 38 hours after exposure. At time of death, although the total white count has usually returned to normal, there is complete absence of lymphocytes. When the radiation dose is 4000 R and above, there may also be a direct cardiovascular component with pronounced hypotension and shock. Therefore, this form is sometimes called the cerebrovascular phase.

Review of the various forms of the acute radiation syndrome indicates that the pattern of response is directly dose-related. The clinical pattern shown results from the most severely damaged organ system with the shortest response time to the radiation. The latent period between the time of exposure and onset of the full clinical manifestations of the damage varies with the system involved. With moderate doses of radiation, the predominant symptoms relate to the hemopoietic system with clinical manifestations reaching maximum severity at approximately four weeks after the exposure. With increasing dose, the gastrointestinal system becomes the organ system of concern, with the clinical effects being manifest at nine to ten days after the exposure. With massive doses of radiation, the central nervous system and cardiovascular system show the most severe response, with death occurring within 24 to 48 hours. Though the hemopoietic system is the most sensitive organ group to radiation exposure, the other systems with shorter latent times supersede the hemopoietic system as the cause of death as the radiation dose increases above 600 R.

E. Cutaneous Syndrome

The skin may also show reaction to acute radiation exposure. The cutaneous syndrome has been observed after irradiation of animals and man with superficially penetrating radiations of the electromagnetic spectrum, as well as with protons and electrons. This pattern may be superimposed upon the four forms of the acute radiation syndrome, or it may result from partial body exposure. The clinical picture show by injured individuals resembles that seen in cases of thermal burns. Immediately after exposures above 200 to 500 R, depending upon the quality of the radiation and sensitivity of the individual, a mild erythema may be seen. This initial erythema may fade and then recur. Within the next few weeks, the erythema deepens; this is in turn followed by blister formation which may progress to desquamation, ulceration, and epidermal slough. The denuded areas are invaded by bacteria; clinical and laboratory evidence of infection appears. The white blood cell count is elevated and shows a prominent component of immature forms (a "left" shift). The serum electrophoresis shows a decreased albumin concentration, but the globulin concentration is increased. Deaths result from the same causes responsible for deaths from thermal burns—infection and loss of protein and fluids. When the deeper structures were not irradiated, the classic gastrointestinal and hematologic syndromes do not appear. As a result, larger radiation doses, which can cause very extensive superficial injury, are possible. When superimposed upon the acute radiation syndrome, the damage to vital organ systems frequently produces death before there is full manifestation of the cutaneous syndrome.

9.3 THE PATHOGENESIS OF THE ACUTE RADIATION SYNDROME

The cellular basis for the gastrointestinal and hemopoietic syndromes rests upon the cell renewal process. The cells of tissues such as the bone marrow and gastrointestinal epithelium have very rapid turnover times, which means that a constant source of new cells must be supplied in order to balance the numbers of cells that are lost. The term "cell renewal system" has been applied to the situation in which the population is kept stable by continuous and equal rates of production and loss.

The cellular renewal system depends upon the presence of *stem cells.* These cells divide and give rise to daughter cells. One daughter cell becomes a mature, functioning element, while the other remains within the stem cell compartment. The daughter cell destined for differentiation may later divide one or more times. None of the cells produced by these subsequent mitoses, however, has characteristics of stem cells. Instead, all of them will eventually differentiate and become mature elements. In the bone marrow, the mature elements produced are the cells of the peripheral blood. Similarly, the cells of the epithelium lining the gastrointestinal tract represent the mature elements.

Since normal biologic processes cause loss of mature elements, the repeated division of the stem cells provides the cells to replace those lost. Consequently, any process which inhibits or delays the division of stem cells ultimately will cause destruction of this tissue.

As described in Chapter 6, one of the predominant effects of radiation at the cellular level is to produce a loss of proliferative capacity. The available evidence indicates that stem cells of the bone marrow, gastrointestinal epithelium, and other primordial cell groups respond in a manner qualitatively and quantitatively similar to cultured mammalian cells.

The hemopoietic system provides mature functional circulating elements. Since these have finite life times and cannot reproduce themselves, those lost through natural attrition are not replaced during the time the bone marrow does not function. If the length of time in which the hemopoietic system does not function is too long, the level of vital circulating elements drops too low and the irradiated organism dies.

In the gastrointestinal tract, stem cells located in the crypts of Lieberkuhn of intestinal villi are killed or mitotically inhibited by irradiation. Mature functional cells at the tips of the villi are exhausted at the usual rate and are extruded into the intestinal lumen. If they are not soon replaced, vital functions of the intestine are lost and the irradiated organism dies. The dose range producing this effect in most mammals is between 600 and 1000 R. The mean survival time is between 10 and 14 days. When the radiation dose exceeds 1000 R, the effect on the gastrointestinal tract is superseded by damage to the cerebrovascular system. Mean survival time is not dose-dependent probably because functional intestinal cells die and are shed at a rather constant rate. Intestinal function is lost when a critical number of epithelial cells is lost. About 600 to 1000 R inhibits division or kills enough stem cells so that the vital, critical number of functional cells will be shed and cannot be replaced. Doses of radiation above 1000 R kill or inhibit more stem cells, but death has already been assured after 1000 R has been delivered. As the radiation dose exceeds 1000 R death will occur from effect on the cerebrovasvular system before full effect is evidenced in the gastrointestinal tract.

9.4 PROLIFERATIVE REPAIR

After acute irradiation of a cell system, an important component of the recovery process is proliferative repair of surviving stem cells to repopulate the tissue and resume the tissue's functions.

The response of the bone marrow may be divided into four steps. The time sequence given is for the mouse. First, there is an immediate reduction in stem cell content that is related to total dose and the cellular sensitivity of the stem cells at the time of radiation. Second, within 24 hours sublethal injury has been repaired. Proliferation of surviving previously cycling stem cells proceeds and is accompanied by recruitment of the surviving noncycling bone marrow compartment. This stem cell proliferation proceeds at an extremely rapid rate and initially may produce stem cells in preference to differentiated cell forms. Third, two or three days after exposure the continuing increase in stem cell content is paralleled by an increase in nucleated cell forms in the bone marrow that is soon reflected in the peripheral blood. Fourth, about two weeks after exposure there is an absolute over-shoot of bone marrow stem cells and nucleated cell content which over the next several weeks returns to normal as the steady state is resumed. In man the steps are the same, but there is a longer time sequence for response and repair.

For the gastrointestinal phase of the acute radiation syndrome, supportive therapy has been administered. A recent report based on data from animals suggests that diversion of the biliary products from the gastrointestinal tract may improve survivals. Though the patient might survive the acute phase, long-term evaluation of the effect of this radiation dose on kidneys and other radiation-sensitive organ systems has not been delineated. On a clinical level everyone that has been exposed to doses in the range of the gastrointestinal phase has expired from this level of radiation exposure.

The treatment for the hemopoietic form of the acute radiation syndrome depends on the phase of the syndrome. For the mild phase of the form, supportive measures such as antibiotics administered for specific infections, platelets, and general measures such as mental and physical rest, high protein bland diet, good general hygiene with protective isolation during the severe depression of the hemopoietic system usually provide control of the effects of the radiation. Replacement of electrolytes, water, and red cells are seldom required. For the severe phase of the hemopoietic

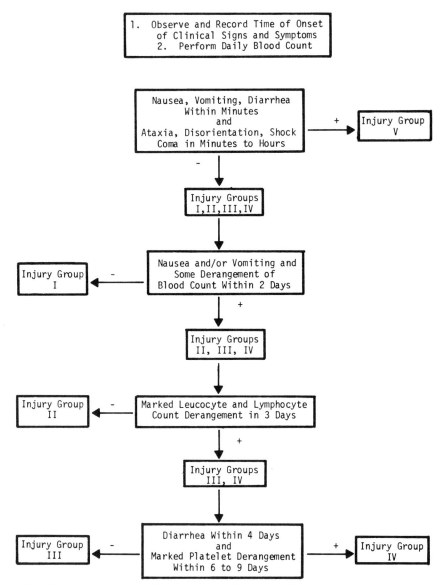

FIGURE 9–2 This flow sheet can be utilized for the rapid sorting of patients into injury groups so that proper follow-up and therapy can be expeditiously instituted. (Reproduced by permission of the Journal of Occupational Medicine.)

form of the acute radiation syndrome, additional therapy such as bone marrow transplantation has been employed. The bone marrow transplants in experimental animals have been of an autologous, isologous, homologous, either adult or fetal, or heterologous form. Other types of treatment that have been tried are administration of splenic cells, either as a cellular fraction or as a humoral fraction. With the bone marrow transplants, there is well documented evidence of take of the bone marrow. In accidental exposure of humans, bone marrow transplants are limited to isologous and homologous marrow. The most successful cases, however, have involved use of bone marrow from a twin of the irradiated individual. Complications of bone marrow transplant are failure of the transplant to take or, if it does take, development of "secondary disease" which has been demonstrated predominantly in experimental animals. Secondary disease is a delayed death after take of a donor bone marrow owing to paralysis of the immunologic defenses of the host. A minor aspect appears to be due to incomplete depression of the host defenses with the host reacting against the donor cells. Of greater importance, the evidence that the donor cells immunologically react against host antigens. This syndrome appears to be due partly to failure to repopulate the lymph nodes.

Transfusion of white blood cells is also a major method of therapy. If equipment for collection of normal white blood cells is not available, transfusion with blood from patients with chronic granulocytic leukemia may be of value. There appears to be little chance of transmitting the disease with these transfusions. E. D. Thomas and associates have suggested cross circulation for the severe hemopoietic syndrome.

In summary, the acute radiation syndrome is a well documented clinical response whose pattern relates to the dose of acute whole body radiation exposure. The knowledge of this syndrome is increasingly necessary because of the widespread use of radiation in industry and increasing development of nuclear power as a source for electricity production. Figure 9–2 provides a simple method for a triage of patients receiving acute whole body radiation exposure with the text outlining the available methods of treatment of the various forms of the acute radiation syndrome.

References

1. Archambeau, J. O., Mathieu, G. R., Brenneis, H. J., Thompson, K. H., and Fairchild, R. G.: The response the skin of swine to increasing single exposures of 250 kVp X-rays. Radiat. Res., 36:299, 1968.
2. Bond, V. P., Fliedner, T. M., and Cronkite, E. P.: Evaluation and management of the heavily irradiated individual. J. Nuc. Med., 1:221, 1960.
3. Bond, V. P., Fliedner, T. M., and Archambeau, J. O. (eds): Mammalian Radiation Lethality: A Disturbance in Cellular Kinetics. New York, Academic Press, 1965.
4. Cronkite, E. P., Bond, V. P., and Dunham, C. L.: Some effects of ionizing radiation on human beings. United States Atomic Energy Commission, Government Printing Office (TID-5358), July, 1956.
5. Gerstner, H. B.: Acute clinical effects of penetrating nuclear radiation, J.A.M.A., 168:361–388, 1958.
6. Hempelmann, L. H., Lisco, H., and Hoffman, J. G.: Acute radiation syndrome: study of nine cases and review of problem. Ann. Int. Med., 36: 279–510, 1952.
7. Knowlton, N. P., et al.: Beta-ray burns of human skin. J.A.M.A., 141:239, 1949.
8. Lushbaugh, C. C., Sutton, J. and Richmond, C. R.: The question of electrolyte loss in the intestinal death syndrome of radiation damage. Radiat. Res., 13:814, 1960.
9. Maxfield, W. S., and Porter, G. H.: Accidental radiation exposure from Iridium-192 camera. Handling of Radiation Accidents: International Atomic Energy Agency. Vienna, 1970. P. 459.
10. Saenger, E. L.: Radiation accidents. Amer. J. Roentgen., 84:715–728, 1960.
11. Thoma, G. E., and Wald, N.: Diagnosis and management of accidental radiation injury. J. Occupat. Med., 1:420–447, 1959.
12. Thomas, E. D., Lochte, H. L., Jr., and Ferrebee, J. W.: Irradiation of the entire body and marrow transplantation: some observations and comments. Blood, 14:1, 1959.
13. The Acute Radiation Syndrome, a Medical Report on the Y-12 Accident June 16, 1958 (ORINS-25) Marshal Brucer (Ed) A.E.C. National Technical Information Service, Springfield, Virginia, April 1959.

Radiation and the Immune Response[*]

Bernard N. Jaroslow, Ph.D.

9.6 RADIATION AND THE IMMUNE RESPONSE

Used as an immunosuppressive agent, radiation is a double edged sword. While it extends survival of organ grafts, it coincidentally renders the recipient more susceptible to infection; many graft recipients contract pneumonia following immunosuppressive therapy. It is particularly noteworthy that radiation, in addition to being an immunosuppressive agent, is also known to be carcinogenic. Recent studies have shown an increased tumor incidence in organ transplant recipients put on an immunosuppressive therapy. In general, radiotherapy for any cause, in doses over 100 R, may have significant effects on immune responsiveness.

An understanding of how immune responsiveness is altered by radiation is vital for maximum therapy with minimum suppression. A whole body dose of radiation depresses both innate immunity and the development of an acquired immunity. If the recipient is already immune to a parasite, irradiation has relatively little effect on his susceptibility to the specific infection. If radiotherapy can be localized or fractionated, immunosuppression is markedly reduced. When appropriate organs are shielded in rabbits, rats, and mice (e.g., spleen and appendix), immunologic capacity is largely retained under massive irradiation. After whole body irradiation, immune responsiveness in laboratory animals can be restored if nucleic acid degradation products are given with antigen. It is likely that under similar conditions of irradiation, the immune response in humans would be similar to those of rats, rabbits, mice, and guinea pigs.

Cellular immunity, which is important in inflammation, many hypersensitivities, and graft rejection processes, responds to radiation injury in much the same way as does humoral immunity (antibody production). Because effects of irradiation on humoral immunity have been more extensively studied and are better understood, antibody production will be emphasized in the following discussion.

9.7 THE NORMAL IMMUNE RESPONSE

The immune response is initiated when antigen (i.e., a foreign protein, a graft, or an infectious agent) enters the body and stimulates cells of the lymphoid-macrophage system, whose primary organs are lymph nodes, the spleen, and Peyer's patches of the intestine. The appendix, thymus, and bone marrow are ancillary organs, essential to the development and maintenance of immune responsiveness. The relative importance of the various organs varies with the animal species and will be mentioned when appropriate to the discussion.

The sequence of cellular events leading to the synthesis of antibodies after the first contact with antigen is as follows. Antigen may or may not be processed by macrophages; that is, particulate antigens require processing, but how soluble antigens are processed is not yet clear. Certain small lymphocytes, derived from bone marrow and pre-programed to respond to the specific antigen (approximately 100 to 1000 cells in mouse spleens, which contain 20×10^6 W.B.C.), are stimulated when they interact with specific thymus-derived cells and antigen to differentiate into large lymphocytes. This is the induction phase. The large lymphocytes proliferate and ultimately differentiate into plasma cells which produce antibody. The interval between antigen injection and the detection of antibody is known as the latent period. (The length of the latent period depends upon the assay procedure, the antigen, and the host.) The antibody rise

[*]Work supported by the U.S. Atomic Energy Commission.

to peak titer in serum is logarithmic for several days before it declines.

The secondary immune response, also called the anamnestic response, has a shorter latent period, an increased rate of serum antibody rise, and a higher peak titer than the primary response. This response is the equivalent of the "booster" injection with a vaccine.

9.8 IRRADIATION AT DIFFERENT TIMES BEFORE AND AFTER ANTIGEN INJECTION

The intensity of the antibody response depends upon the time of irradiation before and after antigen injection. The hemolysin response in rabbits to a single sublethal dose of X-rays is similar to that for rats, mice, and guinea pigs (see Figure 9–3).

Irradiation two days after antigen, during the latent period, delays the appearance of hemolysin and slows its rate of rise in the serum, but it does not depress antibody-forming capacity as judged by normal peak titer. When it is given two hours after antigen (during antigen processing and induction), the process is similarly slowed, but antibody production is significantly enhanced as shown by a higher peak titer. Irradiation during antibody rise or decline

has relatively little effect on the subsequent kinetics of antibody production.

In rabbits immunized from one hour to one day after irradiation all measures of the immune response are depressed. Maximum inhibition of immune responsiveness occurs one to two days after irradiation and its complete recovery time is at least 30 days.

Sensitivity of the secondary response to irradiation is qualitatively similar to that of the primary response. The major differences are that the secondary response is less depressed and recovery is quicker.

The immunosuppressive activity of radiation given before antigenic stimulation is undoubtedly related to destruction of responsive lymphocytes. The lack of depression of antibody-forming capacity when irradiation occurs after immunization appears to be related to rapid proliferation of surviving antigen stimulated cells in competition with slow proliferation of surviving unstimulated cells. The stimulated cells, therefore, have an advantage in repopulating depleted lymphoid organs.

9.9 RADIATION DOSE RESPONSE

After a single exposure to radiation, with antigen given one to two days later (the

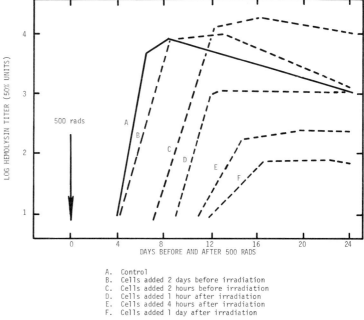

FIGURE 9–3 Hemolysin production in rabbits given sheep red cells from 2 days before to 1 day after 500 rads whole body x-irradiation. Note: Rabbits irradiated after sheep cells were added produced normal or higher amounts of antibody, but the rate of production was slowed, as in curves B and C. Irradiation before immunization, however, decreased as well as slowed antibody production, as in curves D, E and F. After Taliaferro, W. H. et al.

A. Control
B. Cells added 2 days before irradiation
C. Cells added 2 hours before irradiation
D. Cells added 1 hour after irradiation
E. Cells added 4 hours after irradiation
F. Cells added 1 day after irradiation

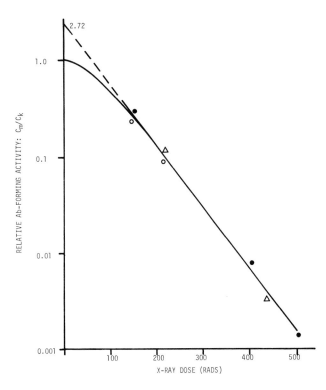

FIGURE 9–4 X-ray inactivation of antibody-forming capacity of mouse spleen cells. ○, 6-day primary antibody response; △, 6-day secondary antibody response; ●, 5-day secondary antibody response. Note that D_{37} for slope is 70 rads; extrapolation number is 2.72. (After Makinodan, T., et al.:

time of maximum suppression of the immune response), the semi-log plot of the serum peak titer versus radiation dose gives a sigmoid curve. The size of the shoulder and the slope varies with the species, but the dose that destroys 90 to 95 per cent of the antibody-forming capacity is sublethal. The X-ray dose response in rabbits gives a shoulder of about 100 R and 90 per cent inactivation with 400 to 500 R. The radiosensitivity of antibody-forming capacity of spleen cells of mice is shown in Figure 9–4. The shoulder of the curve is about 80 R and 90 per cent inactivation occurs at a dose of 250 R. It is noteworthy in regard to appropriate usage of RBE that in mice, which have a higher $LD_{50/30}$ than rabbits, the antibody-forming capacity appears to be more radiosensitive.

Changes in response to radiation dose in the latent period and the rate of serum antibody rise are as expected; the latent period is increased and the rate of rise is decreased.

The radiosensitivity of the lymphoid-macrophage system is in the same range as the hemopoietic system.

9.10 EFFECTS OF FRACTIONATED OR CHRONIC IRRADIATION

Results from experiments using fractionated and low-dose chronic irradiation are more difficult to assess, but, in general, they follow the principles established in studies with single doses.

Fractionated irradiation has less effect than a single acute dose equal to the sum of the fractions. When the fractions are given before and after antigen injection, the dominant effect is the immunosuppression caused by the irradiation given before antigen. Chronic low-dose irradiation, essentially an extreme example of fractionated irradiation, follows the same principles. Dose rate as well as total dose affect the degree of immunosuppression.

9.11 PROTECTION AND RESTORATION OF ANTIBODY-FORMING CAPACITY

Pre-irradiation chemical protection (e.g., cysteine or glutathione) protects immune responsiveness in the same way that it protects any other measure of radiation injury; that is, it reduces the effective radiation dose equally for all measures of the immune response.

Lead-shielding of spleen, appendix, and lymph nodes leads to a very interesting effect. The amount of protection obtained with shielding is directly related to the amount of lymphoid tissue protected and not necessarily to the amount of antibody produced by the organ. This observation is dramatically illustrated in the rabbit immunized with sheep red cells. The spleen normally produces 80 per cent of all the hemolytic antibody during the first two weeks. The appendix, which is not important as an antibody producer, is important in recovery from radiation injury because it contains a large proportion of the lymphoid tissue which is rapidly distributed to the depleted spleen and lymph nodes. Spleen white pulp recovers eight days after irradiation in appendix-shielded animals, as compared to 23 days in rabbits given 500 R whole body of X-rays. Because the appendix contains ten times as much lymphoid tissue as the spleen, appendix-shielded animals recover sooner and produce more antibody than spleen-shielded animals. It is obvious, therefore, that shielding the spleen, Peyer's patches, and the appendix, when clinical radiotherapéutic procedures permit, is important in accelerating recovery of the immune system after treatment.

Restoration of antibody-forming capacity after irradiation, at the time of its maximum suppression, can be accomplished by injecting nucleic acid degradation products at the same time as antigen. (Cytotoxic agents, such as endotoxin or colchicine, may act in the same way by releasing such products from injured cells.) The amount of antibody-forming capacity restored is *proportionately* equal at all doses of radiation that do not completely eliminate it. When no antibody-forming capacity remains, restoration of this type is not possible. *It is noteworthy that the latent period is not shortened, but remains as long as in the untreated irradiated controls.* This observation indicates that the capacity to induce the antibody response is enhanced, but recovery of normal proliferation and differentiation of the induced cells during

the latent period is not accelerated by treatment. The limitation of restoration to the induction period of the immune response is further indicated by the demonstration that restorative agents are effective only when given within a few hours of antigen injection.

9.12 EFFECTS OF LARGE DOSES OF LOCALIZED IRRADIATION

Large doses of localized irradiation inhibit the immediate cellular immune response in the affected area by killing resident immunocytes and by increasing capillary permeability. As a result, invading organisms are not phagocytized or encapsulated by these cells in the normal manner and can disseminate over a larger volume of tissue. The delay in containment of the invaders may tip the balance in favor of a successful infection. This effect of localized irradiation should be considered when planning radiotherapeutic procedures.

The circumscribed destruction of immunocytes attacking a graft can abort a rejection crisis and thereby prolong its survival without a general depression of immunocompetence.

9.13 RADIATION-INDUCED ALTERATIONS IN IMMUNITY TO INFECTION

The antibody response to infectious agents in irradiated animals is similar to the response to nonliving antigens. In infections in which the antibody response plays a dominant role, an immune host retains its capacity to control the infection even though it has been irradiated (see earlier discussion of irradiation of immune recipients, Section 9.8). Animals irradiated shortly after infection may succumb to the infection because of the delay in the production of antibody, despite their potential to produce normal amounts of antibody.

A major contribution to increased susceptibility to infection by nonvirulent parasites is the rapid and extensive breakdown in the humoral and cellular aspects of innate immunity. Within a few days of irradiation there is a major decrease in normal bactericidal activity of serum.

Compounding this, the phagocytic activity and assimilative potency of macrophages are drastically reduced. The end result is lethal septicemia by an otherwise innocuous organism.

The scenario for these events has been well documented. After a large dose of irradiation there is an increase in the normal rate of flow of intestinal bacteria through the wall of the intestine. The bacteria are phagocytized in the mesenteric lymph nodes, but the irradiated macrophages are unable to kill and digest them. They escape into the blood stream after several days and are trapped again by the macrophages of the spleen and liver. After the impotent macrophages have been overcome, the bacteria enter the blood stream and establish an overwhelming septicemia that kills the host.

9.14 SUMMARY

Radiation is an immunosuppressive agent when given before antigen. Irradiation after antigen injection, but before the end of the latent period, does not decrease antibody-forming capacity. This capacity may be restored by the presence of relatively large amounts of nucleic acid degradation products from killed lymphocytes, which have been shown to have adjuvant action if present at the same time as antigen during initiation of the immune response. When irradiation is given during the latent period, one to three days after antigen, the proliferating antibody-forming cells and their precursors have a marked advantage over the relatively inactive unstimulated

lymphocytes in repopulating the lymphoid tissues. These findings are generally applicable to cellular and humoral responses in acquired immunity.

Radiation damage to the immune system that is most significant for survival is probably the destruction of innate immunity. Large doses of radiation dramatically increase host susceptibility to nonpathogenic as well as pathogenic organisms. In many instances, the radiation-induced delay of antibody production is sufficient to prevent recovery.

Radiotherapeutic procedures should be conducted in recognition of their effects on immunologic responsiveness with respect to potential pathogens in the patient's environment and the recent knowledge that patients given a long course of immunosuppressive treatment have a higher incidence of neoplasia.

References

1. Leone, C. A. (ed.): *Ionizing Radiations and Immune Processes.* Gordon and Breach, New York, 1962.
2. Makinodan, T., and Gengozian, N.: *In* Hollaender, A. (ed.): *Radiation Protection and Recovery.* New York, Pergamon Press, 1960.
3. Micklem, H. S., and Loutit, J. F.: *Tissue Grafting and Radiation.* New York, Academic Press, 1966.
4. Penn, J., and Starzl, T. E.: Malignant lymphomas in transplantation patients: a review of world experience. Int. J. Clin. Pharmacol., *1*:49, 1970.
5. Simić, M. M., Sljivić, V. S., Petrović, M. A., and Ćirković, D. M.: *Antibody Formation in Irradiated Rats.* Belgrade, Boris Kidrić Institute, 1965.
6. Taliaferro, W. H., Taliaferro, L. G., and Jaroslow, B. N.: *Radiation and Immune Mechanisms.* New York, Academic Press, 1964.
7. Van Bekkum, D. W., and deVries, M. J.: *Radiation Chimaeras.* New York, Academic Press, 1967.

Chemical Protective Agents

George J. Kollmann, Ph.D.

9.15 CHEMICAL PROTECTIVE AGENTS AGAINST IONIZING RADIATION

Chemical agents which protect against ionizing radiation have been actively

sought since the discovery of the injurious effects of these rays. The early theories of the mechanism of radiation injury postulated that ionizing radiation acted by direct hit on vital cell molecules. The interposition of an agent, other than a lead wall, between the ionizing rays and vital molecules seemed impossible. Later work showed that some and possibly the greater part of radiation damage was mediated by radiation-produced decomposition of water. Some of the destruction or inactivation of vital cell molecules was produced by the highly reactive decomposition products of water. The possibility that chemical agents could intercept the breakdown products of water and prevent their molecules gave a a more hopeful aspect to the problem.

Actual chemical protection of living animals was achieved in the late 1940's and early 1950's using nonlethal doses of cyanide, cysteine, and glutathione. The successful application of these chemicals has initiated a new field of research in radiation biology, one which is being pursued today as one of the promising areas of endeavour.

Research in radiation protective agents has the obvious aim of finding an agent which can be administered safely and conveniently to human beings to protect them from death and the injurious effects of exposure to ionizing radiation. Such exposure might come from the detonation of nuclear weapons, travel in outer space, travel in nuclear-powered vehicles, employment in nuclear power installations, employment in installations utilizing radiation for medical or industrial purposes, or subjection to medical diagnostic or therapeutic procedures employing radiation or radioactive isotopes. Perhaps there are injurious effects even from the low level of everyday exposure to cosmic radiation and radiation from naturally occurring radioisotopes in the ground and in our bodies. Research in radiation protective agents also has as its aim the elucidation of the mechanism of action of ionizing radiation. Chemical protective agents are excellent tools for studying the means by which ionizing radiation produces its effects.

Research in radiation protective agents has followed three main pathways: (1) the testing of various agents for radiation protective effectiveness, (2) pharmacologic and toxicologic studies of the effects of known protective agents, and (3) studies on mechanism of action of known protective agents.

The testing of various agents for radiation protection has included thousands of compounds ranging from simple (e.g., heavy water, ethyl alcohol, carbon monoxide, and ammonium chloride) to the most complex (e.g., nucleic acid derivatives, vitamins, hormones, and synthetic polymers). Agents have been tested at many dosage levels, by several routes of administration, in several chemical forms, and with various timings relative to the radiation exposure. Agents have been tested with several types of ionizing radiation, at various dose rates and total doses, using one or more exposures, and exposing at different time intervals. Agents have been tested in pure chemical systems, in biochemical preparations such as enzyme systems, in single and multicellular organisms, in a variety of animals, under many different environmental conditions, and with exposure of all or part of the test object. Agents have been evaluated by a great variety of criteria, including the percentage of subjects killed within a fixed time interval, survival time in days after irradiation, peripheral blood cell count, physiologic function of various systems, histologic changes, genetic effects, chromosome aberrations, number of mitoses, biochemical changes, changes in membrane characteristics, changes in viscosity of fluids, changes in molecular structure, and many others.

The most commonly used criterion for protection in mammals is the dose of radiation which will result in death of 50 per cent of the animals within the first 30 days after exposure. This is known as $LD_{50/30}$. The ratio of $LD_{50/30}$ in the protected animals to the $LD_{50/30}$ in the unprotected animals is known as the dose-reduction factor (DRF). DRF values can also be obtained using other criteria (e.g., dose required to inactivate all but 37 per cent of enzyme activity in protected versus control systems).

The pharmacologic effects of some protective agents are well known because of their prior use for other purposes. The pharmacology of some of the newer agents is not well known. These studies provide clues to mechanism of action and also to the nature of toxicity. Reduction or blocking of toxicity may permit administration of larger and more effective doses, provided that the mechanism of protection and the mechanism of toxicity are not the same.

Studies on the mechanism of action of radiation protective agents have been made at all levels. Helpful information has been derived from electron spin resonance data, which indicate the site of injury on the molecule and alteration of the injury in the presence of protective agents. The radiation chemistry of some of the protective agents in aqueous solution has been studied, and it has been demonstrated how they may interact with the products of water decomposition, a possible means of protection. The distribution and metabolism of some of the agents have been studied, and it has been shown where and in what form the agent exists in the animal at the time of protection; the protective form of the agent may be different from the administered form. Distribution studies sometimes show why some tissues are better protected than others.

Testing studies also may give information on mechanism. The effect of different chemical structure on protective efficacy provides clues to protection. Knowing the effect of different types of radiation on protection by a single agent is also helpful. Information on the amount of protection afforded to different tissues (e.g., bone marrow damage and intestinal mucosa damage) by an agent also helps elucidate mechanism. Abolition of protection by concomitant administration of other agents or by variation in environmental conditions has provided evidence on mechanism.

Pharmacologic studies may also indicate mechanism of action. Correlation between a particular pharmacologic effect (e.g., change in blood flow to an area) and protection suggests involvement of the effect in protective action. The blocking of protection by an antagonist or inhibitor of one of the pharmacologic effects of an agent implicates this pharmacologic effect.

A. Classes of Radioprotective Compounds

The following is a discussion of some important drugs from each of the several classes of protective compounds.

Aminoalkyl-Thiols and Their Disulfides. Since the discovery of the protective effect of cysteine, a large number of these compounds have been tested. Among these the best agents are cysteine, cysteamine (mercaptoethylamine or MEA), cystamine (the disulfide of MEA), mercaptoethylguanidine (MEG), and guanideothyl disulfide (GED). (MEG is usually obtained from S-[2-aminoethyl] isothiuronium bromide hydrobromide [AET] by dissolving AET in aqueous solutions at neutral pH. Most protective studies reportedly using AET have actually used MEG, MEG-GED mixtures, or GED. See Figure 9–5.)

An extension of these drugs is the newly recognized class of aminoalkylphosphorothioates. The simplest of these is the aminoethylphosphorothioate (MEAP).

$$H_2N—CH_2—CH_2—S—PO_3H_2$$

MEAP

These compounds have been synthesized in recent years and have been found to be as effective as their free sulfhydryl or disulfide counterparts. They are, in actuality, potential sulfhydryl compounds since the phosphate group can be removed by hy-

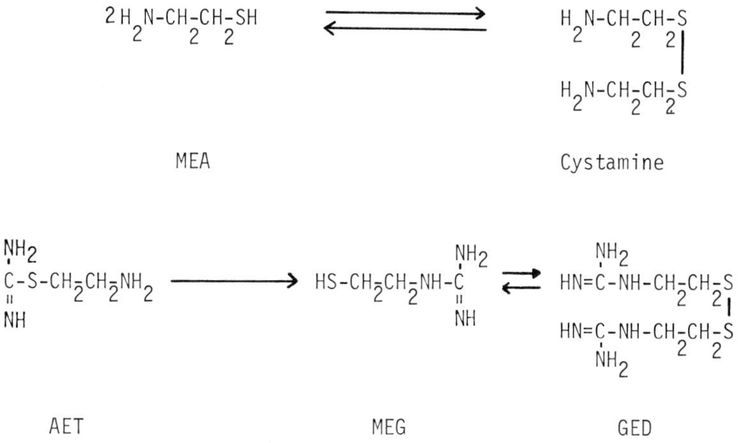

FIGURE 9–5 Reactions of some radioprotective compounds.

drolysis or by enzymatic action and thereby creating an aminoalkylthiol. The advantage of the phosphorothioates is their moderate toxicity compared to the thiols.

Other Sulfur Compounds. Thiols other than aminoalkyl-thiols show small protective ability. Thiourea and its derivatives give some protection. Dimethylsulfoxide has moderate protective effect. Perhaps the best group in this category is the dithio-carbamates. Dimethylammonium diethyldi-thiocarbamate was reported to be particularly successful, approaching the activity of the aminoalkyl-thiols.

Cyanide and Organic Nitriles. Cyanide in toxic doses has been reported to be protective in mice. Detoxification is extremely rapid and parallels the protective activity; therefore, protection disappears in a few minutes. Hydroxyacetonitrile has been reported to be effective in mice against fast neutron irradiation.

Amines. A number of amines have been shown to be protective in mice. Histamine and other amines such as epinephrine, tyramine, and hydroxyphenylethylamine are fair protective agents. The most promising one of this group is 5-hydroxytrypta-mine (serotonin). Its antagonists have been reported to block protective action. Serotonin has been successful not only in mice but in other mammals such as monkeys. Several of its derivatives have been reported to have the same protective effect. Another amine, which has shown significant protection, is p-aminopropiophenone (PAPP).

Chelating Agents. Some chelating agents have been tested, the best known of which is EDTA (ethylenediaminetetraacetate sodium salt). They have shown some protection in rodents.

Other Compounds. There is a large list of additional compounds that have shown some protection in rodents but do not show particular promise for the future. Some protection is provided by drugs that protect by altering the physiologic state of the organism. Compounds that induce hibernation and various hormones may be included here. ACTH, oxytocin, and putressin are somewhat protective. Various adenine nucleotides have been shown to give some protection. The mechanisms of protective action are unknown.

Mixtures of Protective Agents. There has been a great deal of interest in testing mixtures of protective agents. It is done with the hope that the protective action of the different agents will be additive. When one uses compounds that act by different mechanisms, the possibility of additive protection is good. Combination of anoxia and radioprotective drugs have given good results.

B. Mechanisms of Radiation Protection

Mechanism studies of aminoalkyl-thiols have been oriented about seven major theories of mechanism of radiation protection.

The Scavenging of Water Decomposition Products. The decomposition of water by irradiation results in the production of hydrogen, hydroxyl, and hydroperoxyl radicals, as well as hydrogen peroxide. Some or all of these highly reactive species may be responsible for cell damage. Reaction with the radical or hydrogen peroxide could be a means of protection. It has been shown that such interactions can take place during irradiation of MEA, cystamine, MEG, or GED in aqueous buffered solutions. However, the extent of this interaction in living cells or animals is questionable. Although thiols have a great affinity for radicals they are present in such small concentrations in the tissues that they would lose out in the competition with other molecules which are also able to interact with radicals. This has actually been demonstrated *in vitro* in irradiated protein solutions containing a protective agent in which the proteins appeared to protect the protective agent and no oxidation products of the protective agent were observed. Although scavenging of water radicals seems unlikely, there may be very localized sites in the tissues where conditions are suitable for a scavenging and where such a reaction may have protective significance.

The Removal of Oxygen. Thiols are readily oxidized and in the tissues can combine with several moles of oxygen to form sulfate (via sulfinic and sulfonic acids). Since it is known that anoxia increases radiation resistance, this is a conceivable mechanism of protection. Tissue oxygen tension measurements have not supported this theory, and protection with amino-thiols has been demonstrated with normal or increased tissue oxygen tension. In both *in vitro* and *in vivo* systems, additional protection by thiols has been demonstrated even when irradiation took place under hypoxic conditions. In metabolism studies of MEG and GED only small amounts of protective agent are oxidized in the tissues. It is interesting that the thiols are good protective agents against oxygen poisoning, which bears some similarity to radiation injury. It is possible that some oxygen trapping by thiols occurs at a critical tissue site.

The Donation of Hydrogen to Neutralize the Radical Formed on Vital Macromolecules. According to this theory, during irradiation the target molecule is hit directly by radiation or is attacked by radicals formed during the radiation decomposition of water. The loss of a hydrogen atom and the formation of a radical on the target molecule results. Unless this radical can be neutralized by abstracting a hydrogen from some non-essential molecule, the target molecule will react with oxygen to form peroxides or will decompose or cross-link with other important molecules. The protective agent is said to act as a hydrogen donor to prevent these damaging reactions. Evidence for this theory is found in electron spin resonance studies and in studies with bacteriophage particles, which indicate competition between oxygen and thiols for injured sites in the phage. This theory explains much of the observed effects of oxygen and protective thiols. However, in the case of AET, the free protective agent in the tissues of mice is in the disulfide form at the time of protection. The protective disulfide may donate half of its molecule to the macromolecular radical:

$$(\text{macromolecule})\cdot + \text{RSSR} \longrightarrow$$
$$(\text{macromolecule})\text{SR} + \text{RS}\cdot$$

There is evidence for this in the increased protein binding of GED during irradiation of pure protein solutions.

The Sulfhydryl Shielding Theory. It has been proposed that important target molecules are sulfhydryl-bearing and that no matter where those molecules are hit, the damage migrates to the thiol group. According to this theory, if the molecules are attacked by radicals, it is primarily the sulfhydryl groups of the target molecules

that are attacked. Under these conditions, the critical thiol group may be shielded by being bound in mixed disulfide linkage with a protector molecule, and there is a correlation between ability of a thiol to form mixed disulfides with glutathione and protective ability. It is true that thiols are more sensitive to radiation than are disulfides. It is also of interest that 50 per cent of the protective agent is protein-bound in the tissues of a protected animal. It was shown that the mixed disulfide bond between MEA and the thiol group on papain, a sulfhydryl-dependent enzyme, will protect the thiol of papain against radiation destruction. However, there is, in urease solution, evidence that a protective agent bound to an enzyme by mixed disulfide bonds does not protect it.

Metal Chelation As Protection For Certain Enzymes. The fact that sulfhydryl compounds are often good chelating agents suggested to some workers that chelation might be the means by which the thiol-disulfide protection works. Specifically, chelation of copper in copper enzymes was postulated as protecting by preventing radiation oxidation of the cuprous copper. Other workers have shown a correlation between the instability constant of the copper(II) complex and protective capacity of some of the protective agents — substances which form the most stable complexes with copper(II) are the most protective. There is, however, no direct evidence for this hypothesis.

The Alteration of Tissues to a More Resistant State. Lower metabolic states (hibernation, hypothyroidism) seem to increase radiation resistance. There have been many reports of enzyme-inhibiting effects of thiol protectors on tissue enzymes *in vitro* and *in vivo*. The obvious sick state exhibited by animals during the period of protection also suggests the presence of profound metabolic alterations in these animals.

Localized Radical Scavenging. DNA has been implicated as the main target molecule at least in the so-called mitotic death. Recently, it was shown that DNA can be protected very effectively *in vitro* with GED, cystamine, and with Actinomycin D. Although Actinomycin D is not an amino-alkyl-thiol, it is an excellent protector *in vitro* because of its ability to bind to DNA. GED binds to DNA by virtue of its guanido groups at both ends of the molecule. These groups in a neutral, buffered solution are positively charged, and therefore can act as counter-ions for the negatively charged phosphate groups in the backbone of DNA. GED molecules act as a shield for the DNA by being bound to a great extent, and can react through their disulfide groups with radicals that otherwise would react with the DNA. Since they are not homogeneously distributed in the solution but are in the direct vicinity of the DNA, they act as localized radical scavengers. The same applies to Actinomycin D to an even greater extent because of its great affinity for DNA. The difference between Actinomycin D and GED, as radical scavengers, is that Actinomycin D has no disulfide groups, but can react with radicals through its oligopeptide chains which shield parts of the DNA chain from incoming radicals.

Aminoalkyl-Phosphorothioates. The mechanism of protection by these compounds seems to be the same as for aminoalkyl-thiols. Once administered to animals, they are rapidly dephosphorylated and then act as amino-thiols. The difference in toxicity may be explained on the basis of different distribution. These molecules, being phosphorylated, are distributed differently from aminoalkyl-thiols in the various organs and even in the various organelles of the cells.

Other Sulfur Compounds. The pharmacology of dimethylsulfoxide shows that in protective doses, it reduces oxygen tension in the spleen of mice. Presumably protection for some members of this group is effected by oxygen deprivation, but this may not be the whole picture.

Cyanide and Organic Nitriles. Cyanide produces cytotoxic anoxia by reversibly inhibiting cellular oxidizing enzymes, particularly cytochrome oxidase. The mechanism of protection may be oxygen deprivation. Organic nitriles are only protective when they can liberate cyanide *in vivo*.

Amines. The pharmacology of the amines discussed earlier had been thoroughly studied prior to the discovery of their radiation protective action. They all have the common effect of producing hypoxia in the tissues although the mechanisms are different. Epinephrine produces vasoconstriction, histamine vasodilation, and PAPP methemoglobinemia. The pharmacology of serotinin is complex, but it too is a vasoconstrictor. Actual measurements of splenic oxygen tension have shown reduction after epinephrine and after histamine. Serotonin partly prevents the rise in subcutaneous oxygen tension in rats breathing oxygen at pressures up to 60 p.s.i.

The mechanism of radiation protection by the amines is most likely oxygen deprivation. The fact that serotonin protects *in vitro* suggests some additional mechanism of action. PAPP may also have some additional mechanism of action since sodium nitrite, which produces methemoglobinemia of the same degree, does not show similar protection.

C. Conclusion

The foregoing discussion gives support to the optimistic belief that some degree of radiation protection by chemical agents will be achieved in man. The degree of protection is not likely to exceed a dose-reduction factor of two to three. Protective agents must be given prior to exposure and must be of limited duration. Chronic use of protective agents does not seem possible. Despite these limitations, there may be some practical applications of protective compounds. When a necessary, dangerous, acute radiation exposure of predictable magnitude can be foreseen, the administration of protective agents, when they are safe to use in man, may have value.

One possible solution to the problem of toxicity may be the chemical protection of local areas or specific tissues. If protective agents which protect at the cellular level can be delivered locally to the critical tissue, it may be possible to use amounts of the protective agent large enough to provide a protective level while temporarily confined to the local area and yet small enough to be nontoxic when gradually diluted through the whole body. Local protection may be important in radiotherapy of cancer, since parenteral administration of protective agents may result in protection of the cancer as well as of normal tissues. Work is being done to determine whether these protective agents can be used to obtain differential protection between normal tissues and malignant growths. Phosphorothioates are the most likely candidates for such research because it seems necessary to dephosphorylate (partially metabolize) them in the tissues and cells in order to obtain the protective forms. This partial metabolism takes place at different rates in the different organs, and therein lies the possibility for protection of normal tissues with little or no protection of tumors.

References

1. Bacq, Z. M.: *Chemical Protection Against Ionizing Radiation.* Springfield, Ill., Charles C Thomas, 1965.
2. Kollmann, G., Castel, N., and Shapiro, B.: Further studies on protection of DNA against ionizing radiation. Int. J. Radiat. Biol, 18:587–594, 1970.
3. Kollmann, G., Martin, D., and Shapiro, B.: The distribution and metabolism of the radiation protective agent aminopentylaminoethylphosphorothioate in mice. Radiat. Res., 48:542–550, 1971.
4. Leon, S. A., Kollmann, G., and Shapiro, B.: *In vitro* protection against radiation damage to template activity in DNA synthesis. Int. J. Radiat. Biol., 20:337, 1971.
5. Shapiro, B.: Research in agents to protect against ionizing radiation. Med. Clin. N. Amer., 48:547–561, March, 1964.
6. Shapiro, B., and Kollmann, G.: Mechanism of protection of macromolecules against ionizing radiation by sulphydryl and other protective agents. Vienna, International Atomic Energy Agency, 1969.
7. Shapiro, B., Kollmann, G., and Martin, D.: Mechanism of action of radiation protective agents: *In vivo* distribution and metabolism of cysteamine-s-phosphate (MEAP). Radiat. Res., 44:421–433, 1970.

Bone Marrow Transplantation

G. David Ledney, Ph.D.

For the severe phase of the hemopoietic form of the acute radiation syndrome, additional therapy such as bone marrow transplantations has been employed.

In clinical situations several factors influence the recovery produced by hemopoietic tissue grafting subsequent to radiation-induced hemopoietic aplasia. These factors include the following: the depth of the immunologic suppression produced in the irradiated recipient, the type of hemopoietic tissue grafted, the genetic nature of the recipient with respect to the cells of the donor, and the number and condition of the transplanted cells. The successful engraftment of hemopoietic cells in irradiated patients is related to the depth of immunologic suppression. Physical factors of radiation known to influence immune suppression include total absorbed dose, dose rate, and type of radiation. It is generally acknowledged that a take of allogenic marrow is not likely unless the recipient receives about two times (900–1000 R) the total body LD_{50} dose of X- or γ-irradiation or some combination of immunosuppressive agent.

Because of physical limitations on radiation production, most clinical total body irradiation has been delivered at about 5 to 10 R per minute. There are some experimental and clinical data indicating that chances for successful engraftment are improved when the dose rates for total body X- or γ-radiations are increased to about 70 R per minute. Experimental evidence supports the idea that neutrons have a greater RBE on the immune system than do electromagnetic radiations. It is reasonable to assume, then, that neutrons might be of greater clinical benefit than X- or γ-radiation in suppressing the immune system and subsequently allowing for hemopoietic restoration by a marrow transplant.

All tissues that contain hemopoietic stem cells have potential value in restoring radiation-induced bone marrow aplasia. Most clinical hemopoietic transplantation is done with bone marrow, although some attempts have been made to use fetal liver cells, which are of limited value because of the physical problem involved in collecting and storing sufficient numbers of cells necessary for one transplantation.

9.16 TYPES OF TRANSPLANTS AND THEIR EFFECTS

Useful clinical bone marrow transplants are of three genetic types. They may be autologous (self to self), syngeneic (two genetically similar individuals as in maternal twins), or allogeneic (two genetically dissimilar individuals of the same species). The most successful recorded cases of marrow grafting have involved autologous and syngeneic donor-recipient situations. Because man is an out-bred creature, the greatest number of marrow transplants have been done in the allogeneic donor-recipient situation.

The number of marrow cells necessary to effect restoration of radiation-induced aplasia is related to the genetics of the donor-recipient combination, to the use of fresh or frozen (stored) cells, and to the use of whole-marrow cell populations or stem cell concentrates. In genetically similar combinations, 1 to 2×10^8 whole-marrow cells per kilogram are considered adequate to promote restoration. In allogeneic combinations, 2 to 4×10^8 whole-marrow cells per kilogram are sufficient to promote engraftment.

In instances in which the number of marrow cells derived from one donor was insufficient to produce a take, freezing has been employed in order to accumulate sufficient cell quantities. However, frozen cells are not as effective as fresh cells in restoring radiation-induced aplasia. In any donor-recipient combination, the number of grafted frozen marrow cells is doubled over that prescribed for a fresh marrow transplant.

The application of hemopoietic stem cell concentrates is a new development in clinical bone marrow transplantation. Although adequate information is not available, it can be assumed that the number of cells—fresh or frozen—necessary to effect restoration will be reduced as compared to their whole-marrow cell counterparts.

The cells of a bone marrow graft may be considered to belong to two general groups —hemopoietic stem cells and immunocompetent lymphoid cells. If the graft takes, the stem cells are responsible for restoring hemopoiesis and hence preventing death from radiation-induced aplasia. The lymphoid cell component of the proliferating foreign graft is responsible for mounting a rejection reaction against the host's tissues. This immunologic reaction is known as "graft versus host disease" or secondary disease and is directed mainly against the epithelial tissues of the host: the lining of the intestinal tract, the skin, liver, and lymph nodes become foci of immunologic destruction. Coincident with injury to these organs are microbiologic infections which complicate chemotherapeutic efforts designed to modify or prevent secondary disease.

The untreated severe graft versus host reaction will result in death, even though hemopoietic restoration can be observed. A number of immunosuppressive agents are used for the prevention of secondary disease. Some of the best known include cyclophosphamide, methotrexate, azathioprine, and antilymphocytic serum. These agents act by selectively killing the immunocompetent cell portion of the graft. Similar to radiation, these substances can also induce hemopoietic aplasia, hence care is taken in their use not to destroy the proliferating hemopoietic elements of the transplant. Immunosuppressive therapy designed to prevent secondary disease is attended by systemic infections which result in the death of the patient from infection and not from secondary disease. This problem remains as a stumbling block in efforts designed to obtain long-term survival after marrow transplantation.

New developments in transplantation research have allowed for cautious optimism concerning long-term survival after radiation and marrow transplantation. These include the previously mentioned stem cell concentrate and immunosuppressive drugs. Improved donor selection employing the matching for major HL-A (histocompatability leucocyte-antigens) similarities and differences will certainly result in improved survival times. Advances in these three areas will surely be related to future successful endeavors in the matter of restoring hemopoietic function in lethally irradiated persons. Germane to either accidental or intentional exposure to immune suppressants, such as radiation, radiomimetic, and other chemical agents, is the problem of toxic side effects. Specifically, when physical or chemical agents are used to promote survival from the graft rejection reaction in marrow grafted individuals, care must be taken to employ substances which have specificity or selectivity for the immunocompetent lymphoid cells over that of the hemopoietic stem cells. Additionally, the dose and time scheduling of the drug should be adjusted so as not to re-induce marrow aplasia but to prevent rejection of the graft.

In all cell, tissue, and organ grafting the use of immunosuppressive agents can result in the induction of new, or the promotion of existing, malignancies. Indeed, reports are available where patients died not as a result of the surgical procedure and concomitant drug therapy, but as a consequence to malignant growth.

Physiologic toxicity to immune suppressants at the level of the organ and its vital functioning has also been recorded. Probably the most outstanding of these occur subsequent to therapy with cyclophosphamide and antilymphocyte serum therapy. In the former, fatal myocardial damage was associated with large dosages of the drug, while in the latter, immune complexes can impair normal renal functioning.

Lastly, microbiologic infections are a real problem which may limit the clinical use of immunosuppressive agents. Indeed, many successful cell, tissue, and organ transplants have resulted in death not so much from any of the previously mentioned difficulties, but from infections made difficult to manage by the tenuous circumstances leading to the grafting procedure and the postoperative immunosuppressive therapy.

Reference

1. Balner, H. A., van Bekkum, D. W., and Rapaport, F. T. (eds.): *Proceedings of the Third International Congress of the Transplantation Society, September 7–11, 1970. The Hague, Netherlands.* New York, H. M. Stratton, 1971.

Some Physiologic Effects of Radiation

Glenn V. Dalrymple, M.D.

This section considers radiation effects which involve the interaction of several cellular types, tissues, organs, and so forth. Because of frequent multisystem relationships, absolute classification of the information frequently is difficult.

9.17 ENERGY METABOLISM

One of the fundamental precepts of biology is that all living things must have energy to survive. Recall from biochemistry that the primary biologic carrier of energy is adenosine triphosphate (ATP). ATP has the ability to supply energy for many biochemical reactions because of its pyrophosphate bonds. In a very real sense ATP represents one of the keystones of life. Again from biochemistry (and without going into great detail), we recall that two primary biochemical processes responsible for the generation of ATP are (a) anaerobic glycolysis and (b) aerobic oxidative phosphorylation. While anaerobic glycolysis occurs in the absence of oxygen, it is inefficient with respect to generation of ATP as compared to the more efficient aerobic oxidative phosphorylation. This latter process, which occurs primarily in the mitochondria, uses the cytochrome system to link electrons (obtained by glycolysis and the Krebs citric acid cycle) with oxygen, and by this means oxidizes ADP to ATP.

Drugs such as 2,4-dinitrophenol (DNP) produce what has come to be known as "uncoupling" of oxidative phosphorylation. In this situation, the uptake of O_2 is "uncoupled" from the generation of ATP. As a result, the cell still takes up O_2 (respiration), but the generation of ATP is inhibited. Or in the biochemists' words, respiration is "uncoupled" from the formation of ATP. The intracellular ATP levels, then, drop sharply because the cell consumes ATP at a very rapid rate.

Radiation experiments with whole-body irradiated rats showed that uncoupling of oxidative phosphorylation occurs in mitochondria isolated from radiosensitive tissues such as spleen and thymus. This phenomenon has some interesting aspects. Uncoupling after irradiation occurs *only* in the radiosensitive tissues—it has not been found in mitochondria isolated from radioresistant tissues, such as liver and muscle. Also, the uncoupling in the radiosensitive tissues can be detected only if the tissues are irradiated *in vivo*, and *then* the mitochondria removed. Irradiation of mitochondria *after* isolation produces no uncoupling.

The next point to consider is that, if ATP is necessary for most biologic processes, a cell rendered deficient of ATP (by radiation or by drugs such as DNP), should be less able to repair radiation injury than a cell possessing normal intracellular ATP levels. Since we would think that the repair of any

injury should also be compromised, and since radiation produces uncoupling (and presumably a depression of intracellular ATP levels), the effect would seemingly have importance. Experiments, however, have not borne out this hypothesis. Actually, DNP-treated cells survive the effects of radiation *better* than untreated cells; in fact, paired-dose experiments have shown DNP-treated cells to be able to repair sublethal injury as well as (and in some cases better than) cells with normal ATP levels. Consequently, the phenomenon of uncoupling of oxidative phosphorylation does not seem to influence the cell's ability to withstand radiation injury.

9.18 STRESS REACTIONS

There are several stress-related phenomena that have been observed after irradiation. One of the earliest findings was that radiation caused a depression of adrenal cholesterol during the first few post-irradiation hours. Irradiation of hypophysectomized animals, however, did *not* produce this depression. On the other hand, liver glycogen levels followed the opposite pattern after irradiation: the livers of irradiated rats had a higher glycogen content than the livers of control rats. As with adrenal cholesterol, this phenomenon does *not* occur in irradiated adrenalectomized (and/or hypophysectomized) animals treated with adrenal steroids. Recent histochemical experiments have indicated increased secretory activity of cells in the hypothalamic-pituitary axis in both whole-body and head-only irradiated animals. These findings support the notion that radiation has the ability to trigger the stress mechanism. The stress-related phenomena (such as uncoupling of oxidative phosphorylation), while a consequence of irradiation, do not, however, represent the primary radiation "lesion."

9.19 ENZYME RELEASE

The release of enzymes after irradiation has been observed in many systems. The effects of radiation on the serum lactic dehydrogenase (LDH) levels of irradiated monkeys will serve as an example. During the first three days after a lethal dose of radiation, the LDH concentration increases to levels three to 10 times greater than normal. After this period, though, the LDH concentration returns to normal. The explanation is based on the notion that, for a period of time after exposure, LDH leaks from cells — this accounts for the rise. The subsequent fall of LDH levels occurs because of the physiologic clearance of LDH from the plasma. A similar effect has been observed for SGOT (serum glutamic oxaloacetic transaminase).

Although once thought to represent the key to the radiation "lesion," these enzyme changes are probably not of primary importance. They may, however, be valuable as a clinical diagnostic tool. In the absence of a clear history of irradiation, the diagnosis of "radiation sickness" can be very difficult. Elevated LDH and SGOT levels may be of real value in these patients.

References

1. Bacq, Z. M., and Alexander, P. (eds.): *International Series of Monographs on Pure and Applied Biology; Fundamentals of Radiobiology*, Vol. V. London, Pergamon Press, 1961.
2. Dalrymple, G. V., Lindsay, I. R., and Ghidoni, J. J.: The effect of 2 MeV whole-body X-irradiation on primates. Radiat. Res., 25:377–400, 1965.
3. Klouwen, H. M.: Radiosensitivity of nuclear ATP synthesis and its relation to inhibition of mitosis. *In* University of Texas M. D. Anderson Hospital and Tumor Institute (Houston): *Cellular Radiation Biology*. Baltimore, Williams and Wilkins, 1965.
4. Shapiro, B.: Biochemical mechanisms in the action of radiation. *In* Schwartz, E. E. (ed.): *The Biological Basis of Radiation Therapy*. Philadelphia, J. B. Lippincott, 1966.

10 LATE EFFECTS

Radiation Carcinogenesis

Arthur C. Upton, M.D.

10.0 INTRODUCTION

In the half century which has elapsed since the carcinogenic action of ionizing radiation was first recognized, radiation carcinogenesis has been studied extensively in human and animal populations. Within recent decades, interest in the subject has been intensified because of the proliferation of radiation sources in the modern world, to the extent that there is now growing concern over the possibility that small increases in environmental radiation might augment the risk of cancer.

Although precise estimates of the risks to man can be derived only from comprehensive dose-response data for human populations, such data are fragmentary as yet. Moreover, a full understanding of the induction of cancer by irradiation will require systematic study of the nature and mechanism of the process in laboratory animals and model systems. For this reason, relevant experimental studies, as well as human studies, are discussed.

Any consideration of radiation carcinogenesis in human populations is complicated by at least six difficulties. (1) Large populations must be studied so that precise data on the incidence of neoplasms at any given site can be derived. (2) Few populations exist which are sufficiently large and exposed to a significantly high and quantifiable dose to yield dose-incidence data.

(3) The long latent period, intervening between irradiation and the appearance of neoplasia, complicates the follow-up of exposed individuals in prospective studies and complicates evaluation of their exposure history in retrospective studies. (4) Because of the long latent period and the limited follow-up of irradiated populations to date, it is not yet possible to estimate the risks of radiation-induced cancer for the entire life span. (5) Many of the existing data are based on patients who were exposed to radiation for medical purposes and in whom the effects of radiation may be complicated by the effects of other treatments or of the underlying disease itself, complicating the applicability of such data to the general population. (6) The probability of the natural occurrence of cancer varies widely from one organ to another and is influenced by genetic background, age, sex, geographic location, diet, socio-economic factors, and other variables, the action of which is not yet understood. Based on experimental results with laboratory animals, and on the limited empirical data available from human populations, it seems probable that susceptibility to radiation-induced cancer in man varies likewise under the influence of many of these, and possibly other, variables. Hence, dose-incidence data derived from any one population may not be entirely applicable to another. Because of these difficulties, the existing information

on radiation carcinogenesis has limitations which should not be forgotten while considering the data summarized in the following pages.

10.1 SKIN CANCER

In 1902, the first neoplasm attributed to radiation injury was reported: an epidermoid carcinoma on the hand of a radiologist. It was soon followed by reports of similar cases among pioneer radiation workers, who exposed their hands repeatedly to radiation when using their primitive equipment. The development of injury in many of these victims began with reddening and blistering of the skin, often within a few weeks after exposure. Whether or not exposure was then discontinued, the lesions frequently remained painful and were followed within a few years by atrophy of the epidermis, ulceration, and ultimately malignant change. The cancers arising in this way were frequently multiple and occurred on both exposed hands. Within 15 years after Roentgen's discovery of X-rays, nearly 100 such cases of skin cancer had been reported in America, England, and Germany, half of them in physicians and the other half in X-ray technicians.

In nearly all reported X-ray-induced cancers, antecedent radiodermatitis and a relatively long latent period have been observed to separate the time of initial irradiation from the clinical onset of neoplasia (Figure 10–1). The majority of the cancers have been squamous cell and basal cell carcinomas, but fibrosarcomas also have been reported.

The relation between the risk of cancer and the radiation dose to the skin is not known. Since the evolution of modern safety standards, however, epidermoid carcinoma has ceased to be an occupational disease of radiologists, although there continue to be reports of radiodermatitis and cancer among dentists and others using radiation equipment without strict adherence to contemporary protection guides. It is generally postulated that the probability of cancer varies with the severity of antecedent radiodermatitis and that the acute radiation dose required to cause cancer exceeds 1000 R. Some evidence indicates, however, that prolonged exposure to less than four R per day may culminate in neoplasia. Recent reports have described tumors occurring at the site of irradiation in skin that appeared clinically normal. Nevertheless, the absence of a manifestly increased incidence in atomic bomb survivors, irradiated spondylitics, and children irradiated therapeutically

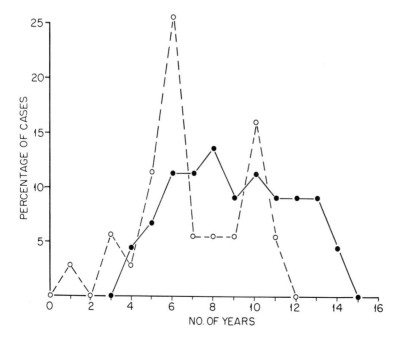

FIGURE 10–1 Latent period in radiogenic skin cancer of man. Circles indicate time after onset of radiodermatitis; dots indicate time after first irradiation. (From Upton, A. C.: Comparative observations on radiation carcinogenesis in man and animals. *In* University of Texas, M. D. Anderson Hospital and Tumor Institute: *Carcinogenesis; A Broad Critique.* Baltimore, Williams and Wilkins, 1967.)

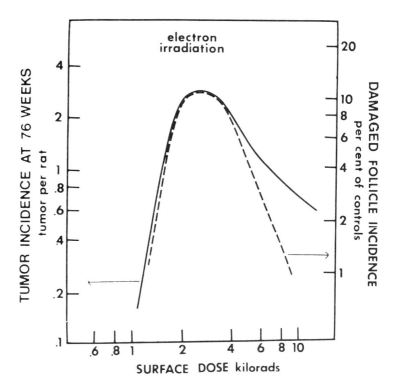

FIGURE 10-2 Cumulative incidence of skin tumors and abnormal hair follicles in rats irradiated with alpha particles. (From Burns, F. J., Albert, R. E., and Heimbach, R. D.: The RBE for skin tumors and hair follicle damage in the rat following irradiation with alpha particles and electrons. Radiat. Res., 36:225, 1968.)

over the mediastinum in infancy supports the tentative conclusion that the risk per unit dose is relatively low in comparison with the risk of other neoplasms.

In experimental animals, cutaneous carcinogenesis induced by ionizing radiation has been studied extensively. Tumors of the skin caused by radiation vary in character with host factors and with the conditions of irradiation. A high incidence of neoplasia generally requires doses of radiation that cause ulceration with residual vascular changes and scarring, or permanent damage to hair follicles. The ensuing neoplasms appear to arise from proliferating epidermal cells or fibroblasts at the margins of the ulcers or in irreparably damaged hair follicles. Nonulcerating doses also have been found to be weakly carcinogenic, however, even in the absence of obvious radiodermatitis or residual damage.

As yet, it has not been fully possible to define the relation among the factors influencing the development of cutaneous neoplasia (i.e., total radiation dose, dose rate, area, and depth—number of epidermal and dermal cells irradiated) and physiologic condition of the host. It would appear, however, that the effects of radiation may be enhanced by croton oil, chemical carcinogens, and conceivably by irradiation of distant parts of the body. In rats, a dose correlation has been noted between the yield of tumors and the frequency of irreparably damaged hair follicles, tumor induction being maximal when the follicles are irradiated throughout their length and at doses ranging from 2000 to 4000 r (Figure 10–2). At doses below this range, radiation apppears to be less effective, presumably because of failure to induce permanent damage to the hair follicles. At doses exceeding the optimal range, radiation loses effectiveness presumably by leaving too few surviving follicular cells capable of proliferation.

10.2 LEUKEMIA

A. Human Data

The leukemogenic action of ionizing radiation was first noted in 1911, in a report of 11 cases in radiation workers which suggested that their occupational exposure might have been of significance. Since then, an association between leukemia and radiation exposure has been amply documented by epidemiologic studies of exposed populations. Such populations include American radiologists, Japanese atomic bomb survivors, patients treated with X-rays for rheumatoid spondylitis, and children irradiated over the mediastinum in infancy for thymic enlargement or other diseases. Intra-uterine and preconceptual irradiation, as a result of diagnostic X-ray examination of the mother, also have been tentatively implicated in the pathogenesis of childhood leukemia by certain retrospective population surveys; other studies have suggested that additional factors are involved and that radiation acts merely as a co-factor under these circumstances.

The precise relation between incidence and dose is not evident from the available data, owing to statistical limitations and to the paucity of cases at low dose levels. It is clear, however, that acute whole body irradiation, or exposure of the major part of the hemopoietic marrow to a dose in the range of 50 to 1000 r, increases the incidence of the disease. The dose-response relation is consistent with a linear regression, but the existing data are also compatible with other dose-response functions (Figure 10–3). A risk of one to two cases of leukemia per million person-years at risk per rad was estimated for the Japanese atomic bomb survivors at doses between 100 rads and 900 rads, based on the excess incidence averaged over the period of 1945 to 1958. A more recent study, based on new estimates of dose (1965) and the leukemia incidence to 1966, suggests that the risk for survivors in Hiroshima may be slightly higher, conceivably because of the neutron component of their exposure, if the neutron RBE is assumed to be greater than 1.0. A similar, if slightly lower, risk estimate $(0.5/10^6/\text{year}/\text{R})$ has been derived for fractionated therapeutic spinal irradiation of patients with ankylosing spondylitis in Great Britain, based on the excess incidence of leukemia averaged over about seven years after exposures of 300 to 1500 R.

In both atomic-bomb survivors and spondylitics, the excess incidence of leukemia appeared within one to two years, reached a peak after five to seven

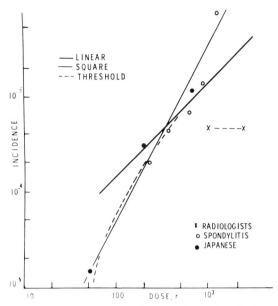

FIGURE 10–3 Dose-incidence relationship for leukemia in radiologists, irradiated spondylitic patients, and Japanese atomic bomb survivors. (From Brues, 1959, cited in Upton, A. C.; Comparative observations on radiation carcinogenesis in man and animals. *In* University of Texas, M. D. Anderson Hospital and Tumor Institute: *Carcinogenesis; A Broad Critique.* Baltimore, Williams and Wilkins, 1967.)

years, and declined after 15 years following irradiation, but as yet there is no conclusive evidence that it has disappeared entirely.

Some justification for assuming that leukemia may be caused by low doses is provided by evidence that prenatal exposure to one-to-five rads in diagnostic procedures is associated with an increased incidence in leukemia and other cancers in childhood. Based on these data, the risks of prenatal irradiation are greater than those for postnatal irradiation, by a factor ranging between two and ten. As in the case of ankylosing spondylitics, however, there is the possibility that the irradiated individuals may not be representative of the general population and that etiologic factors other than radiation have not been excluded. This possibility is further suggested by the fact that no association between prenatal exposure and childhood leukemia has been detected in Japanese atomic-bomb survivors.

In 425 death certificates of radiologists dying between the ages of 35 and 74 years during a 14-year period (1948 to 1961), 12 cases of leukemia were observed, as compared with four cases expected, which corresponds to an excess incidence of $168/10^6$/year. All 12 cases of leukemia were of hematologic types known to be increased by irradiation (i.e., other than chronic lymphocytic). In addition, there were five deaths from multiple myeloma, as compared with one expected; and four deaths from aplastic anemia, as compared with 0.2 expected. On the other hand, for Hodgkin's disease, lymphosarcoma, and lymphoblastoma, the observed numbers of deaths were in reasonable agreement with the expected numbers.

Little is known about the doses received by the radiologists, especially those practicing in the early days of radiology, but the average exposure accumulated by these radiologists may have amounted to 100 R per year, while with recent standards of protection the yearly exposure is about one R. Since the excess incidence of leukemia in the radiologists corresponds to that which would result from a single whole body dose of about 100 rads, based on the risk estimates for leukemia in Japanese atomic bomb survivors (one to two cases/10^6/year/rad), the data suggest that long-term radiation exposure is less effective than short-term exposure in inducing leukemia. It is doubtful, however, that the radiation was uniform or consistently involved the whole body. Hence, the possible influence of these other variables must be taken into account.

Although partial body irradiation is clearly leukemogenic when a large volume of hemopoietic tissue is irradiated, as in the spondylitics and infants irradiated therapeutically over the mediastinum, there is no evidence that exposure of a small volume of hemopoietic marrow is leukemogenic in patients treated with radiotherapy for cancer. Radiotherapy from ^{131}I in patients treated for thyroid cancer and from ^{32}P in patients treated for polycythemia vera has been reported to be followed by leukemia in a few cases, but in these patients the whole marrow was exposed. A few cases of leukemia have also been reported in association with high radium burdens and after intravenous injection of thorium dioxide (thorotrast). No evidence of leukemogenic effects have been detectable, on the other hand, in patients treated with radioiodine

for thyrotoxicosis, which involves an estimated dose of seven to thirteen rads to the bone marrow.

When considering the induction of leukemia, it is necessary to distinguish between different hematologic types of the disease, since the incidence of the various types differs both with age and with irradiation. There is no evidence to date that the incidence of chronic lymphocytic leukemia is affected at all by irradiation, whereas the combined incidence of all other types of leukemia increases with age at irradiation in adult life (Figure 10–4). The types of leukemia chiefly responsible for the excess in adults are the acute myeloid and the chronic myeloid types. On the other hand, susceptibility to the induction of acute lymphatic, or stem cell, leukemia appears to be highest in childhood and to decrease sharply during maturation, as judged from findings in atomic bomb survivors. In view

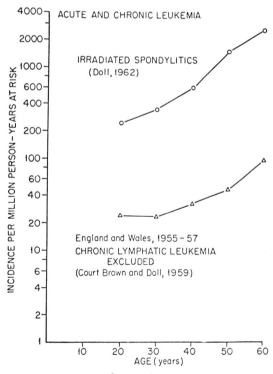

FIGURE 10–4 Incidence of acute and chronic leukemia, chronic lymphatic excluded, in irradiated spondylitics in relation to age at time of irradiation. (From Upton, A. C.: Comparative observations on radiation carcinogenesis in man and animals. *In* University of Texas, M. D. Anderson Hospital and Tumor Institute: *Carcinogenesis; A Broad Critique.* Baltimore, Williams and Wilkins, 1967.)

of these differences in susceptibility, it is clear that numerical risk estimates must be considered no more than crude approximations. Whereas such estimates may have some use in evaluating overall risks to the population at large, it is clear that the risks to individuals may differ drastically and defy characterization at present.

Using the assumption of a linear dose-incidence relationship as a base, it can be estimated by extrapolation from the effects of large doses that natural background radiation might account for roughly one-tenth of the "spontaneously occurring" cases of leukemia. If, however, the incidence were assumed to vary as a quadratic function of the dose, the proportion of "spontaneous" leukemias thus attributable to natural background radiation would be far lower (i.e., less than 1 per cent) (Table 10–1). To explore the possible existence of a correlation between background radiation and the "spontaneous" occurrence of leukemia, the incidence of the disease in populations inhabiting areas differing in background radiation has been analyzed. Such studies have failed to demonstrate a systematic correlation between the level of background radiation from terrestrial or cosmic sources and the incidence of leukemia among populations in different areas. Interpretation of these findings is complicated, however, by the possible effects of variables other than background radiation on the leukemia rates in question.

B. Animal Data

Lymphoma. If we turn to animal studies for experimental and theoretical data to strengthen our concepts of human dose-effect relationships, an extensive body of information is available. The most widely studied experimental leukemia is a lymphosarcoma of the mouse thymus. This neoplasm may be induced in many strains of mice by a variety of agents. Its induction by irradiation is inhibited in the presence of intact hemopoietic tissue; that is, by shielding spleen or marrow from radiation or by infusion of nonirradiated hemopoietic cells after whole body irradiation. Moreover, nonirradiated thymic tissue may be rendered neoplastic by implantation into an irradiated recipient, thus conclusively demonstrating the role of host injury in the pathogenesis of this disease.

The relation between the incidence of the disease and the dose of radiation is complex, depending on time-intensity factors as well as the total dose. In general, a given dose of low LET radiation (but not of high LET radiation) becomes less leukemogenic as the duration of irradiation is increased (Figure 10–5). However, the

TABLE 10–1 ESTIMATED INCIDENCES OF LEUKEMIA INDUCED BY LOW LEVELS OF RADIATION*

Radiation	Dose-Rate Assumed (rems/yr)	Duration of Exposure (yrs)	Estimated Incidence (No. of Cases) of Radiogenic Leukemia**		
			Linear Theory (After Lewis, 1957)	Present 'Two-Hit' Theory Possible Range	
Natural					per 50 million persons in 70 years (as compared with nearly 200,000 "natural" cases)
Background	0.1	70	25,000	1.0 to 100	
Fallout	0.01	70	2500	0.2 to 20	
Maximum					in a population of 4000 over a lifetime of occupational exposure (as compared with 15 "natural" cases)
Permissible		5.0	40	32	0.1 to 10
Occupational					
Exposure					

*(From Burch: Radiation carcinogenesis: A new hypothesis. Nature, *185*:135, 1960.)
**Estimates based on "linear theory" are derived essentially by extrapolation of "linear" curve in Figure 10–3; estimates based on "two-hit theory" are derived essentially by extrapolation of "square" curve in Figure 10–3.

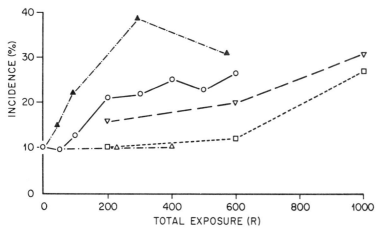

FIGURE 10–5 Dose-incidence relation for lymphomas in whole-body-irradiated female RF mice, as influenced by protraction or fractionation of irradiation. (All mice were 10 weeks old at start of irradiation.) ○, single acute exposure to ^{60}Co gamma-rays at 7 rads/min. △, daily exposure to ^{60}Co gamma-rays at 0.005 rads/min. ▽, two exposures to 3000-kVp X-rays at 75 rads/min, with 270 days elapsing between exposures. □, 10 exposures to 300-kVp X-rays at 75 rads/min, 30 days elapsing between successive exposures. ▲, daily exposure to fast neutrons at 0.0006 to 0.006 rads/min. (From Upton, A. C.: Comparative observations on radiation carcinogenesis in man and animals. *In* University of Texas, M. D. Anderson Hospital and Tumor Institute: *Carcinogenesis; A Broad Critique.* Baltimore, Williams and Wilkins, 1967.)

same dose may be even more leukemogenic if given in several properly timed fractions than if given in a single exposure.

The duration of the mean induction period in experimental animals is inversely related to dose. Relatively few neoplasms are evident clinically within 100 days after irradiation, and a few appear late in life, the peak mortality from the disease occurring 150 to 400 days after a single exposure.

Susceptibility to induction of the lymphoma varies with strain, sex, and age. Female mice are generally more susceptible than males, and this difference is lessened by gonadectomy. With involution of the thymus in adult life, susceptibility diminishes in both sexes. Irradiation does not greatly increase the incidence or reduce the induction period in mice of high lymphoma strains.

Complete characterization of the mechanism of leukemogenesis is not possible at this time, but filterable leukemogenic agents have been repeatedly extracted from thymic tumors in irradiated mice, suggesting that the induction of this neoplasm depends on the activation of a latent leukemia virus. The nature of this effect, its relation to the dosage of radiation, and the mode of action of conditioning physiologic and genetic variables remain to be elucidated.

The production of an irreversible "initiating" or "priming" effect by irradiation, which may be subsequently promoted by various agents, and the inhibition of leukemogenesis by testosterone or corticoids even administered after irradiation, suggest that the evolution of neoplasia in the thymus is a multistage process. This inference is supported by the stepwise progression of autonomy in such growths, as judged on serial biopsy and transplantation. The action of radiation may, therefore, include various combinations of "initiating," "promoting," and even "inhibiting" effects, depending on the dose and conditions of exposure.

Myeloid Leukemia. The induction of myeloid leukemia by ionizing radiation has received less study than the induction of thymic lymphomas, probably because myeloid leukemia is uncommon in most laboratory animals. As in the genesis of thymic lymphoma, however, the induction of myeloid leukemia is conditioned by physiologic variables (i.e., species, age, sex, hormonal activity, and other factors) and is inhibited by shielding part of the body. In the mouse it has also been associated with the appearance of a filterable leukemogenic agent in the affected tissues, suggesting a viral mechanism in its pathogenesis.

Dose-incidence relationships for experimental myeloid leukemia have been studied systematically only in mice of the RF strain. In these animals, the incidence is maximal after 200 to 400 r acute whole body radiation. The shape of the curve below 100 r is uncertain but appears curvilinear within the limits of experimental error. The decline of the curve above 300 r cannot be explained but is a feature characteristic of many other neoplasms. It may conceivably reflect excessive injury to hemopoietic organs and to the host at high radiation dose levels. The induction of leukemias is decreased at low dose rates of low LET irradiation as is the induction of lymphomas and other neoplasms.

Myeloid leukemias and other myeloproliferative disorders have been observed in dogs, rats, and swine exposed to chronic irradiation of the marrow by ^{90}Sr and other internally deposited radionuclides. Systematic dose-response data for these species are, however, lacking as yet.

10.3 OSTEOSARCOMA

A. Human Data

Several decades ago the occurrence of osteosarcomas in more than 40 clock dial painters, who had inadvertently ingested radium and mesothorium in the application of luminous paint to clock and watch dials, called attention to the carcinogenic risks of internal emitters. In addition to osteosarcomas, fibrosarcomas have been seen in these workers, as well as carcinomas of epithelial cells lining the paranasal sinuses and nasopharynx. Hence, although radium dial painting began around 1915, it was not until the period 1925 to 1927, after serious injury had been encountered among workers, that adequate occupational safety measures were taken.

In these and other populations (Table 10–2) the incidence of bone tumors has been interpreted to vary approximately as the square of the terminal concentration of radium in the skeleton (see United Nations, 1964; Mole, 1969), a relationship which is consistent with that observed in experimental animals (Mole, 1969). Such populations, which are comprised of several hundred persons, have failed to

TABLE 10–2 INCIDENCE OF BONE CANCER IN RELATION TO SKELETAL RADIATION DOSE*

Skeletal Dose†	No. of Persons	Incidence per 10^5 per year	
		Male	Female
10.8	30	—	1900
5.2	19	—	1336
3.0	19	—	493
0.26	10^3	—	6.20
2.2×10^{-3}	10^5	1.77	2.53
1.0×10^{-2}	4×10^6	1.91	1.62
9×10^{-4}	3.5×10^6	1.97‡	1.59‡

*From Marinelli: Radioactivity and the human skeleton. Am. J. Roentgen., 80:729, 1958.
†Skeletal dose in units equivalent to 1 μc ^{226}Ra + 0.3 μc daughters permanently fixed in skeleton.
‡Data for population of Chicago, 1940–1950 (excluding cancer of jaw).

disclose evidence of tumor induction associated with terminal body burdens of less than 0.5 microcuries of ^{226}Ra or its equivalent, although the incidence exceeds 20 per cent at levels of 5 microcuries or more. Expression of the dose-incidence relation in rads is complicated by the inhomogeneity of the radiation dose in space and time, radium localizing in "hotspots" where the dose may be an order of magnitude higher than in surrounding bone. Furthermore, the amount of radium present in the skeleton at the time the tumors have been detected has invariably been only a small percentage of the amount present earlier. The latent period for induction of tumors appears to vary inversely with the radium content of the skeleton, being as short as 10 years in patients with 6 to 50 mg of radium, but averaging about 25 years in those with smaller radium burdens.

Osteosarcomas have also been reported sporadically following radiotherapy with penetrating external radiation. The doses in such cases invariably have been large, ranging from 3000 to more than 15,000 rads. The latent period of such tumors have averaged nine years, and the ages of the affected patients have ranged from less than 10 years to more than 60 years.

In addition to osteosarcomas, benign tumors have been noted. These are comprised chiefly of osteochondromas, developing after radiotherapy to the mediastinum in infancy, and exostoses in children injected with radium. The interval between irradiation and histologic diagnosis in these cases has averaged roughly 11 years and the radiation dose less than 500 rads. The lower doses associated with these neoplasms, as compared with the osteosarcomas, imply that susceptibility to induction of bone tumors may be appreciably higher in children than in adults, and that the corresponding tumors induced by irradiation during childhood are predominantly benign, whereas those induced by irradiation in adult life are predominantly malignant.

B. Animal Data

A variety of bone tumors have been induced in experimental animals. Most of the available data come from experiments with internally deposited isotopes; in these cases evaluation of dose-effect relations and mechanisms of tumorigenesis is complicated by the following: (1) nonuniformity in the deposition of radioisotopes within the skeleton, the dose in "hot spots" being higher than that in surrounding bone, possibly by a factor of ten or more; (2) changes with time in the distribution and concentration of radioactivity in bone

owing to metabolic turnover and excretion of the radioelement and its decay daughters; and (3) progressive diminution in the dose rate of the emitted radiation with physical decay of the emitter.

The comparative tumorigenic activity of various bone-seeking radionuclides has been studied in several animal species. Differences in tumorigenic potency have been observed (Figure 10–6) which reflect differences in the quality of the emitted radiation (i.e., energy and charge), as well as in the uptake, distribution, and retention of the radionuclide within the skeleton. Possibly because of differences in the geometry of the radiation between the mouse and larger animals which hinders escape of penetrating radiation from larger bones and makes for less "wastage" of the total emission, the dog has been observed to be several times more susceptible than the mouse to the same injected dose of ^{90}Sr. The sensitivity of the whole endosteum to tumor induction may, however, be similar in humans and in the several animal species studied to date, including the mouse. The probability of tumor induction in the mouse and the dog has been esti-

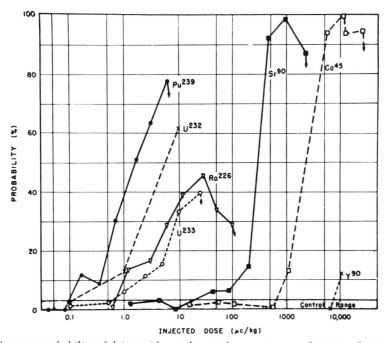

FIGURE 10–6 Average probability of dying with a malignant bone tumor as a function of isotope dose in mice. (From Findel, 1959, cited in Upton, A. C.: Comparative observations on radiation carcinogenesis in man and animals. In University of Texas, M. D. Anderson Hospital and Tumor Institute: *Carcinogenesis; A Broad Critique*. Baltimore, Williams and Wilkins, 1967.)

mated to be directly proportional to the square of the number of beta particles liberated in the skeleton per kilogram of body weight, but in all animal species studied thus far, the dose-incidence curves obtained with alpha emitters, such as radium, imply a more nearly linear dose-effect relation and hence a relatively high RBE for alpha particles.

10.4 THYROID TUMORS

The incidence of thyroid tumors has been observed to be increased in children subjected to external radiation therapy in the neck region in infancy, in Marshall Islanders accidentally exposed to nuclear fallout in childhood, and in Japanese atomic bomb survivors. In these populations the growths have included carcinomas, adenomas, and hyperplastic nodules, developing after a latent period which has averaged 10 to 20 years.

None of the populations surveyed to date has contained enough cases to indicate the dose-incidence relation precisely, but it has been estimated from pooled data that the incidence of thyroid cancer after therapeutic irradiation of the neck in childhood approximates one case per 10^6 person-years at risk per rad during the first 15 years after exposure to a dose of 100 to 300 rads. This estimate may need to be re-evaluated, however, after allowances for variation in irradiation technique, since the dose to the thyroid may vary appreciably with beam direction and port size.

In the Marshall Islanders, the incidence of thyroid nodules among heavily exposed children who were under ten years of age at the time of irradiation increased from 0 to more than 80 per cent between 8 and 16 years after exposure (51 cases/10^6/rad/year). Two of the affected individuals showed evidence of hypothyroidism. The radiation dose to the thyroid was estimated to approximate 700 to 1400 rads from internally deposited radioiodine and 175 rads from external γ rays. Less than 10 per cent of those exposed similarly at ages older than 10 years, and none of 200 individuals in an unexposed control group, have shown comparable lesions.

Tumorigenic effects of therapeutic irradiation of the thyroid gland in adolescence or in adult life have been suggested,

but not proved, in patients treated with ^{131}I for thyrotoxicosis and patients treated with external irradiation for thyrotoxicosis, cervical lymphadenitis, or other lesions occurring in the vicinity of the thyroid.

Observations in animal populations are consistent with those in humans. A number of investigators have reported induction of thyroid tumors in rats, mice, and sheep. The neoplasms, which resemble the papillary and follicular growths resulting from prolonged administration of goitrogens or iodine-deficient diets, show an optimal radiation dose range. Thus, investigators have on occasion failed to induce such tumors by administering too much radioiodine, thereby essentially destroying the gland. Based on the amount of radioiodine needed to "initiate" neoplasia in rats treated with methylthiouracil, it is estimated that 30 mg of ^{131}I corresponds to 1100 rads of X-rays applied externally to the thyroid gland.

10.5 PULMONARY TUMORS

Carcinoma of the lung, long an occupational disability of pitchblende miners in Saxony and Bohemia, has only recently been attributed primarily to occupational irradiation in this population. Uranium miners in the United States also show an elevated incidence of pulmonary carcinoma, the rate increasing with the duration and intensity of exposure, even after correction for such variables as age, cigarette consumption, heredity, urbanization, self-selection, diagnostic accuracy, prior hard-rock mining, and nonradioactive-ore constituents including silica dust. There is evidence, however, that cigarette smoking contributes significantly to the observed risk.

Carcinoma of the bronchus has also been observed in excess among irradiated spondylitics. Since the bronchi were customarily included within the radiation field in these patients, the excess may be tentatively attributed to irradiation. Among Japanese atomic bomb survivors, there is evidence suggesting an increased incidence of lung cancer, but the data are inconclusive as yet.

In miners, determination of the dose-incidence relation is complicated by uncertainties inherent in the circumstances of irradiation. The average duration of exposure among affected miners is 15 to 20 years. The cumulative dose received by any given individual in this time is highly uncertain, but estimates of the average dose to the bronchial epithelium vary from about one rad per 40-hour week to values one to two orders of magnitude lower. Meaningful dose-incidence regressions for bronchial cancer in the other irradiated populations are not available as yet.

In laboratory animals alveolar and bronchial neoplasms have been reported following local irradiation from external and internal sources under a variety of circumstances; however, systematic data on dose-incidence relationships and mechanisms are not yet available.

10.6 OTHER NEOPLASMS

A variety of neoplasms other than those mentioned above have been reported to be induced by irradiation, but the evidence for this is less quantitative or less conclusive than for the neoplasms already discussed. These tumors and the populations affected are as follows: lymphomas, in atomic bomb survivors and irradiated spondylitics; tumors of the pharynx, after therapeutic external irradiation in spondylitics and in patients treated for thyrotoxicosis or other lesions in the neck; tumors of the stomach and pancreas, in irradiated spondylitics; cancer of the uterus, in atomic bomb survivors; cholangiomas and hemangioendotheliomas of the liver, in patients injected intravascularly with thorium dioxide (thorotrast); cancer of the breast, after multiple fluoroscopies for pulmonary tuberculosis and in atomic bomb survivors; salivary gland tumors, after therapeutic external irradiation of the head and neck in infancy; and miscellaneous neoplasms of other types and sites, after intensive localized irradiation.

Such a wide variety of other neoplasms has been reported in irradiated animals that radiation must be considered to be potentially carcinogenic to nearly all tissues under the proper conditions of dosage and host responsiveness. This does not mean, however, that all types of tumors will be induced in any given population under normal circumstances.

The diversity of observed neoplasms in human and animal populations points to the general susceptibility of different tissues of the body to radiation carcinogenesis, but it is not yet possible to specify the relative susceptibility of each organ in quantitative terms. The comparatively long latent period of solid tumors, as compared with leukemias, and the relatively short follow-up of most of the irradiated human populations investigated to date make it likely that further observation will significantly extend existing data. Thus far, the findings in humans are consistent with observations in experimental animals, implying that the carcinogenic effects of radiation will not be fully manifest in a given population until all members of the population have been followed until death, particularly after irradiation at low dose levels. From existing data, some tissues appear to be more susceptible than others, but no final conclusions will be possible without more complete information.

10.7 DOSE-RESPONSE RELATION

Theoretically, cancer may be envisaged to occur through a series of events occurring at any time from before conception (inherited changes) until the appearance of the disease. Any or all of these events may be postulated to be caused by radiation, in which case the dose required for induction of cancer in a given individual may be conceived to vary, depending on the extent to which the necessary changes occur through mechanisms other than radiation. It is evident that under certain conditions ionizing radiation can increase the probability of neoplasia in many organs, but quantitative data concerning the relation between tumor incidence and radiation dose are scanty, particularly at low doses (less than 50 rads) and low dose rates. Although the incidence of leukemia in atomic bomb survivors and of thyroid cancer in patients irradiated therapeutically in childhood is consistent with a linear function of the radiation dose, the data are also consistent with other relationships. Moreover, the bulk of available evidence argues against the hypothesis that the neoplastic transformation is a simple "one-hit" process and, therefore, a linear function of dose. On the contrary, there are grounds for postulating that radiation may influence the process of carcinogenesis through a variety of effects, depending on the particular conditions in a given case, with the dose-response curve varying accordingly.

In general, experimental dose-incidence data reveal several noteworthy features. (1) In the high dose region the dose-incidence curve tends to plateau or even to decline with increasing dose, owing to excessive injury. (2) In the intermediate dose region the curve tends to be steeper than at lower or higher dose levels, owing to optimal interaction of the combined effects of different types of radiation reactions influencing tumorigenesis. (3) With decreasing dose and dose rate the curve tends to become less steep, at least in the case of low LET radiation, presumably because of the influence of repair of some of the radiation injury, "wastage" of radiation, and the absence of enhancing effects that are exerted at higher dose levels.

Whatever the shape of the dose-incidence curve at high doses and high dose rates, the shape of the dose-incidence curve at low doses and low dose rates is a matter of speculation, involving assumptions concerning the mechanisms of carcinogenesis, the influence of dose rate, the distribution of individual dose thresholds in a population, and the latent period for the neoplasm in question.

If, for purposes of radiation protection, estimates of the risk of induction of cancer by low level radiation are to be made, an acceptable, safe hypothetical dose-incidence relationship must be assumed for extrapolation. There are cogent reasons for adopting the linear dose-effect hypothesis for this purpose, since it permits the selection of a single value for characterizing the exposure of a group (mean accumulated tissue dose), the integration of partial body or partial organ exposure, and the neglect of dose rate. By contrast, the use of a non-linear dose-incidence hypothesis requires allowance for the influence of each of these variables, the action of which is not yet adequately known.

Apart from the epidemiologic data reviewed in the preceding, the elevated frequency of chromosomal abnormalities in radiation workers, their inducibility by small amounts of radiation, and their possible significance in the etiology of cancer argue for a conservative approach to the estimation of the hazards of low level radiation.

10.8 POSSIBLE MECHANISMS OF RADIATION CARCINOGENESIS

Because of the mutagenic potency of ionizing radiation, it has long been postulated that radiation-induced somatic mutations play an etiologic role in radiation-induced cancer. Furthermore, the recognition that the induction and expression of point mutations in animal germ cells do not usually follow one-hit kinetics serves to reconcile the mutation hypothesis with the existence of time-intensity and quality effects which have been observed in the experimental induction of neoplasms and the dependence of the neoplasia in certain instances on hormonal stimulation or other conditioning factors. Nevertheless, since neoplasms seem generally to evolve through a stepwise succession of changes, it is unlikely that carcinogenesis results from a single mutation. If, however, cancer arises as the final result of a series of successive alterations, some of which may be mutations, it is conceivable that a single radiation-induced mutation might contribute to the neoplastic process in a suitably conditioned individual. Consistent with this interpretation are preliminary data on the age-specific incidence of malignant growths among Japanese atomic bomb survivors and spondylitics, in whom the numbers of leukemias induced by irradiation apparently vary in relation to age at time of exposure (Figure 10–4).

The indirect induction of neoplasia in unirradiated tissue by effects of radiation on other parts of the body, which cannot be ascribed to mutagenic effects in the ordinary sense, has been amply documented in the experimental induction of thymic lymphomas and pituitary tumors in mice. In the case of mouse lymphomas, osteosarcomas, and certain leukemias, tumorigenesis involves the activation of a latent leukemia virus. The mechanism of this process and the possible role of viruses in the pathogenesis of other radiation-induced neoplasms remains to be determined.

In induction of mouse pituitary tumors, neoplasia results in some instances from hormonal disturbances caused by radiation injury of target organs, such as the thyroid. Likewise, interference with hormonal regulation has been implicated in the pathogenesis of tumors of other endocrine tissues. Other types of indirect effects, mediated through derangement of hemostatic control mechanisms (e.g., cell population kinetics, immunologic surveillance) have also been implicated in certain experimental neoplasms. In considering possible mechanisms of carcinogenesis in any given situation, therefore, a diversity of effects must be contemplated, including indirect as well as direct effects, the nature and relative importance of which may be expected to vary with the type of neoplasm in question and with the conditions of irradiation.

Too little is known at this time about the cancer process to allow precise and detailed statements concerning mechanisms of carcinogenesis for any human neoplasm, or concerning the risks of cancer induction by low level irradiation for any particular site. From limited empirical evidence, however, it would appear that susceptibility may vary appreciably among the different organs of the body, for reasons which remain to be disclosed. In the absence of more complete information, further inferences about the mechanisms of these differences and their implications for radiation protection remain highly speculative.

References

1. Cole, L. J., and Nowell, P. C.: Radiation carcinogenesis; The sequence of events. Science, *150*: 1782–1786, 1965.
2. Furth, J., and Lorenz, E.: Carcinogenesis by ionizing radiations. *In* Hollaender, A. (ed.): *Radiation Biology.* New York, McGraw-Hill, 1954.
3. Furth, J., and Tullis, J. L.: Carcinogenesis by radioactive substances. Cancer Res., *16*:5–21, 1956.
4. Hemplemann, L. H.: Risk of thyroid neoplasms after irradiation in childhood. Science, *160*: 159–163, 1969.
5. International Commission on Radiological Protection: Radiosensitivity and spatial distribution of dose. ICRP Publ. 14. Oxford, Pergamon Press, 1969.
6. Miller, R. W.: Delayed radiation effects in atomic bomb survivors. Science, *166*:569–574, 1969.
7. Mole, R. H.: Endosteal sensitivity to tumor induction by radiation in different species; A partial answer to an unsolved question. *In* Mays, C. W., Jee, W. S. S., Lloyd, R. D., Stover, B. J., Dougherty, J. H., and Taylor, G. N. (eds.): *Delayed Effects of Bone-Seeking Radionuclides.* Salt Lake City, University of Utah Press, 1969.
8. United Nations Scientific Committee on the Effects of Atomic Radiation Report. General Assembly, Official Records: 19th Session, Suppl. No. 14 (A/5814). New York, 1964.
9. Upton, A. C.: Comparative observations on radiation carcinogenesis in man and animals. *In* University of Texas M. D. Anderson Hospital and Tumor Institute: *Carcinogenesis: A Broad Critique.* Baltimore, Williams and Wilkins, 1967.
10. Upton, A. C.: Effects of radiation on man. Ann. Rev. Nucl. Sci., *18*:495–528, 1968.

Radiation Life Shortening

Howard H. Vogel, Jr., Ph.D.

10.9 INTRODUCTION

For more than thirty years it has been known that X-irradiated animals have a shorter life expectancy than unirradiated controls. This late appearing syndrome, radiation-induced aging, has stimulated research in both radiobiology and gerontology.

Studies have not yet unequivocally shown whether radiation primarily accelerates the aging process or whether it shortens the life expectancy by some as yet unknown and unrelated process. Autopsies of irradiated animals show that death is usually caused by the same diseases that kill control animals. The evidence indicates that radiation hastens the appearance of several degenerative and neoplastic diseases, cardiovascular disease, and the acquirement of autoimmune diseases. In addition, analysis of the distribution of survival times of whole body irradiated animals and control animals supports the idea that the average duration of life in an irradiated population is reduced by some general action of radiation which shortens the life of each individual in it. Thus, there may be a single cause common to both aging and the effects of radiation. To test for a nonspecific deleterious effect of radiation (i.e., one which shortens life by some mechanism other than the induction of particular diseases) assessment must be made of the quantitative effect on the actual life span of each individual of all the different induced lesions which it may carry. At present, there is no general agreement about the magnitude of these effects in experimental animals.

10.10 ANIMAL EXPERIMENTS

A. Radiation-Induced Life Shortening Versus Age at Exposure

Over the past two decades a large amount of experimental work has shown that acute radiation sensitivity is not the same for each developmental age. Some data from Reincke *et al.* (1968) are illustrated in Figure 10–7. Noninbred Wistar rats were subjected to whole body radiation or sham irradiated from ages five days to one day before birth and on the day of birth up to 300 days after birth. Radiation doses, chosen to allow 50 per cent 30-day survival of each group, varied from 220 to 700 R of X-rays (or 214 to 580 rads midline dose). Clearly, radiosensitivity varies with age at the time of exposure, the earlier stages being less sensitive to radiation-induced life shortening than the later stages.

It should be pointed out that the life-shortening response to radiation at different ages may vary among animal species. The very high acute radiosensitivity reported for newborn Wistar rats is not observed with newborn FAS/4 mice or with beagles, Analysis of the effect of age on radiation-induced lethality is further complicated by evidence for different age-dependent changes in sensitivity for marrow and intestinal injury after acute exposure of mice.

B. The Dose-Response Curve for Life Shortening

It has been established in several laboratories that even small doses of radiation,

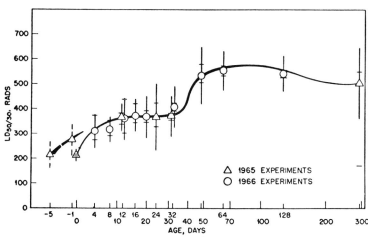

FIGURE 10–7 $LD_{50/30}$ values in Wistar rats between −5 and 280 days of age. The age on the abscissa is shown on a logarithmic scale originating at the day of conception. The indication of age, however, is given in days after birth. The 95 per cent confidence limits of the $LD_{50/30}$ are indicated with horizontal bars. The difference between LD_{16} and LD_{84}, which is reciprocal to the slope of the regression curve, is drawn on a vertical line. This line is broken when the slope was not significantly different from zero. (From Reincke, U., *et al.*: Zur altersabhängigen Strahlenempfindlichkeit weisser Ratten. 3. Bestimmung der $LD_{50(30)}$ während der Säuglingszeit und im Wachstumsalter. Strahlentherapie, *136*:349–359, 1968.)

in the range of 50 to 100 rads, may shorten the life expectancy of animals. The dose-response curve for radiation-induced life shortening in experimental mammals is, however, still a controversial subject. Ten years ago, in a well controlled study, Lindop and Rotblat in England observed that this response is linear in mice. However, other investigators using other strains of mice favored a curvilinear model. That dose response can indeed vary with strain has been shown by Yuhas (1969). He reported that life shortening is a linear function of radiation dose in the A/J strain of mice in the low dose range and plateaus in high dose range. In contrast, $C57B_1/6J$ mice show life shortening as a curvilinear function of radiation dose. It is always extremely difficult to prove that a dose-response curve is truly linear, and opponents can always argue that the response is curvilinear with a very shallow slope and that the sample sizes are insufficient to demonstrate the deviations from linearity.

C. Dose Rate and LET Effects

Some interesting differences have been noted between acute and chronic radiation and between varying dose rates and LET values. An acute dose of gamma rays (low LET) may be as much as four times as effective as an equal dose of the same radiation administered chronically at a much lower dose rate. However, for neutrons (high LET) chronic and acute administration are equally effective. For low LET radiation there seems to be some repair of the radiation injury, depending in part on dose and dose-rate. In contrast, none of the radiation damage caused by neutrons appears to be reparable.

A linear relationship of single sublethal doses of fission neutrons (36 to 275 rads) to the length of life has been shown in irradiated mice (Figure 10–8). In the CF No. 1 female mouse there appears to be 0.22 per cent life shortening per rad of fission neutrons. This effect on mouse longevity is approximately five times higher than that per rad of X-rays, gamma rays, or thermal neutrons. The decreased longevity following single doses of fission neutrons was obtained even when dose rate was changed by a factor of approximately 50. This demonstrates the dose rate independence of fission neutrons compared with either X- or gamma rays. In general, acute radiation with neutrons is approximately twice as effective as gamma radiation for shortening of the mouse life span. However, the RBE may increase to eight or more for chronic exposures (see Figure 10–9). (In this Figure, note the different

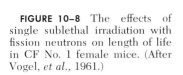

FIGURE 10–8 The effects of single sublethal irradiation with fission neutrons on length of life in CF No. 1 female mice. (After Vogel, *et al.*, 1961.)

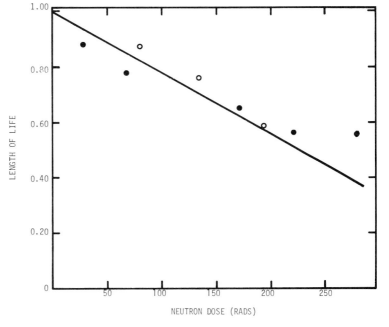

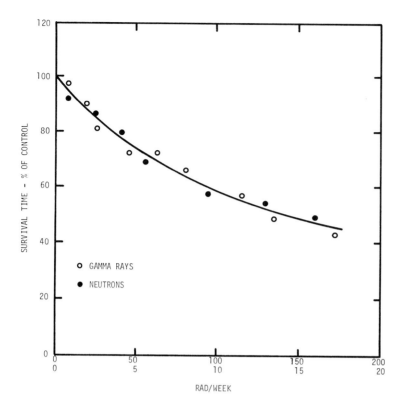

FIGURE 10–9 Survival time for mice as a percentage of control plotted against dosage rate in rads/week for chronic irradiation with either gamma-rays or neutrons. (After Vogel, *et al.*, 1961.)

scales for dose rate used for the two radiations, reflecting an RBE of 10.)

D. Somatic Mutation Theory

The somatic mutation theory of aging states that both natural and radiation-induced aging are caused by spontaneous and radiation-induced mutations, respectively, in the somatic cells. The theory has been examined by the partial hepatectomy technique for unmasking chromosomal damage. The liver is representative of those organs whose cells do not normally undergo divi-

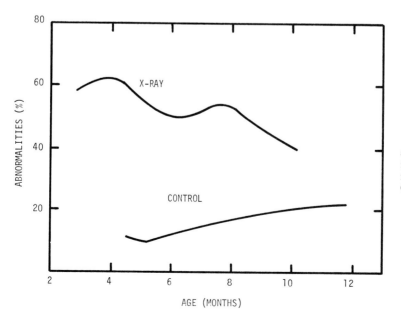

FIGURE 10–10 Chromosome aberrations in liver cells of mice following a single dose of 700 rads of X-rays. (Modified from Curtis, 1969)

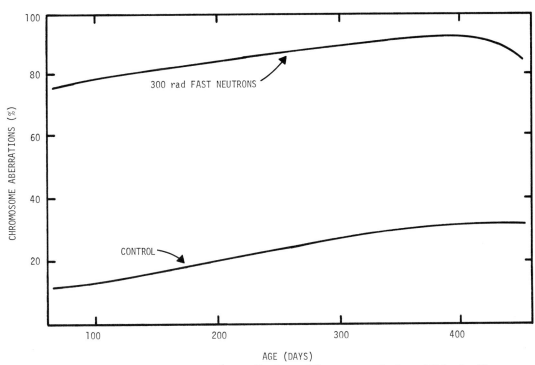

FIGURE 10–11 Chromosome aberrations in liver cells of mice following a single dose of 300 rads of fast neutrons. (The mice were of a different strain from those shown in Figure 10–10, so absolute values cannot be compared between these two experiments.) (Modified from Curtis, 1969)

sion. The frequency of chromosome aberrations (mainly bridges and fragments) in liver cells of mice has been determined after administration of chronic and acute doses of gamma rays and thermal neutrons. In all cases the percentage of aberrant cells is proportional to the shortening of the life span produced by the treatment. Further, acute and chronic neutron irradiation are equally effective in producing chromosome aberrations, but acute irradiation with gamma rays may produce four times as much chromosomal damage as chronic irradiation. It is believed that there is some repair of chromosomes after small doses of gamma rays, but that there is no chromosomal healing following neutron irradiation.

The chromosome aberrations in liver cells of mice after a single dose of 700 rads of X-ray is shown in Figure 10–10; those produced after a single dose of 300 rads fast neutrons are shown in Figure 10–11. Since the mice used in these two experiments were of different strains, absolute values cannot be compared. The recovery of chromosome abnormalities clearly is different following the two radiations. The RBE

for induction of chromosome aberrations is the same as for life shortening. These results support the somatic theory of natural and radiation-induced aging. Further, the data support the concept that organs which continually exhibit cell division, such as bone marrow, eliminate many or most of their defective cells by division and thus do not contribute to aging. However, organs such as the brain, whose cells never or rarely divide, cannot eliminate aberrations and thus contribute to aging. Organs with dividing cells are more likely to contribute to life shortening through carcinogenesis. One could argue that there is no cause-effect relation between chromosome aberrations and life span shortening, but the weight of evidence suggests a real relationship.

10.11 LONGEVITY

A. Longevity and Body-Brain Size

Investigators have tried for years without success to correlate longevity with meta-

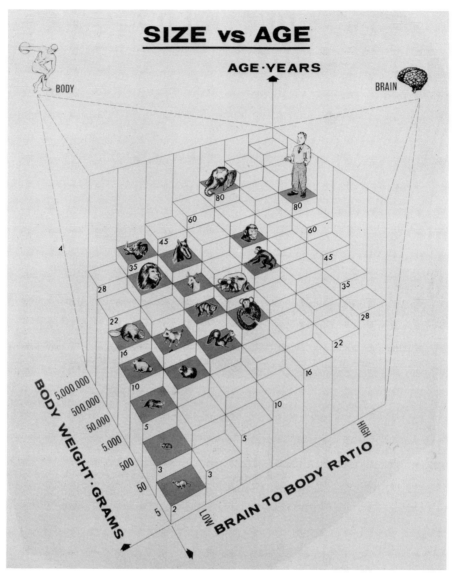

FIGURE 10–12 Diagram showing possible relationships between body size, brain size, and longevity in a number of mammalian species. (After Sacher)

bolic rates, body size, thyroid gland activity, single organ weight, and other factors. In 1959, George Sacher of the Argonne National Laboratory demonstrated that longevity is related to at least two factors: body size and brain size (Figure 10–12). Recently he has shown that the introduction of metabolic rate as a third factor improves the longevity prediction significantly. Analysis of life span for at least 254 species of mammals has led him to conclude that, "for the major orders considered separately, as well as for the overall relationship between orders, there is a single consistent formula governing the relation of life span to brain and body weight. This formula indicates that life span is positively correlated with brain size when body size is held constant" (Sacher, 1970).

Sacher's work suggests that the longevity of a mammalian species is an evolved characteristic based on the evolution of a larger, and presumably better, nervous system, together with the sensors and effectors requisite for improved adaptation and control. This hypothesis is now being tested with the order Rodentia. In this mammalian group animals having approximately the same body size may have significantly different brain sizes. In short, a squirrel with a larger brain, and therefore presumably more integrative nervous organization, would be expected to live longer than a smaller-brained rat of the same body size — and it does.

B. Human Longevity

The human evidence that exposure to radiation has a general deleterious effect, in addition to tumor induction, comes from analyses of the age at death and of the certified cause of death of radiologists. When allowance is made for changing age-distribution of American radiologists, during the period 1930 to 1959, an excess of deaths as compared with other American medical men is found. The numerical excess of deaths in radiologists was least for leukemia and highest for renal and cardiovascular disease, with other cancers and all other causes in an intermediate position. This was taken as evidence for a nonspecific life shortening effect of occupational exposure.

It is of interest to note that the excess mortality found among radiologists has decreased with time in all but the oldest groups. No excess mortality was demonstrable during the period 1945 to 1958 in the youngest age group. These data suggest that life shortening need not be regarded as one of the hazards of occupational exposure for radiologists at the present dose limits. However, a more recent study (1970) indicates that there is still an increased risk of leukemia and myeloproliferative diseases among radiologists. Continuing studies on this group of occupationally exposed individuals are needed. The conclusion of the International Commission on Radiation Protection (Publication 8, 1966) is still true: "The sum of the present

evidence is, therefore, inconclusive. The possibility that small doses of radiation have a nonspecific and deleterious effect on life expectancy is not excluded; but the weight of evidence in favor of such an effect is not sufficient to justify making any quantitative estimate of the risk."

References

1. Curtis, H. J.: The nature of the aging process. *In* Bittar, E. E., and Bittar, N. (eds.): *The Biological Basis of Medicine*, Vol. I. New York, Academic Press, 1969.
2. Fry, R. J. M., Grahn, D., Griem, M. L., and Rust, J. H. (eds.): *Late Effects of Radiation.* London, Taylor and Francis, 1970.
3. International Commission on Radiological Protection: Radiosensitivity and spatial distribution of dose. ICRP Publ. 14. Oxford, Pergamon Press, 1969. (See especially pp. 17–19: Life shortening and generally deleterious effects.)
4. Lewis, E. B.: Ionizing radiation and tumor production. *In Genetic Concepts and Neoplasia.* 23rd Symposium on Fundamental Cancer Research. M. D. Anderson Hospital and Tumor Institute. Houston, 1969. Baltimore, Williams and Wilkins, 1970.
5. Lindop, P. J., and Sacher, G. A. (eds.): *Radiation and Aging.* A colloquium held in Semmering, Austria. London, Taylor and Francis, 1966.
6. Sacher, G. A.: Allometric and factorial analysis of metabolic and constitutional variables in mammals: Relation to longevity. AIBS Meetings, Indiana University. Abstract 415, 1970.
7. Seltser, R., and Sartwell, P. E.: The influence of occupational exposure to radiation on the mortality of American radiologists and other medical specialists. Amer. J. Epidem., *81*:2–22, 1965.
8. Storer, J. B., Rogers, B. S., Boone, I. U., and Harris, P. S.: Relative effectiveness of neutrons for production of delayed biological effects. II. Effect of single doses of neutrons from an atomic weapon on life span of mice. Radiat. Res., 8:71–76, 1958.
9. Vogel, H. H., Jr.: *In* Katz, J., and Crewe, A. (eds.): Radiation and aging. *Nuclear Research USA: Knowledge for the Future.* New York, Dover Publications, 1964.
10. Vogel, H. H., Jr., Frigerio, N. A., and Jordan, D. L.: Life shortening in mice irradiated with either fission neutrons or cobalt-60 gamma rays. Radiology, 77:600–612, 1961.
11. Warren, S.: The basis for the limit on whole-body exposure — experience of radiologists. Health Physics, *12*:737–741, 1966.
12. Yuhas, J. M.: The dose response curve for radiation-induced life shortening. J. Gerontol., *24*:451–456, 1969.

Radiation Cataracts

Howard H. Vogel, Jr., Ph.D.

10.12 INTRODUCTION

The word cataract is used to describe any detectable change in translucency of the optic lens. These changes may vary from tiny granules, usually observed at the posterior portion of the lens, to conditions of complete opacity. The most common cataract is one associated with aging in man. Cataracts are also associated with metabolic conditions, such as diabetes, and more recently radiation cataracts have been described in man.

Radiologists have known for many years that the lens of the human eye is a radiosensitive organ. One of the complications of radiation therapy (X-, beta, or gamma radiation) in the region of the orbit is damage to the lens. Opacities in the human lens may often be minor and may even disappear. Usually eyes are examined for radiation cataracts by means of an ophthalmoscope or a slit-lamp microscope. It should be emphasized that the methods for detecting lens changes are very sensitive and that the murine optic lens is highly radiosensitive, compared to the human lens.

10.13 CAUSES OF RADIATION CATARACTS

The changes in the lens after exposure to radiation apparently are due to damage to individual cells of the lens epithelium. There is a decrease in mitotic activity of the germinative cells with abortive attempts to form fibers of the lens. Abnormal cells and resultant debris accumulate at the poles of the lens. The first opacities are usually visible, by slit-lamp examination, at the posterior pole. The lens is a peculiar structure, enclosed in a capsule and characteristically avascular. The major metabolic activity, particularly oxidative respiration, occurs within the layer of the epithelial cells located only in the anterior subcapsular region extending toward the equator. The lens is located at least 2 mm from any blood supply. Latent periods for cataractogenesis in different species appear to be related to the length of time it takes the damaged epithelial cells to grow around to the equator of the lens where they "turn in" to form lens fibers. The latent period between radiation and opacity varies from months to years.

The majority of experimental work with radiation cataracts has been carried out on rodents — especially rats and mice — and rabbits, which seem to be very sensitive to this somatic effect of radiation. These species are particularly sensitive to high LET radiation, such as neutrons, for the formation of complete opacities of the lens of the eye.

10.14 RADIATION CATARACTS IN EXPERIMENTAL ANIMALS

Bateman and his colleagues at Brookhaven National Laboratory have been studying radiation cataract formation in mice. Careful comparison has been made of mice exposed to neutrons of 0.43 MeV, 1.8 MeV, and 14 MeV. The influence of radiation quality on RBE is clearly shown between neutrons of these three energies tested. When comparing neutrons and X-rays, extremely high RBE's have been obtained. In some cases, opacities of the mouse lens can be obtained following a dose as low as a fraction of one rad of neutrons. The higher RBE's obtained from these experiments cannot, however, be extrapolated directly to man, since such low doses have not caused detectable effects in the human lens.

The data in Table 10–3 show comparative doses for X-rays and neutrons required to produce lens changes in a series of experimental animals and in man.

TABLE 10–3 LOWEST SINGLE EXPOSURES* TO LOW OR HIGH LET RADIATION FOR PRODUCTION OF LENS CHANGES

Species	Grade of change in lens**	Low LET Radiation (R)	Fast Neutrons† (rep or rads)	RBE††
Mouse	d	33	1·3	9
	m			5
	d	50	1	10
Rat	d	240	12–37	20+
	m			2–3
Guinea pig	m	<120	<90	2–3
Rabbit	d	>333	>37	
	d	75	2–7§	20+
	c	500	54	9
Dog	m	>300		
	m		300	
Monkey	d		150§§	
	d	500	75	
	c	<1000	250	4
Goat	m	>400	466	
Man	d	200		
	c		epilatory	

*Lens or whole-body dose as cited by authors.

**d, change detectable with the slit-lamp but not of a degree to impair vision; m, marked change easily recognizable with the ophthalmoscope; c, opacification sufficient to interfere with vision.

†Fission neutrons usually.

††Derived from papers and therefore not necessarily in agreement with ratios of columns 3 and 4.

§These authors imply that the effect of 17 millirads was just detectable.

§§Plus an approximately equal exposure to gamma rays.

A. Experimental Fractionation Studies in Cataract Formation

Fractionation of X-ray dose has a marked effect on cataract induction. Figure 10–13 shows the percentages of rats with cataracts of two plus and three plus severity after 2000 rads of 200 KeV X-rays delivered in a single dose (S) or in three equal fractions (D) in six days. It is obvious that fractionation delays the onset of cataracts considerably. In this study the investigators distinguished five observational stages of increasingly severe opacity in the rat lens, ranging from no opacity to completely opaque lens (0 to 4+).

B. Protecting the Irradiated Lens by Partial Shielding

There is a direct relation between radiation dosage and its effect on the lens. Injury to the lens epithelium is directly related to cataractous changes. The mitotically active lens epithelial cell is more sensitive to radiation than the mitotically inactive epithelial cell. Species variation in response to irradiation is wide.

Several different research groups have demonstrated prevention of the development of complete cataracts after irradiation of rabbit eyes by *partial* shielding of the lens. This type of shielding was accomplished by inserting a half-oval lead corneal contact lens under the eyelids. Other investigators have concluded that the transparency of the lens of the rat eye is maintained after an overwhelming exposure to radiation if only one-half the lens is shielded. Protective effects are also evident on the lids, conjunctiva, and cornea. These results indicate that partial shielding of the human lens may be useful in radiotherapy, when eyes are exposed, since such procedures may increase the ability of the ocular structures to maintain their integrity after high radiation doses.

There is experimental evidence that some of the radioprotective drugs (such as cysteine and AET) may protect against some late effects of radiation, such as cataractogenesis.

10.15 HUMAN RADIATION CATARACTS

In 1949, Abelson and Kruger first reported cataracts in the lenses of ten cyclotron workers, thus indicating that human lens opacities might result from occupational irradiation. For decades the lens of the eye had been observed to be a highly radiosensitive structure, but neutrons had not been recognized as having a specifically high relative biologic efficiency for this somatic effect. The report of the cyclotron workers' cataracts in the United States was followed by similar cases among cyclotron workers in other countries, among survivors of the atomic bombs in Japan, and among certain victims of reactor accidents in the United States.

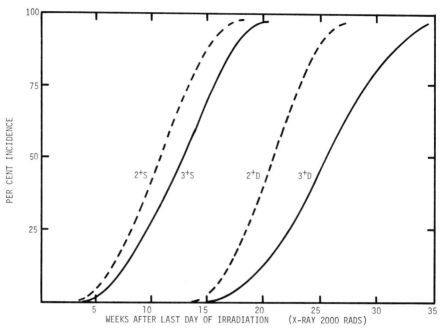

FIGURE 10–13 Broken curves show percentage of rats that have reached 2+ or higher cataracts with 2000 rads delivered in a single dose (*S*) or in three equal fractions (*D*) in six days. Solid lines show incidence of 3+ or greater cataracts for the same two groups of rats. The fractionation delays onset of the cataracts considerably. (Modified from Focht, E. F., *et al.*: A method of radiation cataract analysis and its uses in experimental fractionation studies. Radiology, 87:465–474, 1966.)

Radiation Dose to the Human Lens (Therapy)

Several British investigators examined 104 patients treated for 106 eyelid tumors during the periods 1952 to 1953 and 1957 to 1958. During these periods about 700 patients had been treated for squamous or basal cell carcinoma on or adjacent to the eyelids. Superficial X-ray therapy was given with a 140 kV unit at a half-value thickness of 3 mm aluminum; the cornea was protected by lead shields 1 mm thick which transmitted about 0.7 per cent of the radiation delivered. Typical minor congenital and senile cataracts were noted in several cases, as were a few nonspecific opacities. Radiation cataracts were, with one exception, seen only in eyes treated with radon gold seed implants. Such implantation work is rarely done in the United States, so this late radiation effect should be rare. The exception was in a 69 year old man who received a single dose of 2250 rads for a basal cell carcinoma in the right inner canthus. A typical posterior cortical radiation cataract was found in the inner quadrant of the left eye 10 years after treatment. In this case the lens dose was calculated to be about 950 rads. Of 14 cataracts considered to be caused by radiation from radon gold seed implants, five were of classic appearance and affected all or nearly all of the lens. In eight patients segmental or sector-shaped areas of the posterior lens cortex showed vacuoles and granular opacities, but no significant visual loss occurred in these cases. No radiation cataract developed with an edge dose below 2000 R, whereas a cataract almost always occurred with a central dose exceeding 4000 R. Major cataracts causing serious visual deterioration occurred only with central doses exceeding 3000 R.

These British authors conclude that "the usual one mm lead protection for superficial X-ray therapy is adequate, but when higher-energy gamma or X-ray therapy or interstitial implantation is contemplated, the radiation dose to the lens should be calculated. Serious radiation cataracts should be expected in most instances after doses of 4000 R in seven days and possibly after 2000 R."

From other studies of X- and gamma irradiation of radiotherapy patients, quantita-

TABLE 10–4 LENS OPACITIES AND DOSE OF LOW *LET* RADIATION IN MAN

Authors	Radiation	Overall duration of exposure	Minimum dose at which lens change was detected R	Grade of change at "minimum" dose	No. of individuals with lens opacities/No. of individuals examined				
					Dose range in fractions of minimum dose for detectable opacification				
					0--	1/2--	1--	1 1/2--	2--
ADULTS (10 years+)									
Cogan and Dreisler (1953)	X	I "Single" exposure	600	Just visible by use of ophthalmoscope or slit lamp		0/1	1/3		1/1
		II 3 weeks–3 months	800		0/20		2/2		1/1
Merriam and Focht (1957)	Mostly radium	I Single exposure	200		0/9	0/8	2/2	2/2	16/16
		II 3 weeks–3 months	400		0/10	0/9	4/4	2/3	25/26
		III Greater than 3 mos.	550		0/1	0/5	2/4	0/1	15/15
Britten *et al.* (1966)	Radon gold seeds		1600	Minor (not noticed by patient)		0/8	2/12	4/7	7/11	Same subjects classified in two different ways
			3100	Major (vision impaired)	0/8	0/18	4/10	1/2	
INFANTS AND CHILDREN									
Merriam and Focht (1957)	Mostly X radium	II 3 weeks–3 months	560	Just visible by use of ophthalmoscope or slit lamp			4/7	13/23	1/1
		III Greater than 3 mos.	550		0/2	0/1	2/3	1/2	11/12
Qvist and Zachau-Christiansen (1959)	Radium		1380		0/52		2/2		2/2

tive dose-effect data for cataract induction for low LET radiation have been obtained (see data in Table 10–4):

1. A dose of 200 to 600 rads of low LET radiation appears to be required to cause detectable changes in the human lens when the dose is given in a single brief exposure.

2. Fractionation or protraction of the dose seems to increase the threshold dose for cataractogenesis. If the dose is given over several months, instead of during a brief single period, two to three times as much radiation may be required before cataracts are observed. However, when the total dose to the lens exceeds 1100 to 1400 rads, there is a high probability of cataract formation, irrespective of the duration of exposure.

3. The time required for appearance of cataracts in man varies in relation to both dose and dose-rate from less than one year to more than ten years. This latent period differs in several mammalian species investigated.

4. The lens opacities may progress, remain stationary, or even regress. As the dose increases, the probability of progression of opacity increases.

5. Not all opacities detectable by ophthalmologic examination as "radiation cataracts" are necessarily severe enough to cause significant impairment of human vision.

Quantitative dose-effect data on cataractogenic effectiveness of high LET radiation are fragmentary. Estimates of the dose to the cyclotron physicists have been consistent with a threshold cataractogenic dose of 70 to 100 rads of fast neutrons. This value would be consistent with the experimental data on the RBE of high LET radiation for producing cataracts in many mammalian species.

Within the past two decades, several surveys have been undertaken by different investigators to determine the relation of the incidence of lens changes in the human eye according to the dose delivered. There is in general a highly sigmoid dose-response for adult eyes. (This S-shaped curve is characteristic of many biologic effects of radiation whether we are considering the incidence of cataracts, or acute lethality or organ weight loss, in a mammal.) The evidence from radiation therapy also points to the fact that there appears to be an apparent threshold dose (about 200 R of low LET radiation) below which we do not find lens opacities.

References

1. Abelson, P. M., and Kruger, P. G.: Cyclotron-induced radiation cataracts. Science, *110*:655–657, 1949.
2. Bateman, J. L., and Bond, V. P.: Lens opacification in mice exposed to fast neutrons. Radiat. Res., 7:239–249, 1967.
3. Bateman, J. L., and Snead, M. R.: Current research in neutron RBE in mouse lens opacity. Symposium on neutrons in radiobiology, ORNL, 192–205, 1969.
4. Ham, W. T., Jr., Geeraets, W. J., Cleary, S. F., Williams, R. C., Mueller, R. S., Berry, E. R., and Guerry, D., III: A study of the comparative effects of ionizing radiation and aging on the mammalian lens of the eye. Health Physics, *13*:687–700, 1967.
5. International Commission on Radiological Protection: Radiosensitivity and spatial distribution of dose. ICRP Publ. 14. Oxford, Pergamon Press, 1969.
6. Lerman, S.: *Cataracts; Chemistry Mechanism; Therapy.* Springfield, Ill., Charles C Thomas, 1964.
7. Merriam, G. R., Jr., and Focht, E. F.: Clinical study of radiation cataracts and the relationship to dose. Am. J. Roentgen., 77:759–785, 1957.
8. National Research Council Committee on Radiation Cataracts Reports. (The NRC has sponsored conferences and research in this field since the early 1950's, and a series of relevant reports are available.)
9. Upton, A. C.: Effects of radiation on man. Ann. Rev. Nucl. Sci., *18*:495–528, 1968.
10. Von Sallman, L.: Further efforts to influence X-ray cataract by chemical agents. Arch. Ophthal., *48*:276, 1952.

11 RADIATION EFFECTS ON BEHAVIOR

Donald J. Kimeldorf, Ph.D.

11.0 INTRODUCTION

Radiation-induced changes in behavior have been observed under a wide variety of circumstances. These observations have been derived principally from an evaluation of symptomatology in man and from controlled experimentation with laboratory animals. The sources of evidence in man include clinical reports of response during radiotherapy, observations on the populations exposed at Hiroshima and Nagasaki, and from accidental exposures. Most animal studies have been made with standardized tests designed to assess some specific aspect of behavior such as learning, retention of learning, motivational strength, emotionality, and perception.

Each source of data contains elements of unreliability that should be recognized. For example, in the therapeutic study situation, radiation-induced behavioral reactions may overlay the psychic anxieties of the patient who is already ill and perhaps fearful about radiation treatment. The observations on the Japanese people are complicated in many cases by thermal and blast injury and by uncertainties with respect to the parameters of exposure and dose. Animal studies can be well controlled, but carry the difficulties of extrapolation both with respect to possible differences in the sensitivity of critical organ systems to radiation and to differences in behavioral repertoire.

Despite these uncertainties, a pattern of behavioral changes has emerged from the observations that can be crudely scaled to dose with respect to the type of change, its latency, severity, and duration. In many cases, the physiologic basis for the behavioral disturbance is reasonably apparent.

For the present purpose, behavior may be considered the total response that an organism makes in any situation with which it is faced. The response may be mediated by both glandular and motor effector systems. As such, changes in behavior may be anticipated if radiation exposure is sufficient to alter the functional state of neural and endocrine integrative systems, sense organs, and muscle systems. Moreover, radiation need not act directly on these systems in order to alter behavior since the nervous system, in its special role as integrator, reacts to damage in other systems. For example, radiation injury to a visceral organ can provoke compensatory responses in cardiovascular, respiratory, and gastrointestinal functions that are mediated by the autonomic neuroregulatory system. These responses can, in turn, become the cause of symptomatic complaint or behavioral disturbances after moderate to heavy exposures. It has been postulated that transient complex symptoms such as malaise, lethargy, nausea, anorexia, and vomiting may occur in this manner without radiation damage to the nervous system and its receptors.

11.1   MASSIVE DOSES OF RADIATION

The behavioral reactions to massive doses (greater than 10,000 rads) are of interest primarily because of the degree of incapacitation produced. High intensity, massive, total body exposure generates a set of symptoms which is indicative of neural damage and terminates in death within a few days.

Shipman (1961) has reported an accidental exposure of a man whose clinical symptoms are primarily those associated with central nervous system damage. The dose to the head was estimated at 10,400 rads while the body received considerably less. Immediately after the accident, the subject behaved in a confused and disoriented manner, and within a few minutes he became ataxic and could not stand unaided. By five minutes after the accident, he was virtually unconscious and in a state of shock that persisted for 20 to 30 minutes. On arrival at the medical emergency room, he was described as semiconscious and incoherent and underwent episodes of retching, vomiting, hyperventilation, and an episode of propulsive diarrhea. During the next 90 minutes, he exhibited coarse purposeless movements of his torso and extremities that necessitated restraint by the nursing staff. During the next 28 hours, there was anorexia, hypotension, and circulatory failure. The terminal phase began with the onset of rapidly increasing irritability and uncooperativeness, bordering on mania, followed by coma and death 35 hours after exposure.

When this case is supplemented by other evidence of massive dose effects, the neurologic signs associated with massive exposure include ataxia, convulsions, hyperirritability, disorientation accompanied by nausea, vomiting, anorexia, lethargy, somnolence, and total incapacitation.

The behavioral changes, neurologic signs, and clinical pattern displayed by diverse animal species after massive exposures corroborate the findings described for man. Species specificity, however, is apparent in the severity and duration of behavioral reactions and, in some cases, includes behavioral changes peculiar to the species. Among the alterations which appear to differentiate species is the sharp epileptoid seizure observed in rabbits, an immediate ataxia in mice and rats, a prolonged muscular rigidity in dogs, a peculiar sensitivity of burros, and the absence of convulsions in the hamster even after exposure to 100,000 R. The symptom of vomiting, prevalent in primates and dogs, does not occur in burros and rodents because they are incapable of emesis.

With respect to the origin of neurologic disturbances at high doses, there is evidence within several species that exposure of only the head is as effective as total body exposure, leading to the conclusion that damage to the brain is the basis for much of the incapacitation. The evidence available from studies with localized exposure in the rabbit and hamster indicates that neurologic signs of postural disturbances, loss of equilibrium, and many of the ataxic maneuvers may be associated with lesions within the vestibulocerebellar system. Other motor signs may represent cerebellar damage since pathologic changes in granule and Purkinje cells have been observed in several species with exposure in excess of 4000 R. Brain damage may be the result of direct neuronal destruction, or it may be secondary degeneration as a result of vascular and glial cell damage within neural structures. The relative importance of these two mechanisms for neural injury is not entirely understood at present.

11.2   DOSES IN THE MID-LETHAL RANGE

In the lethal dose range, involving less than massive doses, most signs and symptoms of immediate nervous system damage disappear, and behavioral changes secondarily reflect the relative severity of the gastrointestinal and hemopoietic syndromes. The course in man usually consists of a prompt transitory prodromal phase followed by a relatively asymptomatic period and then a recurrence of symptoms during the evolution of major illness.

The behavior-related clinical signs and symptoms during the prodromal phase include nausea, vomiting, anorexia, acute mental depression, apathy, fatigue, and weakness. This phase generally commences one to two hours after exposure. Its incidence, severity, and duration is inversely related to dose with an apparent threshold in man at approximately 50 to 100 R. In the exposure range of 50 to 100 R, only an occasional individual will complain of nausea. With exposures approaching 200 R, episodes of nausea, vomiting, and complaints of fatigue occur in the majority of patients, lasting one to two days. With 200 to 400 R, the prodromal phase persists for three days and consists of nausea, vomiting, anorexia, general weakness, fatigue, headaches, and drowsiness. At higher doses the severity of symptoms increases and, with exposures in excess of 600 R, the prodromal phase may merge without much relief into the manifestations of gastrointestinal injury.

It has been suggested that much of the prodromal response is an emotional reaction by the patient to the radiation treatment situation. This was not substantiated in a study on a group of patients that were subjected to an actual therapeutic exposure and to sham exposure in a random sequence. With actual exposure, most patients exhibited the previously described complex of symptoms with a relatively constant latency to reaction. Some complained of mild symptoms during or after sham exposure which in no instance resembled those following X-ray exposure. Furthermore, the patients who reported symptoms during sham exposure did not exhibit comparable reactions during actual exposure. It appears that the major prodromal symptoms are responses to irradiation and can be reasonably differentiated from a psychologic reaction to the treatment under these circumstances. It is likely the symptoms of the prodromal phase are manifestations of transient autonomic disturbances of visceral functions. Some investigators believe that the triggering mechanism for autonomic reaction may be circulating toxic histamine-like substances released during the period of rapid necrosis of radiosensitive tissues following exposure.

The appearance and duration of a relatively asymptomatic period, following the prodromal phase, depends on the radiation dose. With exposures capable of inducing a severe gastrointestinal syndrome, the symptoms present during the initial phase can continue until death. The asymptomatic phase emerges when exposure is reduced to a level at which gastrointestinal injury is minor, and the duration of the phase is a function of the time (one to three weeks) preceding the appearance of hemopoietic deficiencies.

The behavior-related symptoms that occur during the major period of illness include anorexia, fever, lethargy, and complaints of weakness and fatigue. Signs of recovery in man may become evident by eight to ten weeks after exposure (200 to 400 R), although symptoms of fatigue and weakness sometimes persist for several months.

11.3 RADIATION AND VOLUNTARY ACTIVITY

Studies of general or voluntary activity in several laboratory species show that irradiation induces marked depressions in activity that correspond in time and with dose to the early period of gastrointestinal dsyfunction and the later phase of hemopoietic effects. There is a comparability in the sensitivity to exposure for induction of symptomatology in man and the activity depressions in the laboratory rat. Both respond to 50 to 100 R with an early transient reaction and to 200 to 300 R for a later prolonged reaction during the hemopoietic phase. In rats, shielding the abdomen during exposure reduces the early depression in activity, while injection of isologous bone marrow immediately after exposure eliminates the later depression. The general activity and behavior of infra-human primates also reflect the periods of underlying physiologic disturbances much like that predicated for man. Total body exposure of the rhesus monkey (400 to 800 R) induces an immediate depression in activity and some vomiting, followed by relatively symptom-free period of several days and then a period of subdued activity with anorexia and decrements in exploratory behavior and the manipulation of puzzle problems. For survivors, complete recovery in activity may take several months.

The decrements in general activity and in more specific manipulatory task performances appear to reflect a reduction of motivation rather than a physical incapacitation. The tendency to perform in a given situation reflects the animal's motivational state. Motivation can become very intense when the performance is related to drives for food, water, sexual activity, or release from forms of physiologic distress. Curiosity (exploratory and manipulatory drives) has been identified in the behavior of primates and other vertebrates and also serves to motivate behavior. Lightly motivated behavior is readily affected by irradiation, whereas highly motivated behavior is much less affected, if at all. The persistence of intensely motivated behavior has been amply demonstrated in conditioned shock avoidance behavior studies with primates. Monkeys have been trained to avoid brief electric shock by learning to discriminate a specific stimulus and to respond in a given manner when presented with a choice between stimuli. Some of these shock-avoidance tasks have involved discrimination of symbols associated with the correct door to escape electric shock, or escape by movement to the opposite end of the alley in response to a particular sequence of light and sound stimuli, or avoidance of shock by pressing a lever during a specific light signal. After the monkey has learned the task well and exhibits stable behavior, he is exposed to radiation and retested for reliable performance on the task at various times after exposure. It has been found that the performance of these relatively simple discrimination tasks in highly motivated monkeys is relatively stable even after exposures in the kiloroentgen range. Not only is there no appreciable loss in retention of the learned discrimination, but the persistence of the intensely motivated behavior is remarkable. Monkeys exposed to 10,000 R have been known to press a lever to avoid shock for many work sessions despite the occurrence of vomiting, diarrhea, nystagmus, and ataxia.

11.4 RADIATION AND LEARNED BEHAVIOR

A variety of experimental techniques have been employed to determine if irradiation interferes with the acquisition of learned behavior in rodents, rabbits, dogs, and monkeys. For the most part, these studies have revealed no effect or only slight transient effects in the formation of conditioned reflexes, maze problem solving, and in the learning of instrumentally conditioned responses. The retention of learned behavior for simple tasks is also stable after irradiation. When errors in retention have been observed, the amount of exposure typically exceeds that required to produce acute radiation sickness in the species, and the temporal course of transient disturbances corresponds to the periods of severe illness. As suggested previously, the performance decrement may reflect the degree of motivation rather than learning and retention.

It is, however, possible to arrange a very complex discrimination problem and find that the animal changes his performance after irradiation with relatively small doses. This approach has been used frequently by Soviet investigators in studies on rats, rabbits, and dogs. In the standard arrangement, the animal is conditioned to discriminate correctly in a complex serial sequence of visual and auditory stimuli and to respond by a specific reflexive behavior (e.g., limb flexion, salivation), or by pressing a lever, or by other manipulatory responses. The serial discriminations may involve a sequence of five or six stimuli and require extensive schedules of conditioning to achieve a stereotyped response pattern. These are apparently very difficult patterns to learn, sometimes requiring several hundred trials to complete conditioning. After a reasonably stable behavior stereotype has been established, the animal is irradiated and tested for the stability of the conditioned behavior. Breakdowns in the stereotype pattern have been reported in some cases with exposures below 100 R. The basis for the disruptive influences of irradiation under these circumstances is largely unknown. It is possible that the complexity of discrimination may approach the limits of the animal's emotional and perceptual capacities. The performance of such difficult tasks would be influenced by slight emotional or motivational alterations and could provide the most sensitive test of behavior. As yet, this approach has not been utilized successfully in radiation studies by investigators trained outside the USSR.

11.5 RADIATION AND THE DEVELOPING NERVOUS SYSTEM

A. Animal Studies

The nervous system is especially sensitive to irradiation during prenatal development. At no other time in the life of the individual will radiation exposure to less than a few hundred roentgens have greater morphological consequences in the nervous system. The type of malformation and the severity of distortion depend on dose and the stage of development at the time of irradiation. Unfortunately, our present scanty information regarding the behavioral consequences of prenatal exposure is limited largely to two species, man and the rat.

In the rat, neural development commences at nine days and parturition occurs at about 21 days after coitus. Neural development continues for several days after birth. There are no detailed timetables for behavioral effects comparable to those developed in the studies of morphology. Exposures in the range of 50 to 200 R have been found to produce neurologic signs of motor dysfunction after birth. Locomotor coordination defects, ataxia, myoclonus, gait defects, and postural defects have been reported in juvenile animals. Some of these motor problems disappear as the animal matures. The threshold for electroshock-induced convulsive seizure is significantly lowered and suggests a permanent shift in the excitability of the irradiated developing brain. However, only mild changes have been observed in the electrical activity of electroencephalograms of prenatally exposed juvenile animals despite rather drastic distortions in brain morphology.

Insofar as they have been investigated, cognitive (intellectual) functions do not show the dramatic changes in the rat that one might anticipate from the evidence of underlying morphologic changes. Maze learning by young rats is typically deficient after exposure during the middle (gestational days 13 to 14) and late (postpartum days 1 to 4) phases of neural development, but otherwise no marked deficiencies have been uncovered. Several investigators have reported that rats, exposed to less than 200 R between the thirteenth day of gestation and birth, exhibit hyperactivity when placed in a novel environment. Hyperactivity may be considered as an excessive reaction to novel stimuli. It is manifested in terms of heightened, nondirected locomotor activity and slower specific responses towards the novel stimulus. Some investigators have interpreted hyperactivity in a novel situation as an indication of increased "emotionality" or "fearfulness" after pre-

natal irradiation. They point out that heart-rate activity is also increased to novel stimuli, as might be expected if the emotional state were involved.

B. Evidence in Man

In man, studies regarding the behavioral consequences of prenatal exposure have been concerned primarily with the occurrence of microcephaly and severe mental retardation. The induction of these abnormalities was recognized from observations on children who had been exposed *in utero*, mostly unintentionally, within the course of therapeutic radiologic procedures used during the 1920's and 1930's. In one analysis, reviewed in the UNSCEAR 1969 report, 18 of 75 offspring from women irradiated during pregnancy were reported to be microcephalic, while only 3 of 417 offspring from women irradiated prior to pregnancy showed developmental defects involving the nervous system. One of the microcephalic children was described as "mongoloid" and most of them as "idiots" or "imbeciles." Among the microcephalic children, all but one had been irradiated at least once between the second and sixth month of intra-uterine life, the exception having been irradiated during the first month only. These early clinical observations have limited value because of uncertainties regarding the fetal dose and the sampling procedures used in the surveys. The dose appears to have been relatively high in most cases. Also, not eliminated from consideration is a possible association between the developmental defects and the conditions necessitating the irradiation.

The study of children acutely exposed *in utero* to the explosions at Hiroshima and Nagasaki offers an independent source of information. These data are based on larger samples and were more rigorously tested, but may be complicated by other physical trauma that could conceivably contribute to the eventual effect. Mental retardation was diagnosed only if the subject was unable to perform simple calculations, to make simple conversation, to care for himself, or if he were completely unmanageable or had to be institutionalized. When examined at 17 years of age, the children exposed within 1500 meters of the hypocenter displayed the highest incidence of mental retardation. All cases of retardation within 2000 meters were exposed between the sixth and twenty-fourth week of pregnancy. The UNSCEAR Report of 1969 provides a rough estimate of incidence and effective dose. It appears that the frequency of mental retardation with reduced head size is in the order of 10 per cent per 100 rads for doses in excess of 100 rads. There was not a significant difference between the incidences of control groups and those of groups receiving less than 50 rads. The reader is referred to the UNSCEAR report for the qualifications and limitations that must be considered in an analysis of this type.

It is apparent that radiation exposure during certain phases of prenatal development can severely limit behavioral capacities. These problems are presumably related to radiation-induced disturbances in neural development. The occurrence of motor dysfunction in animals and the increased incidence of mental retardation in man with exposures in excess of 50 to 100 R suggests the importance of recognizing the presence of a pregnancy in the consideration of radiotherapeutic treatment wherein the fetus might be accidentally exposed.

11.6 RADIATION AS CONDITIONING STIMULUS FOR AVERSIVE BEHAVIOR

There is yet another action of radiation on behavior that has been uncovered in recent years. It has been found in several species that radiation exposure (or its immediate effects) can serve as a conditioning stimulus to promote aversive behavior towards cuing stimuli associated with exposure experience. For example, if rats taste a distinctively flavored fluid, such as 0.1 per cent saccharin-flavored water, immediately before, during, or shortly after irradiation, they will subsequently display an aversion towards drinking saccharin-flavored water that may persist for several weeks. Saccharin water has been used as the taste stimulus in more than 50 radiation studies simply because rats normally have a high preference for sweet flavored water over tap water; radiation-conditioned taste aversions have been produced towards a variety of substances including ethanol, saline, grape juice, milk, and morphine solutions. Radiation-conditioned taste aversions have

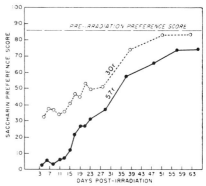

FIGURE 11–1   An example of radiation-induced conditioned behavior in rats. Rats that tasted saccharin during a single exposure to ^{60}Co gamma-rays (30 R or 57 R) exhibited an aversion towards the flavored water that persisted for several weeks after exposure. The preference score is the amount of saccharin fluid in per cent of the total fluid consumed per day with both saccharin water and tap water made available continuously. The pre-irradiation preference score indicates the high preference for this fluid typically exhibited by rats. (From Garcia, J., Kimeldorf, D. J., and Koelling, R. A.: Conditioned aversion to saccharin resulting from exposure to gamma radiation. *Science*, *122*:157–158, 1955.)

been demonstrated thus far in mice, rats, cats, pigs, and monkeys. A remarkable aspect of radiation-conditioned behavior is the effectiveness of small exposures (Figure 11–1). A conditioned reduction in saccharin preference has been demonstrated in rats having received only 10 R, while a strong aversion can be produced with 30 to 60 R. The learned avoidance behavior is not limited to taste stimuli and has been demonstrated towards stimuli associated with the place of exposure. Rats and mice, for example, can be taught to avoid residence in that region of an alley in which they previously experienced irradiation. Radiation-conditioned spatial avoidance generally has required somewhat larger doses than has taste-conditioning to establish reliable avoidance behavior.

The mechanism, or mechanisms, by which radiation exposure in small amounts can lead to conditioned aversive behavior has not been established. Radiation-conditioned behavior has been established with X-rays, gamma radiations, and neutron exposure. The effectiveness of conditioning is more closely related to total dose than to dose-rate. Whole body exposure is most effective in producing aversive behavior; however, abdominal exposure is almost as effective and usually superior to selective irradiation of other body regions. Conditioned taste aversion has been developed in rats after hypophysectomy, adrenalectomy, and ophthalmectomy. It has been found, with much higher doses, that the transfer of blood (by parabiosis) between an irradiated rat and its shielded partner can lead to a conditioned taste aversion if the shielded partner tastes saccharin shortly after the exposure of its partner. This observation suggests that a humoral factor may be involved in the induction of the motivational state, and perhaps it is this humoral factor in blood which is monitored by interoceptors so as to produce aversive behavior toward cueing stimuli.

There have been no published reports as yet concerning the possibility that human behavior can be conditioned by radiation exposure. The evidence for behavior conditioning in other species has been based on relatively recent findings and will require considerably more development before their implications for human behavior can be established. An understanding of the mechanisms involved should contribute to a better evaluation of the role of the nervous system in the biologic effects of low levels of radiation.

The use of radiation as a stimulus to condition behavior has stimulated a re-examination of the potential pathways available to organisms for the detection of ionizing radiations. Ionizing radiation has also been found to be an effective physiologic stimulus for certain receptors of the nervous system. There is no known receptor for which ionizing radiation constitutes the adequate or most efficiently utilized energy form. There is reliable evidence, however, that ionizing radiation can be effective as a physiologic stimulus for at least some of the known receptor systems.

11.7 RADIATION AND SENSORY RECEPTORS

Both visual and olfactory receptors can be excited by X-ray exposures in the milliroentgen range. With respect to visual perception, dark-adapted human subjects will perceive X-ray stimulation of the eye as a light of blue to yellow hues. Lead symbols in the path of X-rays impinging on the retina of dark-adapted human subjects can be described accurately by the subject in total darkness by virtue of the X-ray shadow cast on the retina. Astronauts on Apollo Missions 11, 12, and 14 have reported perceiving occasional flashes of light when situated in the darkened regions of the space craft. It is likely that these are the result of cosmic radiations impinging on the eye. Electrophysiologic studies of both vertebrate and invertebrate (compound) eyes have shown that brief bursts of X-rays, gamma rays, beta and alpha particles can excite the photoreceptor cells. Energetic particles (beta, alpha) may produce fluorescence in the eye sufficient to trigger the retina. With photons (X-rays, gamma rays), fluorescence has not been detected in the exposure range used for retinal stimulation, and direct photochemical excitation appears more likely.

It has been demonstrated in rats, rabbits, dogs, cats, pigeons, and monkeys that the olfactory system is very responsive to small amounts of radiation (Figure 11–2). Evidence for this pathway evolved from the observation that a one second exposure at the rate of 50 mR per second would arouse an ophthalmectomized rat from sleep. The response was dependent on exposure rate rather than total amount. This form of behavioral activation was accompanied by desynchronization of brain wave pattern and was followed by a transient acceleration of heart rate, a pattern indicative of central neural excitation. Subsequently, it was found that removal of the olfactory bulbs from the brain eliminated the behavioral arousal response. Further studies showed that the neurons of the olfactory bulb fired in response to X-ray exposure and that this response could be triggered by introducing a small beta radiation needle into the nasal passages of rabbits.

A more powerful behavioral method, the conditioned suppression technique, has been used to study olfactory detection of ionizing radiations. Animals are trained initially to press a lever for food or comparable reward. They are then subjected to a conditioning phase in which a brief exposure to X-rays is used as a signal to forewarn the animal of impending electrocutaneous shock. After this training, detection of X-ray exposure can be assessed by the occurrence of a disruption in leverpressing behavior when the exposure occurs. Using this technique, it has been

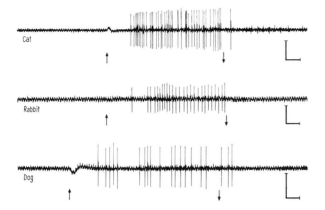

Cat

Rabbit

Dog

FIGURE 11-2 The responses of a single olfactory bulb neuron in the cat, rabbit, and dog to X-ray exposure (250 kVp, HVL = 1.35 mm Cu) at 1 R/sec. In each record, the arrows indicate the onset and cessation of exposure. The spike potential frequency increased markedly within 150 to 200 msec of the onset of exposure. Calibration: 1 mV and 100 msec. (From Cooper, G. P., and Kimeldorf, D. J.: Responses of single neurons in the olfactory bulbs of rabbits, dogs, and cats to X-rays. *Experientia*, 23:137–138, 1967.)

found that the detection exposure rate threshold for conditioned suppression by the rat is about 4 to 5 mR per second, while the threshold for suppression by the rhesus monkey ranges from 3 to 8 mR per second for medium hard X-rays. In the monkey complete bilateral sectioning of the olfactory tracts eliminated the detection response; however, if as little as 20 per cent of the fibers of a single tract remained intact, the animals retained their capacity to detect the radiation.

These findings are very recent and the precise mechanism through which radiation acts to excite olfactory receptors has not been established. In man, no confirmation has been made as yet for olfactory detection. In any event, detection through visual and olfactory receptors appears to be in the physiologic range of stimulation, and no evidence of damage has been found in receptor efficiency, even with an extensive series of repeated stimulation at the levels of exposure normally employed. There is indirect evidence that ionizing radiations may excite other receptor avenues in the absence of visual and olfactory pathways. Thus far, the experiments have not been definitive enough to support more than an admission of this possibility.

11.8 SUMMARY AND CONCLUSIONS

In retrospect, we can consider some conclusions with respect to behavior and radiation exposure. With massive doses, alterations in performance appear to reflect direct radiation injury to the central nervous system, with death occurring within a few days. A complex of neural signs and symptoms are apparent that limit the capacity to perform more than simple, highly motivated tasks. These symptoms generally involve discoordinated motor activity, tremors, convulsions, and disorientation. With less than massive doses, behavioral changes reflect the phases of dysfunction associated with gastrointestinal and hemopoietic injury. There is an early syndrome of neural-mediated changes involving nausea, vomiting, and anorexia which affect the behavior. Phases of lethargy, apathy, and depressed voluntary activity also correlate with the periods of acute sickness. Performance reductions appear to reflect motivational losses for tasks under low levels of drive. However, primates that are intensely motivated by electric shock in a simple avoidance problem can sometimes perform with high efficiency after supralethal doses despite obvious systemic damage. Learning and retention of learning appear to be relatively stable functions except, perhaps, where the performance demands are highly complex, such as in a serial sequential discrimination problem.

It is remarkable that experimental studies of prenatally exposed animals have not yet uncovered marked behavioral changes to correlate with the distortions produced in neural structure. Clinical observations indicate that exposure during neural development in man can lead to an increased incidence of mental retardation.

With small exposures, evidence derived from several animal species indicates that ionizing radiation can be used as a noxious stimulus to provoke a conditioned aversive behavior towards stimuli paired with the exposure experience. Radiation-induced aversive behavior appears highly motivated since a conditioned aversion to a taste stimulus in the rat, produced by only 30 R, may require several weeks to extinguish.

Finally, with exposure rates of only a few mR per second, ionizing radiations may act as an effective stimulus to excite receptors of the visual and olfactory systems. Detection has been demonstrated by both behavioral and electrophysiologic techniques. Other receptors may be excited by ionizing radiation, but the evidence is still indirect and not definitive at the present time.

°The author wishes to acknowledge the support of a U.S. Public Health Service Grant, RL00119-05, during the preparation of this chapter.

References

1. Garcia, J., Buchwalk, N. A., Feder, B. H., Koelling, R. A., and Tedrow, L. F.: Ionizing radiation as a perceptual and aversive stimulus. In Haley, T., and Snider, R. S. (eds.): *Response of the Nervous System to Ionizing Radiation.* Boston, Little, Brown and Co., 1964.
2. Gerstner, H. B.: Acute radiation syndrome in man. U.S. Armed Forces Med. J., 9:313–354, 1958.
3. Kimeldorf, D. J., and Hunt, E. L.: *Ionizing Radiation: Neural Function and Behavior.* New York, Academic Press, 1965.
4. Shipman, T. L. (ed.): Acute radiation death resulting from an accidental nuclear critical excursion. Special Supplement, J. Occup. Med., 3:146–192, 1961.
5. Smith, J. C., and Tucker, D.: Olfactory mediation of X-ray detection. In Pfaffman, C. (ed.): *Olfaction and Taste.* New York, Rockefeller University Press, 1969.
6. Smith, J. C.: Radiation, its detection and its effects on taste preferences. In Steller, E., and Sprague, J. M. (eds.): *Progress in Physiological Psychology,* Vol. IV. New York, Academic Press, 1971.
7. United Nations Report of the Scientific Committee on the Effects of Atomic Radiation: Effects of ionizing radiation on the nervous system. General Assembly, Official Records: 24th Session, Suppl. No. 13 (A/7613). New York, 1969.

12 RADIOBIOLOGIC ASPECTS OF NUCLEAR MEDICINE

Richard L. Witcofski, Ph.D.

12.0 INTRODUCTION

In a relatively short time nuclear medicine has grown from a new clinical science to a major medical specialty. Increasing numbers of humans are being irradiated through the use of radioactive materials localized in organs or distributed throughout their bodies. The dose of radiation received by the patient measures the potential risk he takes and must be weighed against expected advantages the procedure has for him. Since these radiopharmaceuticals are given internally, the many factors that determine the time-course of its distribution make the absorbed dose and patient risk only an estimate. Numerous factors produce uncertainties in dose calculation, particularly when applied to specific patients. These factors include (1) redistribution of radionuclides within the body after administration, (2) inhomogeneous distribution within organs (3) excretion, (4) the effect of illness or pathologic states, and (5) the age of the patient.

12.1 ESTIMATE OF RADIATION DOSE FROM NUCLEAR MEDICINE PROCEDURES

Radiation dose measures potential risk of patients with radioactive materials localized or distributed throughout their bodies.

Two of the most important areas receiving radiation doses are the critical organ (the organ receiving the *highest* dose) and the total body. Typical examples of dose levels from widely used diagnostic studies are listed in Table 12–1.

The values listed in Table 12–1 represent estimates for a standard or average man. The techniques for the calculation of radiation doses are highly developed. The necessary physical information regarding the modes of radioactive decay, the energies of radiations, and their relative numbers are known with great precision for clinically used radionuclides. The problems associated with the calculation of radiation doses in patients relate in the main to biologic variability. The radiation dose to an organ will depend upon the organ's size and the fraction of the administered dose accumulated by the organ. These values will vary considerably even among so-called normal individuals; yet it should be remembered that in many patients the organ under study will undergo some pathologic changes, which may influence the size of the organ as well as its ability to accumulate the radionuclide, resulting in even more variation between individuals. Further, there is scant data on the biologic elimination of radiopharmaceuticals.

Variation in absorbed dose is dependent on the patient's size and age, since organs

TABLE 12-1 ESTIMATES OF ABSORBED DOSES

Radiopharmaceutical	Administered Dose (μCi)	Dose to Critical Organ (rads)		Dose to Total Body in rads
^{198}Au Colloid	150	5	(Liver)	0.4
^{99m}Tc Colloid	1000	0.3	(Liver)	0.02
^{131}I Aggregated albumin	300	1.9	(Lung)	0.1
^{99m}Tc Pertechnetate	10,000	2.7	(Thyroid)	0.1
^{75}Se Selenomethionine	250	6.3	(Liver)	2
^{197}Hg Chlormerodrin	100	1.2	(Renal Cortex)	0.001
^{131}I Sodium iodide	50	50	(Thyroid)	0.02
^{57}Co Cyanocobalamin	0.5	0.01	(Liver)	0.003
^{51}Cr Sodium chromate	50	1.6	(Spleen)	0.01
^{59}Fe Ferrous citrate	5	0.4	(Blood)	0.12

are smaller in infants and children than in adults and the proportionate sizes are also different. Not only do infants and children receive greater radiation doses than adults from given quantities of radionuclides, but their tissues are also more susceptible to deleterious effects of ionizing radiations. Little is known of effective radionuclide half-life in children because of the proper reluctance of investigators to administer radioactive materials in studies of their normal physiologic processes. It is true that in clinical nuclear medicine smaller quantities of radioactivity are used in young patients, yet reduction in the amount based only on their weights relative to those of adults may result in a poor estimate of radiation risk.

When the magnitude of radiation doses delivered from nuclear medical procedures are compared to those from diagnostic X-ray procedures, it should be pointed out that the dose rates are usually much lower from radionuclides. Thus, lower dose rate from radionuclide decay in nuclear medicine might result in less damage from the same radiation dose (as delivered with X-ray) because of the potential for repair. This potential for repair may be reduced with the newer short-lived radionuclides, yet these dose-rates are still lower than those encountered in diagnostic radiology and probably do not represent an undue hazard.

12.2 POTENTIAL RISK FROM DIAGNOSTIC NUCLEAR MEDICINE PROCEDURES

The main concern about the potential hazards of diagnostic nuclear medicine procedures are carcinogenesis, induction of leukemia, and genetic effects. No human studies have shown increases in cancer from doses below 50 rads, although recent studies of atomic bomb survivors have demonstrated increased risk of leukemia for doses as low as 20 rads. On this basis it appears that the risk of cancer or leukemia associated with the low radiation doses delivered by radionuclides *administered for diagnostic purposes* is very small compared to potential benefits. Diagnostic nuclear medicine procedures should be considered to have about the same relatively small potential risk of inducing cancer as procedures in diagnostic roentgenology. The risk, however small, should be weighed against potential benefits to the patient.

Most biologists assume a nonthreshold, linear relationship between dose and genetic damage. This damage usually will be in the form of recessive mutations. Because of the increasing use of radionuclides in medicine, we are approaching a situation in which large segments of the population will be exposed with a resultant increase in the pool of such recessive mutations. As time passes and continued exposure of many generations occurs, the increase in the pool will go on. Eventually these mutations will be expressed, with the possible damaging or weakening of the human population the result. Because of their high reproductive potential, patients under 30 should not have tests involving radiation except in instances where definite medical indications are present.

It is also necessary to question closely women of reproductive age prior to administering radionuclides to be sure they are not pregnant. Irradiation of the sensitive developing embryo may occur from radionuclides concentrated in maternal organs or in the embryo itself when the radionuclide can cross the placental barrier.

12.3 POTENTIAL HAZARDS OF THERAPEUTIC USE OF RADIONUCLIDES

A. Iodine-131

The use of radioactive iodine (^{131}I) for treatment of hyperthyroidism has been widely accepted as a successful means of controlling the disease for over 20 years. Patients treated number in the hundreds of thousands, yet there is no general agreement about its indications and, more important, its contraindications (the potential for induction of leukemia and thyroid carcinoma).

Since radiation is a carcinogen, it may be argued that it is unwise to use radioiodine in treating benign diseases such as hyperthyroidism. At this time, the question cannot be resolved to the satisfaction of all because many feel that insufficient time (at least 20 years) has elapsed since widespread treatment began for late effects to be observed.

There is considerable evidence suggesting that external irradiation of the thyroid gland increases the incidence of thyroid cancer in infants and children. Most of these children received 300 to 600 rads to the area of the thyroid before the age of six years. Although results are not uniform, they demonstrate a history of prior thyroid irradiation in 40 to 80 per cent of these patients with thyroid carcinomas; the period from irradiation to detection of thyroid cancer usually ranges from 5 to 18 years. There is no agreement on a minimum age for ^{131}I therapy for hyperthyroidism, but because of the strong circumstantial evidence implicating therapeutic X-irradiation as an etiologic factor in thyroid cancer in childhood and adolescence, there has been a tendency not to treat the young with radioiodine. Initially, only people over 40 were treated, except where other forms of therapy were considered unwise, but the recent trend has been to lower this age limit to around 20 to 25 years of age.

At present there is no good evidence that cancer of the thyroid is induced in adults by ^{131}I, and too few children and adolescents have been treated for hyperthyroidism to enable radiologists to make sound judgments.

In the treatment of hyperthyroidism the usual dose of ^{131}I delivers about five to 10 rads to the whole body, a level well below those demonstrating increases in cancer induction or leukemia in studies in humans.

In an effort to find a definite answer to the problem of whether leukemia is induced in patients treated with ^{131}I for hyperthyroidism, the U.S. Public Health Service and the Center for Radiologic Health studied a very large group of hyperthyroid patients treated with ^{131}I or with surgery. The patients treated with ^{131}I showed a slight increase in the incidence of leukemia when compared to the normal population, but it was no greater than in the control group of patients treated surgically for the same disorder.

These studies indicate that ^{131}I therapy does not induce leukemia. Nevertheless, they do not totally exclude the possibility, although it does appear remote.

Pregnancy should be considered an absolute contraindication to treatment of hyperthyroidism with radioiodine. Even the relatively small doses delivered to the fetus by general body irradiation is undesirable because of the potential for malformation during early development and the possibility of late effects (cancer) of this radiation. Also, radioiodine passes the placental barrier, so its hazard is increased, because after the first trimester, sensitive fetal thyroid is capable of concentrating radioiodine. In order to prevent treating pregnant women, a careful history should be taken prior to treatment.

In thyroid cancer, in which many hundreds of millicuries of ^{131}I may be given to a patient during the course of therapy, severe suppression of bone marrow may occur because of the high total body radiation dose (a dose of 100 mCi of ^{131}I will deliver 50 to 100 rads to the hemopoietic tissue). These depressant effects on bone marrow are the same as results from total body radiation, as discussed in Chapter 8. Ultimately bone marrow depression is the limiting factor in treatment of thyroid cancer with ^{131}I. During therapy, complete blood counts should be routine.

Because treatment of thyroid cancer involves using large and repeated doses of radioiodine, a few cases of myeloid leukemia may have been reported following ^{131}I therapy. The incidence is well above expected levels and there seems to be little doubt concerning its origin. Yet when one considers that this is therapy for a very serious disease, the risks appear justified.

B. Phosphorus-32

The question of whether the incidence of leukemia is higher in patients treated for polycythemia with ^{32}P (a dose of 4 mCi of ^{32}P delivers about 100 rads to bone marrow, liver, and spleen, while the remainder of the body receives about 10 rads) than in those treated in other ways (alkylating agents) is a statistical question complicated by disagreement on the spontaneous incidence of leukemia in polycythemia. There is evidence to suspect an increased inci-

dence of acute leukemia in patients treated with radiophosphorus for polycythemia, but larger, more carefully controlled studies will be required to answer this question.

References

1. Hagler, S., Rosenblum, P., and Rosenblum, A.: Carcinoma of the thyroid in children and young adults: Iatrogenic relation to previous irradiation. Pediatrics, 38:77–81, 1966.
2. Holcomb, R. W.: Radiation risk: A scientific problem? Science, 167:853–855, 1970.
3. Ishimura, T.: Leukemia in atomic bomb survivors, Hiroshima and Nagasaki, 1 October 1950–30 September 1966. Radiat. Res. 45:216–233, 1971.
4. Silver, S.: Radioactive Nuclides in Medicine and Biology (Medicine). Philadelphia, Lea and Febiger, 1968.
5. United States Atomic Energy Commission: Medical radionuclides: Radiation dose and effects. Conference 691212. June, 1970.
6. Winship, T., and Rosvoll, R. V.: Childhood thyroid carcinoma. Cancer, 14:734–743, 1961.

13 OTHER ASPECTS OF RADIATION BIOLOGY

Radioecology

John P. Witherspoon, Jr., Ph.D.

13.0 INTRODUCTION

Ecology is traditionally defined as the study of the relation of organisms or groups of organisms to their biologic and physical environment. It has also been defined as the study of the structure and function of nature. Radioecology, or radiation ecology, is a newer discipline which is concerned with radioactive substances, radiation, and the environment. The development and subsequent expansion of nuclear energy for military and peaceful uses has been accompanied by many environmental problems; some of these are typical of other facets of industrialization and some are unique to atomic energy. The unique problems primarily concern the fate and ecologic effects of radionuclides released into the environment.

Major environmental problems of the Atomic Age may be grouped into several areas of scientific and public concern. Fallout, reactor development, waste disposal (radioactive and thermal), nuclear war, and technological projects each has an impact upon man and his environment. Understanding the manner in which ecologic systems receive and control radioactive substances, and the effects such substances have on these systems, is the major order of business for the radioecologist.

13.1 RADIOECOLOGY

A. Radionuclides of Ecologic Importance

Radionuclides that are of interest to the ecologist are listed in Table 13–1. These radioactive elements represent the major naturally occurring and man-made sources of radiation in the environment. Principal sources of exposure from background (natural) radiation are represented by the uranium, thorium, and actinium decay series. Internal exposure to man results primarily from ^{40}K, ^{14}C, ^{226}Ra, and ^{228}Ra and their daughter products that are deposited in the body. Radionuclides such as ^{222}Rn and ^{220}Rn and their daughter products represent sources of internal radiation that are inhaled. Exposure for these sources varies greatly and depends upon what one eats and where one lives. Morgan (1963) has estimated the average gonad dose to man from background radiation at about 100 mrem per year with maximum doses up to 1000 mrem per year. Lung exposures were higher with values of 500 to 1000 mrem per year.

TABLE 13–1 RADIONUCLIDES OF
ECOLOGICAL IMPORTANCE

Category	Major Radionuclides	Ecological Importance
Naturally occurring	Uranium Thorium Actinium series elements Potassium-40 Carbon-14	Major contributors to background radiation (long half-lives)
Fission products	Strontium-89, -90, -91 Yttrium-90, -91 Zirconium-95 Niobium-95 Ruthenium-103, -106 Rhodium-106 Iodine-131 Cesium-137 Barium-137, -140 Lanthanum-140 Cesium-141, -144 Praseodymium-143, -144 Neodymium-147 Promethium-147	Enter ecologic systems through fallout or waste disposal (half-lives ranging from a few hours to 30 years)
Radioisotopes of elements essential to organisms	Hydrogen-3 Carbon-14 Sodium-22 and -24 Phosphorus-32 Sulfur-35 Potassium-42 Calcium-45 Manganese-54 Iron-59 Copper-64 Zinc-65 Iodine-131	Used as tracers in studies of both radionuclide cycling and radiation effects in organisms and ecological systems

Radionuclides produced by the fission of uranium (fission products) are of the most concern. With the exception of ^{131}I, these man-made isotopes are not elements essential to organisms, but they constitute the sources of radiation in the environment from fallout or waste disposal from nuclear operations. All these isotopes may enter ecologic systems where they become part of the flux of elements that are being circulated within and among systems.

Some of the fission products which are chemically similar to essential elements are of special interest. Cesium-137 tends to follow the pathways of potassium in living systems. Strontium isotopes are circulated like calcium and, in many food chains, tend to concentrate in the radiosensitive erythropoietic tissue of mammals. This chemical behavior and a relatively long half-life (about 30 yrs) make ^{137}Cs and ^{90}Sr of particular concern as environmental contaminants.

Finally, there are man-made radionuclides which are important because they represent elements which are essential to plants and animals. Some of these may also enter the environment as activation products produced by reactors or nuclear explosives. Use of the isotopes in metabolic studies of organisms, populations, or communities leads to an understanding of regulatory processes and structural characteristics of living systems. Examples of experimental use of radioactive tracers may range ecologically from studying the uptake by corn of ^{45}Ca-tagged fertilizer to following the pathways of ^{32}P in a stream with its associated nonliving and living components.

B. Radioactive Fallout

Fallout is the radioactive material that settles to earth after a nuclear explosion; two forms are recognized. The first is *early* or *local fallout,* which consists of larger particles injected into the atmosphere by the explosion. These particles usually descend to earth within 24 hours near the site of detonation and in areas extending downwind for variable distances. The second form is *delayed* or *worldwide fallout,* which consists of smaller particles that ascend into the upper troposphere and stratosphere. These particles are distributed over a wide area of the earth by circulation of air, and their descent to earth may take weeks, months, or years.

Factors which influence the nature and extent of fallout are the design and energy yield of the nuclear device, the height of the burst, the prevailing meteorologic conditions, and the nature of the surface over or under which the device is detonated.

Nuclear devices which use fissionable uranium or plutonium may produce as many as 200 isotopes of 36 elements. The radioactive half-lives of fission products range from small fractions of a second to about a million years. However, in general, fission product (or fallout) decay may be expressed by the formula

$$I = I_1 \, t^{-1.2}$$

where I is radiation intensity at anytime after a nuclear explosion, I_1 is intensity one hour after the explosion, and t is time in hours from the time of the explosion. This formula is valid for fallout radioactivity arising from fission products for times between 30 minutes and about 5000 hours after the explosion.

Early fallout poses the greatest biologic hazard since it falls within a few hours after a nuclear detonation. Worldwide fallout, on the other hand, loses a great deal of its radioactivity by decay before it falls. While not presenting an immediate biologic hazard, it may be capable of producing long-term effects as it enters food chains.

Of course, radionuclides become concentrated in specific tissues and organisms in the same fashion that elements do. For example, phosphorus is several orders of magnitude more concentrated in the eggs of fish than in the water in which the fish live. Thus, ^{32}P, the radioactive species, shows a similar but lesser concentration in fish eggs than in the surrounding water.

Fallout can enter food chains by many routes. Deposited on edible plants, it can be directly consumed by man. If contaminated vegetation is consumed by animals, the animal tissues and products (e.g., milk and eggs) can be a source of radionuclides in man. Also, the soil may be contaminated so that radionuclides enter plants through the roots. Thus, man may be exposed again by eating plants, animal tissues, or animal products.

Fortunately most fission products decay rapidly. Moreover, only a few are absorbed readily in the human gastrointestinal tract. However, several radionuclides are of particular significance because they are readily absorbed, locate in specific body sites, and thus present potential long-term hazards. Radioisotopes of strontium are deposited in bone tissue. Strontium-89, with a half-life of 51 days, is of concern when fallout is of recent origin. A longer-term problem is presented by ^{90}Sr, which has a 28 year half-life. Iodine-131, with a half-life of eight days, is deposited in the thyroid gland and, like ^{89}Sr, is of greatest concern during the first few days or weeks after contamination. Cesium-137, with a 30-year half-life, is distributed throughout the body primarily in muscle tissue.

Because of their long half-lives, ^{90}Sr and ^{137}Cs are the most important fission products from the standpoint of long-term effects. The biologic fate of ^{90}Sr in food chains depends on the calcium content of foods. While strontium and calcium move together through food chains from soil to plants to animals, relatively more calcium is deposited in bone tissue. Calcium is preferentially utilized relative to ^{90}Sr in nearly every step of a food chain. For example, milk containing ^{90}Sr may represent less of a hazard than some other dietary pathway to man owing to the high calcium content of dairy products.

Uptake of ^{90}Sr from soil by plants depends upon the type of soil, the soil's moisture content, and amount of calcium in the soil. Strontium is more mobile in soil, however, than cesium.

Although a chemical similarity exists between cesium and potassium, the degree of interdependent behavior is not as great as that between strontium and calcium. Cesium-137 tends to bind strongly to soils, and is, therefore, less available for uptake by plants. Thus, direct contamination of edible plants is the major source of entry into food chains. Since the biologic half-life (time required for the body to eliminate one-half of an administered quantity of radionuclide) of ^{137}Cs in man ranges between 70 to 140 days, it does not present as great a hazard as ^{90}Sr, which has a biologic half-life of about 50 years.

The fate of fallout radionuclides in the sea is strikingly different. Elements that form strong complexes with organic matter (^{60}Co, ^{59}Fe, ^{144}Ce, and ^{106}Ru) enter marine food chains, in contrast to the soluble fission products such as ^{90}Sr and ^{137}Cs which are prominent in land food chains.

The importance of fallout as a source of environmental contamination has diminished since the moratorium on aboveground nuclear weapons tests by the major nuclear powers. However, weapons tests by other nations, potential consequences of nuclear war, and future uses of nuclear devices for excavation purposes are study areas that remain important to the environmental scientist.

C. Radioactive Waste Disposal

Most radioactive waste products come from nuclear reactors and associated processing plants. Relatively small amounts, mostly solid wastes, may also come from institutions where use of radionuclides in medicine or other scientific research produces radioactive wastes. These waste products may be released into the environment in a gaseous, liquid, or solid state. The possibility that this radioactivity will contaminate soil or water to a degree that radioactive substances build up to hazardous levels in organisms, including man, represents a potential danger. This hazard has to be considered in any assessment of treatment and control of radioactive wastes. Fortunately, expanding research on development of atomic energy has been accompanied by increased research on disposal of wastes.

Two main procedures have been used for atomic waste disposal: (1) dilution and dispersal and (2) concentration and storage (containment). The first method is suitable for gases or liquids having a low level of radioactivity. These wastes are processed, held for some time to permit decay, and then extensively diluted and dispersed in large volumes of air or water. If the soil has appropriate ion exchange properties, low level liquid wastes may simply be run into the ground. Of course, it is necessary to monitor both the dispersal media and biologic systems in this type of waste disposal operation.

Treatment of liquids of moderate or high level activity is more difficult. Also, there is a greater potential danger if these wastes are released into the environment so that they enter food chains. These wastes are generally concentrated by evaporation or filtering processes and then stored in a manner which prevents their entrance into soil, water, or biologic systems. The practice to date has been to store these wastes as aqueous solutions, or slurries, in tanks. In special geologic situations injection of intermediate level liquid wastes into deep rock strata has been used successfully.

The wastes of primary concern are solid wastes characterized by intense, penetrating radiation, high thermal output, and very long-half-lives. These are principally fission product "ashes" from spent nuclear fuel or solid materials contaminated with toxic plutonium during fabrication of reactor fuel. Since these wastes must be kept out of contact with the environment for literally thousands of years, past practices of storage in tanks or burial will not be adequate in an expanding economy based on nuclear power. Recent research in waste disposal indicates that natural salt formations are well suited to serve as repositories for these high level wastes. Salt formations are free of circulating ground water, protected by impermeable shales, and have good structural and thermal properties. Moreover, these formations are generally located in zones of low seismicity.

The fate of radioactive wastes released into ecologic systems and the effects of such releases are study areas which link many radioecologists to atomic waste disposal operations. Ecologic research in this area is necessary for the proper surveillance of current waste disposal practices and for the development of practical and safe future practices.

D. Radiosensitivity of Ecologic Systems

Although one of our concerns about development of future nuclear power operations is the possible effect of low level, chronic radiation on ecologic systems, there is little information on this subject. Much more is known about the radiosensitivity of organisms exposed to radiation doses which are much higher than we expect to contend with in the normal environment. For example, Table 13–2 gives estimated acute doses of gamma or X-radiation that are necessary to kill 50 per cent or more of the adult members of several groups of organisms. These data should be taken only as an indication of relative radiosensitivity as they represent generalized ranges.

Much more information is needed to obtain a more complete ecologic picture. For example, all organisms have stages in their life cycle which are affected by much lower doses than those necessary to produce lethality. In radioresistant groups such as insects, 10 per cent or less of the lethal dose to adults may produce lethality when critical egg stages are irradiated. In *Drosophila*, the fruit fly, LD_{50} values for acute X-irradiation have ranged from 163 to 100,000 R when a population was irradiated during egg cleavage and as adults, respectively.

In plants and animals the reproductive stages of the life cycle are the most radiosensitive. Even within the reproductive

TABLE 13–2   COMPARATIVE RADIOSENSITIVITY
OF GROUPS OF ORGANISMS

Group	Lethal Dose Range (rads)*
Bacteria	100,000–1,000,000
Insects	5,000– 100,000
Fish	1,000– 3,000
Mammals	300– 1,200
Herbaceous plants	5,000– 70,000
Coniferous trees	800– 3,000
Deciduous trees	4,000– 10,000

*Estimated acute whole body gamma radiation doses required to kill 50 per cent or more of the adult organisms.

stages there are critical phases of short duration during which the organism is most vulnerable. The effects of radiation on a population of organisms, then, would be dependent upon the proportion of the total population in various stages of the life cycle at the time of irradiation.

Effects other than lethality also may be produced by radiation. Aside from genetic or reproductive effects, changes in growth (production), disease resistance, life span or response to environmental factors are of interest to the ecologist. Radiation-induced changes in these parameters can affect an organism's or population's ecologic role. Predator-prey relationships, food chains, transfers of energy and materials, and even the type of ecologic system may be altered.

Responses of herbaceous plants to short-term chronic gamma radiation are shown in Table 13–3. These data show the fraction of the lethal (LD_{100} — usually expressed as

TABLE 13–3   RESPONSES OF HERBACEOUS
PLANTS RELATIVE TO MORTALITY AFTER
GAMMA IRRADIATION*

Response	Fraction of LD_{100} Dose Rate
Normal	0.11
10% growth reduction	0.26 ± 0.02
Failure to set seed	0.31 ± 0.06
50% growth reduction	0.34 ± 0.04
Floral inhibition or abortion	0.44 ± 0.04
Severe growth inhibition	0.58 ± 0.03
LD_{50}	0.75 ± 0.02
LD_{100}	1.00

*Exposure to ^{60}Co from eight to 12 weeks. (Data from Sparrow and Woodwell, 1962.)

LD_{99}) dose rate that is necessary to produce other, less drastic, biologic effects. In the case of whole plant irradiations during plant growth, doses far below those required to produce lethal effects will cause complete failure of sexual reproduction. Plant seed (and spores of some bacteria), however, are relatively radioresistant once they have matured. Doses several times larger than those necessary to kill mature plants are required to prevent seed germination. It is possible, then, depending on the time of irradiation, to kill a plant but retain viable seed.

With plants some ability to predict radiation effects is possible. The meristematic, or growth, regions in vegetating plants are the most radiosensitive tissues. Absorption of radiation energy in these regions alters plant growth and development. Sparrow (1964) demonstrated a linear relationship between interphase chromosome volumes in meristematic tissue and gamma-ray exposures necessary to produce various biologic effects; that is, plant species with large chromosomes are more radiosensitive; those with small chromosomes are more resistant to radiation. In general, this is an extremely useful concept, and it has been used to assess probable radiation effects on vegetation (natural and agricultural) from military uses of nuclear devices. Also, this concept has been used to estimate the relative radiosensitivities of a number of major plant ecosystems, ranging from grasslands to various types of forests (Woodwell, 1966).

Radiosensitivity in animals does not seem to be so closely related to nuclear or chromosome volume. In mammals the concept of "critical organs" is emphasized. These are tissues which are radiosensitive due to high rates of cell proliferation, or they are tissues in which certain radionuclides may concentrate (e.g., iodine in the thyroid).

Some studies on the effects of low level, chronic radiation in the environment have recently been summarized by Auerbach and co-workers (1971). Recent attention to ecologic considerations in reactor power plant sites has reinforced the need for such information. In general, the results of studies to date suggest that no serious ecologic effects are produced where dose to key organisms does not exceed that expected from radioactive wastes released at MPC* levels. However, there is not enough information available yet on the kind and number of radionuclide concentration points in ecologic systems, so the question of whether MPC levels released to the environment are "safe" over a long period of time is still unresolved.

Because some radionuclides do become concentrated in food chains, organisms may be better monitors of contamination than environmental materials (soil and water).

*Maximum Permissible Concentration values for radionuclides are derived for internal exposure of man. The International Commission on Radiological Protection (ICRP), the National Council on Radiation Protection (NCRP), and the Federal Radiation Council (FRC) formulate and review these values.

E. Environmental Fate of Radionuclides

The consequences of releasing radioactivity into the environment depend on how ecologic systems regulate the flow of such releases. These materials may be dispersed and diluted or they may be concentrated. Major ecologic considerations are (1) the dynamics of radionuclides in food chains, (2) the potentials to concentrate at different ecologic levels, and (3) the pathways by which radionuclides may expose individuals or populations, including man.

A considerable body of information exists on the behavior of radionuclides in terrestrial, aquatic, and agricultural systems. These studies have involved both the experimental approach and monitoring opera-

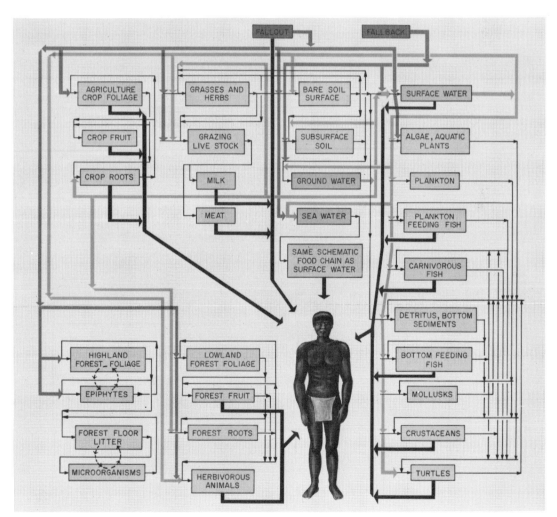

FIGURE 13-1 Food chain pathways for man in a tropical environment. (After Kaye and Ball, 1969.)

tions after atomic wastes or fallout have been released.

Evaluation of these and future studies in terms of risk to man will require some coherent theories which are not yet formulated. One promising approach is the use of predictive mathematical models of radionuclide cycling. The complexity of evaluating or predicting dose to man is illustrated by the number of pathways in which radioactivity can reach man. In some cases simple food chains (e.g., ^{90}Sr → soil → plants → cows → milk → man) are easy to identify, but identification and quantification of all pathways to man can be extremely complex. Figure 13–1 depicts the pathways for transfer of radionuclides to man in a tropical environment. It is apparent that not only geographical differences in man's environment but also cultural differences in diet or habit are important.

The problems of environmental radioactivity will become more critical in the future. What we learn now about the fate of radionuclides and radiation in ecologic systems may help determine (1) whether release or containment of atomic wastes is the better policy or (2) if release practices continue as nuclear power production increases, whether the benefits are worth the risks.

F. Future Research in Radioecology

Like other environmental scientists, the radioecologist of the future will be concerned with providing information necessary for technological assessment of our expanding energy needs. Much more research on the ecologic consequences of chronic, low level releases of radionuclide and thermal effluents is needed to provide the best locational and operational criteria for power reactors.

The continued experimental use of radionuclides as tools to elucidate pathways, food chains, and bioaccumulations in aquatic and terrestrial ecosystems will provide knowledge that is relevant to both radioactive and nonradioactive pollution problems. For example, tracer studies with mercury-203 can be used to determine the rate and extent to which this toxic substance concentrates in aquatic food chains which lead to man.

Thus, the radioecologist will continue to be involved with research that is both practical and basic. It is practical in its concern with the fate and effects of radioactivity in the environment. It is basic in that knowledge of these radioactive substances also help us understand the structure and function of ecologic systems.

SUMMARY

Radioecology is a discipline which is concerned with the distribution and consequences of radiation and radioactive substances released to the environment. Sources of such releases may be natural (background), peaceful or military uses of nuclear explosives, and industrial or technological uses of radioactive substances. The consequences of releasing radioactivity into the environment depend on how ecologic systems (forests, lakes, fields, oceans, etc.) regulate the biologic distribution of radioactivity. Major study areas are (1) dynamics of radionuclides in food chains, (2) identification of pathways by which radionuclides may expose individuals or populations (including man) to ionizing radiation, and (3) determination of the radiosensitivities of living components of ecologic systems.

In addition to considering radionuclides as pollutants, the radioecologist uses them as tools to determine structure and function of ecologic systems. This basic information is necessary for assessing the impact of nonnuclear technologies on the environment.

References

1. Auerbach, S. I., Nelson, D. J., Kaye, S. V., Reichle, D. E., and Coutant, C. C.: Ecological Considerations in Reactor Power Plant Siting. International Atomic Energy Agency SM-146/53, 1971.
2. Fowler, E. B. (ed.): *Radioactive Fallout, Soils, Plants, Foods, Man.* New York, Elsevier, 1965.
3. Hungate, F. P. (ed.): *Radiation and Terrestrial Ecosystems.* Oxford, Pergamon Press, 1966.
4. Kaye, S. V., and Ball, S. J.: Systems analysis of a coupled compartment model for radionuclide transfer in a tropical environment. *In* Nelson, D. J., and Evans, F. C. (eds.): Symposium on radioecology. USAEC Conference 670503, 1969.
5. Morgan, K. Z.: Permissible exposure to ionizing radiation. Science, *139*:565–571, 1963.
6. Nelson, D. J., and Evans, F. C. (eds.): Symposium

on radioecology. USAEC Conference 670503, 1969.

7. Odum, E. P.: *Fundamentals of Ecology*, 3rd ed. Philadelphia, W. B. Saunders, 1971.

8. Packard, C.: The relation between age and radio-sensitivity of *Drosophila* eggs. Radiology, 25:223–230, 1935.

9. Schultz, V., and Kelment, A. W., Jr. (eds.): *Radioecology*. New York, Reinhold, 1963.

10. Sparrow, A. H., and Woodwell, G. M.: Prediction

of the sensitivity of plants to chronic gamma irradiation. Radiat. Botany, 2:9, 1962.

11. Sparrow, A. H.: Comparisons of the tolerances of higher plant species to acute and chronic exposures of ionizing radiation. Japan. J. Genet., 40:12–37, 1964.

12. Woodwell, G. M.: Sensitivity to ionizing radiation. *In* Altman, P. L., and Dittmer, D. S. (eds.): *Environmental Biology*. Bethesda, Md., Federation of American Societies for Experimental Biology, 1966.

Radiation Hazards in Space

Michael A. Bender, Ph.D.

13.2 THE SPACE RADIATION ENVIRONMENT

The radiation background to which people are exposed on the surface of the earth comes partly from decay of radioisotopes in the environment and in their bodies and partly from cosmic radiations. On earth the cosmic ray component is small because of the active shielding effect of the earth's magnetic field, which deflects most of the particles except near the poles, and because of the passive shielding provided by the mass of the atmosphere through which a particle must pass to reach the surface. In addition, most of the radiation reaching the surface from cosmic rays is actually softer secondary radiation from primary cosmic ray interaction with the atmosphere, rather than the energetic primary particles themselves. In deep space, however, the cosmic ray flux is unattenuated, and space travelers may thus receive appreciable doses. In addition, the deflection and consequent trapping of the cosmic radiation flux by the earth's magnetic field results in local high radiation level zones, the Van Allen belts, located some distance from the earth.

The cosmic radiation flux has two distinct components, one from the sun and the other originating outside our solar system. The solar component is very much larger than the so-called galactic component and is composed of electrons and especially protons produced by the sun during solar flare activity. Solar flare activity is relatively unpredictable, although the cycle of flare events has a rather regular 11-year period of maxima and minima. The size of individual flares is also quite variable. Large flares, though infrequent, can produce peak dose rates of as much as 100 R per hour in deep space in the neighborhood of the earth's orbit, even inside a shielding of a few grams per square centimeter of aluminum such as is practical in a spacecraft. The galactic cosmic ray flux is composed mainly of heavy charged particles, the nuclei of various atoms stripped of electrons and traveling with enormous speed. One of these particles thus may have a very large mass, depending on the element involved, and very large energy. Unlike the particles originating from the sun, which tend to be somewhat directional, making "shadow" shielding practical, the galactic cosmic ray flux is omnidirectional; the frequency of galactic particles is quite low, however, and the flux does not change in magnitude appreciably with time.

The charged particles trapped in the Van Allen belt are distributed in fairly discrete bands around the earth's equator. As might be expected, the intensity of the radiation in the belts is somewhat dependent on the level of solar flare activity in the past. In

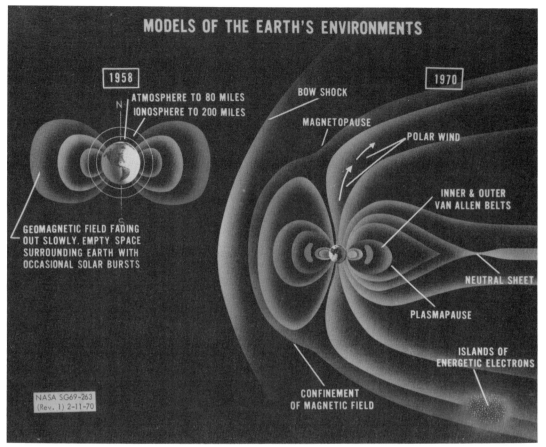

FIGURE 13-2 NASA drawing illustrating the relationship of the earth's magnetic fields and the Van Allen trapped radiation belts.

addition, stratospheric nuclear weapons tests have injected large quantities of particles into the inner belt, thus markedly increasing the flux for a relatively long time. The radiation dose rates in the most intense parts of the Van Allen belts may be of the order of about 100 R per hour. Fortunately, this falls off quite rapidly both with radial distance from the earth and with angular displacement from the plane of the equator.

The possibility of encountering fairly large radiation fluxes in space thus appears quite real, and has been a concern for manned space flight from its earliest planning stages. In addition to these natural sources, man-made radiation must also be considered in assessing radiation hazards in space. Radioactive power generation and fuel gauging devices have been considered for spacecraft and even carried on some of the Apollo Missions. In the future, nuclear power generators and quite possibly nuclear spacecraft propulsion systems will doubtless be used because of their relatively high power yields per unit mass added to the spacecraft. Though more easily controlled, exposures from such sources must also be considered in planning future flights.

13.3 RADIOSENSITIVITY UNDER SPACE FLIGHT CONDITIONS

In considering the radiation hazards associated with space travel one must take into account special conditions that might be expected to modify radiation response. The only obvious example is oxygen tension. Because of constraints on the mass that can be carried on board spacecraft, the crews of the United States' Mercury and Gemini space flights breathed pure oxygen (this does not appear to have been true of any of the Russian manned flights). The oxygen pressure, however, was only about 5.5 pounds per square inch, and the men were thus exposed to partial pressures of oxygen about twice as large as air at sea level pressure. Partial pressures of this order would not be expected to alter tissue oxygenation levels enough to produce notable changes in radiosensitivity.

In contrast to oxygen tension, the effect of which may be tested in terrestrial experiments, there is one factor unique to space flight—a long-term exposure to weightlessness. Weightlessness is produced by either orbital or free fall flight and is thus characteristic of all but the launch, re-entry, and maneuvering phases of most space flights. While brief periods of weightlessness (up to a few seconds) may be produced by free fall or by parabolic flight in aircraft, weightlessness of significant duration can only be produced in space.

Partly because the effects of prolonged weightlessness were unknown, early spacecraft carried various biologic test systems that were later studied and compared with controls that had remained on the ground. Surprisingly, effects usually associated with radiation were reported. The levels of effects observed were often enormously greater than could be accounted for on the basis of the radiation exposure to which the organisms had been exposed during flight. This led to serious consideration of the idea that there might be a synergism between radiation and weightlessness, and to considerable apprehension about the radiation hazards of manned spaceflight. Several series of in-flight experiments were undertaken to test this possibility. Experimental systems commonly used in radiobiology, including human white blood cells, spores of the bread mold *Neurospora*, *Tradescantia* flowers, and adults and pupae of various insects were flown aboard manned and unmanned spacecraft for periods of up to three days. During orbital flight they were irradiated with various carefully measured doses of radiation of known quality and quantity. Following the spaceflights, the samples were recovered, and the levels of various radiobiologic effects, including mutations, chromosomal aberrations, and survival rates, were measured. Although comparison of the results from the materials irradiated in space with those from the control material that remained on the ground did in a few cases appear to suggest that there might be synergism (or even an antagonism for some endpoints), the results from most of the experimental systems suggested no radiation interaction at all, thus refuting the synergism theory.

Some of the materials flown for these experiments were not deliberately exposed to the on-board sources of radiation and thus served as in-flight controls. Comparison of these with the ground controls allowed testing of the possibility that either the ambient radiation encountered during the flight, or some other spaceflight factor such as weightlessness, might produce effects similar to those reported from the early observations that led to the development of the synergism theory. But in most cases no such effects were observed. In a few of the biologic systems observed there did appear to be differences between the in-flight and ground control samples, but these effects were all noted for rather poorly understood endpoints involving cell division and maturation. Such results suggest that the vibration, weightlessness, or some other factor associated with space flight may affect cell division or timing of the cell cycle or differentiation. An effect of this kind, although of biologic interest, appears to have little importance with respect to radiation hazards in space.

Another set of observations tends to confirm the conclusion that there are no special hazards associated with the low doses of ambient radiation received by space crews during orbital or lunar missions. Pre- and postflight peripheral leukocyte samples were obtained from the crew members for all of the Gemini and the early Apollo Missions and used to determine somatic chromosome aberration frequencies. No postflight increases in aberrations that could be attributed to radiation were seen. Small increases in chromatid aberrations (which in this system could not have resulted from radiation exposure) were seen in a few cases, but even these appeared to be unrelated to mission duration, extra-vehicular activity, or other factors associated with the flights. The production of somatic chromosome aberrations is a sensitive indicator of radiation damage. Though the radiation doses received by crew members were quite small (of the order of 50 mR), the leukocyte aberration observations agree with the results of the biologic experiments, so it seems safe to conclude that there are no special radiation hazards associated with space flight.

13.4 RADIATION HAZARDS IN MANNED MISSIONS

Though radiation hazards have not been a real problem in the earth orbital and lunar flights carried out so far, radiation exposures and their possible effects have been a consideration in mission planning. For types of missions being planned for the future, including long stays in orbiting space stations and manned planetary missions of long duration, radiation hazards become much more important and have had to be carefully evaluated.

The philosophy that must be adopted in evaluating radiation hazards for spacecraft crews is obviously very different from that appropriate for considering, for example, the problem of occupational exposures in industry. The question of genetic hazards does not arise at all, both because the population of crew members is so small, and because of their ages. Space flight is an extremely hazardous business at best, and the risks incurred through radiation exposure during a mission must be considered in proportion to the risks from other sources. There is little question that moderate increases in radiation doses will increase an individual's probability of developing various forms of neoplasia, especially leukemia, or will be responsible for nonspecific life shortening. But an increased risk of leukemia of—for example, 5×10^{-6} per year— while clearly unacceptable for other populations, seems insignificant when one considers the orders of magnitude greater risks of sudden death from other sources that must be accepted by space travelers. The practical considerations, then, must be of radiation exposures that might produce high risks of death, either directly or as a result of degrading crew performance enough to significantly jeopardize the mission, or that will produce later clinical effects—cataracts, for example—with high probability. Though such factors as dose

rate and radiation quality must be taken into account, generally such effects require doses of the order of hundreds of rads.

Of the sources of radiation in space already outlined, only two are matters of concern in this regard: the solar flare event and the radiation from nuclear power generators and propulsion systems. Excepting for the moment the relatively rare, high Z, high energy particles, the galactic cosmic ray dose rates appear to be too low to present a real hazard, even for interplanetary flights of very long duration. The radiation trapped in the Van Allen belt, though capable of producing relatively high dose rates, need only be encountered for brief periods during a mission. Earth orbits have generally been roughly circular and well below the intense portion of the inner belt. The orbits for future earth orbital flights, such as for space stations and platforms, can be chosen to largely avoid this hazard, both by selection of appropriate apogee and perigee and by inclination of the orbit from the equatorial plane of the belts. Lunar and interplanetary flight paths can be selected to avoid passing through the belts; and even if the belts are traversed, the time spent at high dose rates is short.

In the absence of solar flare events, the solar cosmic ray flux is relatively small. A large or even a moderate flare event, however, may produce lethal or at least damaging doses in a relatively short period of time. A relatively large portion of the particle flux produced by a flare event is of low energy, and the doses received by crew members are therefore greatly reduced by the light shielding provided by their suits and by the spacecraft itself. The larger spacecraft that might be built for space station or interplanetary use may well provide somewhat greater average shielding, but it seems impossible that enough can be provided to adequately protect crews caught in space during a major flare event. This is, of course, because of restrictions on the mass of the spacecraft that can be accelerated to the necessary velocities with the energy sources available, complicated by the fact that shields become less effective at higher energies because Bremsstrahlung and "build-up" particle production tend to increase dose rate inside the spacecraft.

For the low altitude earth orbital flights made in the past a network of stations observing known predictors of solar flare activity was set up so that missions could be delayed if a flare seemed likely or so that a mission could be aborted before the crew members received an appreciable dose. This approach was also used for the lunar orbiting and lunar landing missions, though it was recognized that the risks were greater because return to the earth's surface could not usually be achieved in a sufficiently short time. Nevertheless, the early warning system would give the crew time at least to return to the lunar landing spacecraft, and possibly to the orbiting Apollo spacecraft, and take advantage of the protection of the additional shielding.

On very long journeys into space the probability of at least one large flare event occurring becomes very high, and the possibility of returning to earth for protection virtually approaches zero. It is apparent that some solution other than adequately increasing the spacecraft's skin thickness to protect the crew must be found. Providing shielding for a small "foxhole" area for the crew, possibly using some of the spacecraft's most massive equipment for a shadow shield, has been suggested as a reasonably practical solution. The crew, given warning from earth, could confine themselves to the protected area and orient the spacecraft so as to minimize their exposure. Another proposal has been to attempt to provide magnetic shielding similar to the earth's, possibly using superconducting coils to generate a field large enough to effectively deflect protons around the spacecraft. Though the method that will be adopted to provide radiation protection for such missions has not yet been decided upon, it seems almost certain that the problem of radiation protection for the crew will have to be solved before these missions are undertaken.

Man-made radiation sources, such as nuclear reactors for propulsion, also pose a serious shielding problem in manned spacecraft. In general, this problem may be somewhat ameliorated by placing the source some distance from the crew, thus taking advantage of both the reduction in dose rates from the inverse square law and also of the reduction in mass required for a simple shadow shield because of the smaller solid angle it must protect.

Another possible, though not very probable, hazard for crews of long duration interplanetary missions may exist. The very heavy, very energetic galactic cosmic ray particles are capable of penetrating most shields and have very long path lengths in tissue. In tissue they produce tracks along which energy is deposited locally in very large quantities. Though the flux of such particles is low, and the dose rate very small when averaged over the body, the local dose rates along their paths are large enough to kill cells. In tissues which are self-renewing, such as bone marrow or skin, the occasional killing of a few cells by a cosmic ray "needle" will clearly be of no consequence. However, in a tissue that cannot replace dead cells, such as brain, it is possible that the gradual accumulation of damage from heavy galactic particles might eventually lead to a dangerous decrement in crew performance. The real extent of this hazard remains a matter of conjecture at this point, but the problem will probably have to be settled before flights of extremely long duration are attempted.

SUMMARY

The radiation environment in space has features that may constitute a hazard to manned spaceflight. Solar flares occasionally produce fluxes that could be hazardous or even lethal to space travelers on long missions far from earth. The steady flux of galactic heavy energetic nuclei may also constitute a hazard if enough brain cells are killed to produce a performance decrement.

References

1. Langham, W. (ed.): *Radiobiological Factors in Manned Spaceflight.* Washington, D.C., National Academy of Sciences, 1968.
2. *Space Biology.* Washington, D.C., Space Science Board, National Academy of Sciences, 1970.

Microwaves

Glenn V. Dalrymple, M.D.

13.5 BIOLOGIC EFFECTS OF MICROWAVES

Microwave radiation represents a form of electromagnetic radiation which does not cause ionization. These radiations are produced by such diverse sources as radar units, cooking ovens, diathermy units, and microwave generators for communication purposes. In radiology, one usually thinks of photon energy in terms of MeV, KeV, and so on. Since the microwave energies are so low (10^{-3} to 10^{-7} eV) these radiations are characterized by their frequencies. The frequencies of greatest biologic interest fall between 100 and 30,000 megahertz.* The photon energy, in fact, is so low that microwaves cannot cause ionization. Instead, when they are absorbed they cause molecules of the absorber to have an increased rate of vibration. The result of this is increased heat production. Most of the observed biologic changes are due to the heating which accompanies microwave absorption. Although some nonthermal effects have been ascribed to microwaves, for our purposes heating will be considered as the major hazard.

The amount of energy absorbed in biologic material is a function of several variables. Such factors as the frequency of the radiation, the intensity of the beam, the thermal conductivity of the tissue, and the depth of the target beneath the surface greatly affect the eventual result of irradiation. The frequency dependence of the absorption of microwaves is, in a sense, reversed from that of ionizing radiation. The lowest energy microwaves (below 150 MHZ) pass *through* biologic material without being absorbed. As the frequency increases from 150 to 1000 MHZ, the energy is absorbed by deeper tissues within the human body. The result is heating of deeper structures, while relatively little heating of the skin thermal receptors is produced. This situation becomes particularly ominous because the individual can receive a great deal of damage to his viscera while not sensing that anything is wrong. As the frequency increases, the range in tissue *decreases.* As the frequencies increase above 3000 MHZ, the depth of penetration becomes so reduced that the effects are similar to those of infrared. In this instance, the individual being irradiated senses the heating.

For a given beam at a given intensity and frequency, not all of the microwaves are absorbed. Depending upon certain physical conditions, some of the microwaves are reflected, transmitted, or absorbed. For those microwaves that are absorbed, the amount of *energy* absorbed varies with the tissue type. Experiments have shown that microwave absorption increases with an increasing water content. Since skin, muscle, and the viscera have a high water content, they absorb microwaves more effectively than fatty tissue and bone, which have a lower water content.

As in the case of the more familiar ionizing radiations, the biologic hazard depends not only upon the energy (frequency) of the microwave radiation, but also upon the intensity of the beam and the length of exposure. Consequently, the combined effect of these factors must be considered. If the body cannot dissipate the heat, the temperature will rise and severe injury can result.

Under usual conditions the human body can dissipate some 10 mW per cm²; this is equivalent to .0024 calories per sec per cm².* If an individual is total body irra-

---

*The term "hertz" is synonymous with cycles per second. A 100-megahertz (MHZ) frequency then equals 10^8 cps. The energy of the microwave beam can be calculated from the relation: $E = h\nu$, where E is the energy in ergs, ν is the frequency (in hertz) and h is Planck's constant.

---

*The dissipation of heat can be stated in many ways. Recall from elementary physics the following relations:

$$1 \text{ watt} = 1 \text{ joule/sec}$$
$$1 \text{ calorie} = 4.186 \text{ joules}$$

Therefore, $10 \text{ mW} = .01 \text{ W} = .01 \dfrac{\text{joules}}{\text{sec}} \times \dfrac{1}{4.186} \dfrac{\text{calories}}{\text{joules}}$
$= .0024$ calories/sec. Since this is also a function of surface area, 10 mW/cm² = .0024 calories/sec/cm².

diated with a beam of sufficient intensity such that the input of heat exceeds 100 mW per cm² (this is assumed to be the maximum rate of heat dissipation), the body temperature and the basal metabolic rate will rise. If carried to an extreme, this can result in prostration, heat stroke, and death. The pathologic changes produced are indistinguishable from those produced by severe fever of any origin.

Experimental evidence indicates that the eyes, testes, the gallbladder, the urinary bladder, and the gastrointestinal tract are the regions most sensitive to microwaves. The basic lesion probably concerns the ability of the tissue in question to dissipate the heat. The eye is so constructed that the lens represents an Achilles' heel. It is avascular and enclosed in a capsule. Not only does it lack a cooling system, but it also lacks macrophages to remove dead cells. The result of sufficient microwave irradiation is cataracts, and at higher doses damage to the conjunctiva and cornea can occur. The primary microwave frequencies causing these changes fall between 1000 and 3000 MHZ.

The testes are sensitive to the microwave irradiation because even a modest elevation of temperature causes degenerative changes in the seminiferous tubules and the spermatozoa. The normal testicular temperature remains 2 to 3° C below body temperature. When the testicular temperature becomes elevated to body temperature, the spermatozoa exhibit abnormalities, and sterility may result. Low power densi-

ties of microwaves, 0.01 W per cm² given as a continuous exposure, is thought to represent the threshold for causing testicular damage.

The primary microwave frequencies causing testicular damage and damage to internal organs fall between 150 and 1200 MHZ. Frequencies above 3500 MHZ produce heating of the outer layers of the skin and the lens of the eye. Frequencies above 10,000 MHZ cause heating of the skin surface; no significant penetration to the deeper structure occurs.

On the basis of experimental and clinical evidence, the permissible continuous exposure level for microwaves has been set at 10 mW per cm². Greater intensity (up to 100 mW per cm²) is allowed for short periods of time, however.

References

1. Moore, W., Jr.: Biological aspects of microwave radiation; A review of hazards. Washington, D.C., U.S. Department of Health, Education and Welfare, Consumer Protection and Environmental Health Services, National Center of Radiological Health, 1968.
2. Barron, C. I., and Baraff, A. A.: Medical considerations of exposure to microwaves. J.A.M.A., 168:1194, 1968.
3. Cleary, S. F. (ed.): Biological effects and health implications of microwave radiation. Symposium proceedings. Washington, D.C., U.S. Department of Health, Education and Welfare, Public and Environmental Health Services, 1970.
4. Deichmann, W. B., Bernal, E., Stephens, F., and Landeen, K.: Effect of chronic exposure to microwave radiation. J. Occup. Med., 5:418, 1963.

Lasers

A. J. Moss, Jr., Ph.D.

13.6 BIOLOGIC EFFECTS OF LASERS

The laser is a device capable of amplifying electromagnetic radiations which fall in that portion of the electromagnetic spectrum occupied by microwaves and visible light. The development of the optical laser arose from the concept of stimulated

emission for microwave amplification, first suggested independently during the period from 1953 to 1954 by Weber at the University of Maryland, by Townes at Columbia University, and by Basov and Prokhorov in the Soviet Union. The optical laser, developed by Maiman in the latter part of 1960, provided for the first time a light beam having characteristics commonly associated with microwave radiation. Today, lasing action has been exhibited in a variety of solids, organic liquids, gases, and vapors, resulting in a variety of wavelengths from the near ultraviolet to the infrared.

Light is an electromagnetic radiation that exhibits properties which may be described by classic optics. A characteristic of all common sources of light (such as the light produced by incandescent bulbs) is the *lack* of coherence of light emanating from different points of a radiating source. The term coherence is used to describe a correlation between the phases of monochromatic radiation emanating from two different points. Consequently, light from common sources is "spatially incoherent." This term means that the light emerges randomly in an array of separate waves which may either reinforce or cancel each other in a random fashion. This results in the production of wave fronts which are random and change from one moment to the next. Such a phenomenon may be visualized by throwing a large number of pebbles into a pool of water at one time. If only a single pebble is thrown, however, a coherent circular wave front is produced.

On the other hand, light produced by the laser is coherent. Thus, any point on these fronts exhibits identical characteristics. As the wave fronts pass a point in space the field strength rises and falls smoothly in phase, oscillating from maximum to minimum.

Stimulated emission, which is the basis of laser action, is the reverse of the process in which electromagnetic radiation, or photons, are absorbed by atoms. When electromagnetic energy is absorbed by an atom, changes occur in the energy configuration of the electron shells surrounding the nucleus. The energy of the absorbed photon is converted into internal energy of the absorbing atom. Under the proper conditions of absorption, the atom is raised to an "excited" quantum energy state. The "excited" atom, however, now exists in an unstable state and at some later time may radiate this energy spontaneously by emitting a photon. The atom then reverts to the "ground" state or to some state intermediate between the excited and ground states. During the period in which the atom is still excited, it can be stimulated to emit a photon if it is struck by an outside photon

having precisely the energy of the one which would otherwise be emitted spontaneously. In this process, the released photon falls precisely in phase with the wave that triggered its release, resulting in the emission of two photons of the same wave length with the previously excited atom returning to the ground state.

A major concern in laser design is the production of an active material in which most of the atoms can be raised to an excited state so that electromagnetic radiation of the correct frequency passing through them will stimulate the release of an avalanche of photons. There must be an excess of excited atoms to enable stimulated emission to predominate over absorption. Atoms are raised to an excited state by introducing into the system electromagnetic radiation at a wavelength different from the stimulation wavelength. This process is known as "optical pumping." Once the active medium has been prepared, it is enclosed in a structure with two small mirrors facing each other. When photon emission occurs, the resulting wave starts out near one mirror and travels along the axis of the system. Along its path the wave grows by stimulated emission until it reaches the other mirror. There it is reflected back into the active material so that growth can continue. Provided that the gains on repeated passages exceed the losses at the mirrors, a steady wave is formed. One of the mirrors is semi-transparent so that a portion of the wave can escape and pass to the exterior. This outlet provides the output of the laser.

The light generated by the laser is directional, powerful, and essentially monochromatic and coherent. The output is directional since the only waves emitted must have repeated passages and monochromatic because stimulated emission is a resonant process and takes place most strongly at the center of the band of frequencies that can be emitted by spontaneous radiation. These selected frequencies, in turn, cause emission at the same frequency; thus, the wave contains only an extremely narrow range of frequencies. The output is also spatially and time coherent since all wave fronts are perpendicular to the direction of propagation and there is a fixed phase relationship between the portion of the wave emitted at any instant and the wave emitted after a fixed time period.

A variety of lasers have emerged since the

initial development of the first ruby laser. Currently a wide range of lasers are available covering a multiplicity of operating characteristics. Both pulsed and continuous wave lasers are available which provide a wide range of frequencies and power levels.

The response of tissue to laser light varies and depends upon a number of factors; however, temperature transmission and absorption appear to be the most critical considerations. In addition, secondary effects such as tissue ionization, alterations in cellular physiology, and so on, are important. These tissue alterations depend in a large part upon such factors as energy density, the wavelength of the laser beam, and the type and mode of energy delivery. Tissue destruction appears to be directly related not only to the degree of pigmentation, but to the size of the area to be treated and the cellular consistency of the exposed tissue.

The most critical organ, as far as biologic effects are concerned, is the eye. Both the cornea and the lens are highly transparent to wavelengths in the visible region. As the wavelength of incident light is increased, significant absorption becomes apparent at wavelengths longer than 10,000 Å in the lens and in the cornea at wavelengths greater than 14,000 Å. On the other hand, the absorption of the pigment epithelium of the retina and the choroid is significantly greater in the visible portion of the spectrum. The absorption ranges from a maximum at 4500 Å to a minimum at 7000 Å. The power density required to reach the threshold for retinal injury increases with a reduction in pulse duration. Presently, many investigators feel that the effects produced by pulses of a nanosecond or shorter may be explained on the basis of absorbed thermal energy.

The retinal injury threshold is defined as that energy or power density required to produce a barely observable lesion after a period of five minutes or more post-exposure. This threshold region lies in the range of several tenths of a joule per cm² for pulsed white light (xenon laser) and pulsed ruby systems. A number of patients with eye disorders have been treated with the ruby laser photocoagulator.

In addition to ophthalmological uses, lasers are also finding use in dermatology, surgery, and cellular biology. Dermatologic uses of the laser may generally be divided into two areas: applications requiring moderate exposure levels and applications requiring massive doses. The first area includes exposure doses an order of magnitude above the minimal reactive dose for skin. Such exposures are useful for the removal of foreign pigments in the skin, the treatment of vascular disorders, and the removal of various skin lesions. Generally, these moderate doses are delivered with pulsed ruby and neodymium lasers operating in the long pulse mode. The second area of use deals with the treatment of surface skin cancers. In this respect, massive doses are delivered with pulsed ruby and neodymium lasers.

High power continuous laser systems have been applied to the area of surgery. With high power beams the primary reaction with tissue is thermal. When the beam is focused on a tissue surface, the absorbed radiation rapidly increases the temperature of a small volume of tissue causing vaporization and ablation of the region. Since the thermal response is very rapid, the beam may be moved across the surface, resulting in a continuous cut, spontaneously coagulating small capillaries present and thereby eliminating bleeding. For this application, initial studies have included the argon and carbon dioxide lasers.

For biologic and cellular research the instrumentation includes a small pulsed or continuous laser in conjunction with a microscope. For these investigations, the beam is focused at the microscope stage. In this manner focal sizes in the range of 1.0 to 5.0 μ in diameter have been used for cellular irradiation.

The development and utilization of lasers in medicine and biology has greatly increased since their inception. As the number of different lasers increase and biologic effects become more fully understood, lasers will assume an increasingly important role in the biomedical field.

References

1. Goldman, L.: *Biomedical Aspects of the Laser.* New York, Springer-Verlag, 1967.
2. Lengyel, B. A.: *Lasers—Generation of Light by Stimulated Emission.* New York, John Wiley, 1962.
3. McGuff, P. E.: *Surgical Applications of Laser.* Springfield, Ill., Charles C Thomas, 1966.

14 RADIATION DETECTION AND PROTECTION

Gail D. Adams, Ph.D., and Aaron P. Sanders, Ph.D.

14.0 INTRODUCTION: DETECTION

Radiation detectors altogether present as great a diversity as the radiations to be measured. There is no one kind suited to all purposes. At low radiation levels one uses counters (devices which provide one response for each triggering event). The Geiger-Mueller counter produces a charge avalanche in a gaseous atmosphere whenever triggered; the size of the avalance is determined by counter characteristics, not by the initiating particle. When counting charged particles, the efficiency of the G-M counter can approach 100 per cent; when counting photons, the efficiency approximates one per cent.

Solid scintillation counters are widely used now, mostly NaI(Tl), and particularly when photons are to be counted. The NaI(Tl) is a transparent crystal and can readily be obtained in sizes measured in inches. For such sizes, there is a large probability of interaction by any incident photon. An initial interaction will normally be either by photoelectric or Compton effect. If the former, substantially all of the energy of the incident photon will be deposited near the interaction site. If Compton, the energy given to the electron will be deposited locally, and the secondary photon may escape the crystal or may suffer another interaction, photo or Compton, with the same considerations. Any photon whose absorption history in the crystal ends with a photoelectric interaction deposits substantially all of its energy in the crystal. This particular crystal is chosen because (a) the interaction probability with photons is relatively high, (b) the energy deposited produces a light flash, or scintillation, (c) the amount of light so produced is almost exactly proportional to the amount of energy deposited, and (d) the wavelength (color) of this light is suited to efficient detection by a multiplier phototube. The phototube converts this light flash through a series of steps to a voltage pulse, the height of which is proportional to the energy deposited in the crystal. The use of an electronic circuit called a pulse height analyzer is the key to the special utility of this counting system. Counts recorded can be segregated into pulse height groupings. In particular, one commonly chooses a small pulse height group with a central value corresponding to the energy of an incident photon of concern. This technique is particularly useful to minimize the effect of background radiation or to discern the quantity of one radionuclide present when others are also in the same sample.

Liquid scintillation systems are used primarily where the radionuclide of concern emits only a β of relatively low energy.

Counting becomes reasonably efficient, perhaps even possible, in this system, because attenuation in a container wall is avoided. Notable radionuclides are $^3_1$H, $^{14}_6$C, $^{35}_{16}$S, and $^{45}_{20}$Ca. In some suitable fashion, the radionuclide is dispersed in the liquid (toluene or p-dioxane plus additives), and the light is proportional to energy deposited. Although not quite as clean as for photons, separation of mixtures of β-emitters is possible when the energy maxima of the β spectra are substantially different.

There are also solid state detectors [Ge(Li) or Si(Li) crystals] which have excellent energy resolution but low efficiency and, hence, are little used biomedically.

At high radiation levels, the count rate becomes so large that individual pulses cannot be detected as entities. In such circumstances, one tends to use some form of ionization chamber. This is a contained volume of gas, most frequently air, with two electrodes (one +, the other −) exposed. The interactions of the incident radiation with the walls and with the gas in the chamber results effectively in the production of ionization of the gas molecules. Positive ions migrate to the − electrode, negative ions to the + electrode. The current so formed may be amplified and read, as in the survey instrument called "Cutie Pie." Or, the total charge transfer in a given exposure may be measured, as in the condenser R-meter. These instruments may be, and frequently are, calibrated so that radiation amounts can be read for specific exposure circumstances in terms of recognized units, notably the roentgen.

14.1 DOSIMETRY

Measurements of quantity of radiations are included in the term "dosimetry." Diversity again requires us to mention various situations. In general, when energy is deposited in a medium some changes are made. Many of these changes are quite detectable. A good detector will exhibit a response which is reproducible, discernible at useful radiation levels, and proportional to the amount of radiation.

For charged particle beams the primary measurement is normally related to the number of particles in the beam. The detector involved is a Faraday cup, which absorbs the particle beam and gives an external electron current equal to that absorbed. This typically would be used to calibrate a transmission ionization chamber which then could be used to monitor the beam intensity.

The rate at which energy is deposited in a medium by a beam of charged particles, in principle, may be either calculated or measured. For example, the total beam energy in a given exposure might be measured with a calorimeter. A second similar exposure, but with a layer of absorbing material interposed, would reduce the energy available to the calorimeter by an amount equal to that removed by the absorber.

When the beam is of uncharged particles, a secondary production methodology must be employed for measurement. In the case of photons, the method involves the ability of the radiation to ionize air; the quantity measured is called exposure and the unit is the roentgen (1 R = 2.58×10^{-4} coulomb/kilogram). For neutron beams, one uses the neutron spectrum and the number of particles involved to predict the energy deposition pattern.

But no matter what method is used to assess quantity for the incident radiation, the measurement of effect is uniformly agreed to be in terms of energy deposited. The name of the quantity is "absorbed dose" (now shortened to "dose") and the unit is the rad (1 rad = 100 ergs/gram = 10^2 joule/kilogram). Energy deposition has been assessed with a wide variety of instrumentation. Examples are microcalorimeters, chemical systems, thermoluminescent materials, small ionization chambers, and so forth. The steps needed to assure or calibrate any particular measurement in energy units are not within the scope of this presentation.

In the case of radionuclides incorporated in the medium, simple calculations may be valid. When the radionuclide distribution is reasonably uniform, the absorbed dose rate is available. For a β-emitter, when the radionuclide concentration is c microcuries/gram and the average energy of the β's is E_βMeV, the average dose rate is $R_\beta = 2.13\ c\ \overline{E}_\beta$ rad/hour. If the radionuclide emits photons, $R_\gamma = 2.13\ c\ E_\gamma$ rad/hour would be correct if a volume involved had dimensions very large compared with the

HVL of the photons. Very often this is not true, so a more complex argument is needed accounting for the geometrical distribution of any particular volume.

As a matter of fact, radionuclide dosimetry frequently entails a rather complex detailed analysis. Certain questions are pertinent:

a) Is the exact decay scheme known? Are the branching ratios and correct particle energies understood?

b) What fraction of gamma rays interacts with orbital electrons of the emitting atom? (This process, known as internal conversion, ejects from orbits internal conversion electrons, which are followed by characteristic X-rays.)

c) Have all sources of characteristic X-ray production been recognized, and in due proportion?

d) What fraction of these characteristic X-rays interacts with orbital electrons (ejecting Auger electrons)?

e) What is the effect of the particular geometrical distribution? What is the edge effect?

14.2 MAXIMUM PERMISSIBLE DOSE

The concept of the maximum permissible dose (MPD) is based upon the idea that maximum radiation exposure levels should be established, both for radiation workers and for the general population. These levels are kept well below the level at which adverse effects may be expected to occur. In the radiation work, as well as in the general population, the concern is to minimize the possibility of genetic damage and carcinogenesis. The recommendations for MPD have been established by the National Council on Radiation Protection and Measurements and by the International Commission on Radiological Protection. The values for MPD do not include any dose received by any individual as a patient or the dose from natural background radiation.

Although levels are quoted for MPD, it should be recognized that this set of values represents the best-educated guess derived from information obtained on overexposure of workers in X-ray departments and in the atomic energy field and from animal experimental data. Consequently, one should always strive to keep the radiation exposure as low as possible while taking into account the practical side of the operation of any radiation facility. The current recommendations for MPD are shown in Table 14–1. It should be noted that occasional deviations from the maximum in a short time interval should not be considered as significant in that the overall averaging of

TABLE 14–1   MAXIMUM PERMISSIBLE DOSE EQUIVALENT VALUES (MPD)[a]

	Average Weekly Dose[b]	Maximum 13-Week Dose	Maximum Yearly Dose	Maximum Accumulated Dose[c]
	rem[d]	rem[d]	rem[d]	rem[d]
Controlled Areas				
Whole body, gonads, blood-forming organs, lens of eye	0.1	3	—	5 (N − 18)[e]
Skin of whole body	—	10[f]	30[f]	—
Hands and forearms, head, neck, feet, and ankles	1.5	25	75	—
Non-Controlled Areas	0.01	—	0.5	—

[a]Exposure of patients for medical and dental purposes is not included in the maximum permissible dose equivalent. From NCRP Report No. 33, Appendix B, Table 1.
[b]For design purposes.
[c]When the previous occupational history of an individual is not definitely known, it shall be assumed that he has already received the full dose permitted by the formula 5 (N − 18).
[d]The numerical value of the exposure in roentgens for the purposes of this report.
[e]N = Age in years and is greater than 18.
[f]Amer. J. Roentgen., 84:152, 1960.

exposure is more important from the individual standpoint.

The values that are shown in Table 14–1 are for radiation workers and do not include the general population. The radiation exposure levels for the general population should be maintained at a level of less than 10 per cent of that indicated for the radiation worker. Currently there is a widespread belief that even the general population should be subdivided into two groups, i.e., those who work in the vicinity of radiation departments but are not truly classified as radiation workers, and the remaining population. Those non-radiation workers who work in areas adjoining radiation departments should have their radiation exposure maintained below 10 per cent of that of the radiation workers. In contrast, for the remaining general population, it is believed that the exposure levels should be maintained at less than 1/30 of the MPD equivalent for radiation workers. In all instances, the MPD equivalent should be taken as a guideline for upper limits, and lower levels should always be aimed for wherever practical.

14.3 BACKGROUND RADIATION

All life is subjected to a continuing source of background radiation which comes from cosmic radiation, from the sun, and from the natural radioactive elements that are present in the earth, in building materials, in the body of each individual, and so forth. Such background radiation levels will vary with altitude and will vary with the locale due to variations in the soil of the naturally occurring radioactive materials. The higher the altitude, the greater is the contribution from the cosmic radiation.

Wherever radiation facilities are to be established, a record of the natural background radiation should be obtained for a period of six months to a year to give an indication of the natural levels prior to the installation of a radiation facility. This would give a record against which to measure subsequently whether or not the radiation facility contributes to increasing background levels. Such background radiation surveys should include levels of radioactive materials in streams, in the air, and elsewhere. In recording radiation background levels it should be noted such levels may vary markedly with the time of day. For example, in the early morning hours air temperature inversions frequently occur when the ground air becomes cooler than the upper air. Under such conditions, the ground air remains quiet, with little mixing with surrounding air. Thus, as radon and thoron gases escape from the earth, they will build up higher concentrations than during the day due to the stationary air from the temperature inversion. These conditions may increase background radiation levels as much as three- or fourfold during such intervals.

It must be emphasized that the background radiation levels should be maintained as close as possible to the natural conditions that exist prior to the installation of any radiation facility, be it an atomic energy plant of some sort or a medical radiographic or radiotherapeutic facility.

14.4 SHIELDING CRITERIA

The shielding of any radiation facility must be such that the areas occupied by an individual, whether he be radiation or non-radiation worker, are shielded and the exposure levels conform to the recommended MPD levels. This means that the shielding for areas where radiation workers are involved will be shielded for one level of radiation as delineated in the MPD values. Those for the general population will be shielded for a different exposure level.

When calculating shielding for any area where radiation workers will be working, the occupancy factor must always be taken as one, i.e., radiation workers will be considered to be in potential radiation zones at all times during a work day. However, in those areas where non-radiation workers are involved, it is possible to take advantage of occupancy factors which are based upon possible time of occupancy for any given individual in the area to be shielded. Table 14–2 indicates the general criteria that one can use in assigning occupancy factors to those areas surrounding a room where non-radiation workers are involved. Similarly, a use factor can be employed, i.e., the percentage of time that a machine might be operational. However, again, a use factor

TABLE 14–2 OCCUPANCY FACTORS*

Full Occupancy (T = 1)

Control space, offices, nurses' stations, corridors, and waiting space large enough to hold desks; darkrooms, workrooms, shops, restrooms, and lounges routinely used by occupationally exposed personnel; living quarters, children's play areas, and occupied space in adjoining buildings

Partial Occupancy (T = 1/4)

Corridors too narrow for desks, utility rooms, restrooms, and lounges, not used routinely by occupationally exposed personnel; wards and patients' rooms, elevators using operators, unattended parking lots, and patients' dressing rooms

Occasional Occupancy (T = 1/16)

Closets too small for future conversion to rooms for occupancy, toilets not used routinely by occupationally exposed personnel, stairways, automatic elevators, sidewalks, and streets

*For use as a guide in planning shielding when complete occupancy data are not available. The maximum permissible dose levels, summarized in Table 14–1, are computed on the basis of the integration of doses received over a period of a year. Therefore, the degree of occupancy of an area should be considered in terms of the time which may be spent in that area by any one person over a period of a year.

cannot be considered to be less than one for a radiation worker since a radiation worker might be working in one radiation zone part of the day and another radiation zone during a later period. Thus, if one took a use factor and an occupancy factor into account in shielding each area, the radiation worker might receive excessive exposure. The work load in roentgens per week at one meter may also be utilized in shielding for the general population. This may not be used in shielding for radiation workers for any given room; the same rationale as stated above applies. In all shielding of radiation installations one must take into account the leakage radiation coming directly through the sides of tube housings and such containment structures: for example, in an X-ray facility or through the shielding for cobalt teletherapy heads. Similarly, one must take into account scattered radiation from patients or equipment when calculating secondary barriers. Primary barriers, of course, are calculated upon the maximum primary beam being directed toward a wall, floor, ceiling, or such. In all instances, where radiation workers are concerned, occupancy factors and use factors must be considered as one.

Similar criteria apply when shielding for storage of radioactive materials, as in radioisotope laboratories. Again, all radiation exposure levels must conform to the MPD as recommended by the National Committee on Radiation Protection and the International Committee on Radiation Protection.

14.5 METHODS OF DOSE REDUCTION TO THE POPULATION BY PHYSICIANS

Considerable progress has been made in the development of radiographic and fluoroscopic X-ray equipment which has led to reduction of the radiation dosage being delivered to patients receiving X-ray examinations. All diagnostic tube housings must now conform to the requirement that leakage through the side of the tube cannot exceed a dosage rate of 100 milliroentgens per hour at a distance of one meter from the target. Primary X-ray beams must now be filtered with a minimum of 2.5 millimeters of aluminum equivalent filtration (preferably three millimeters aluminum filter). The use of such filtration in the primary beam leads to a reduction of radiation dosage by a factor of three to seven (dependent upon the kVp) when compared to the non-filtered X-ray beam. In addition, X-ray equipment with higher kVp outputs are available so that the use of the high-kVp techniques, where applicable, leads to considerable reduction in the radiation dosage to the patient when compared to the low-kilovoltage techniques used in diagnostic radiology.

The use of high-speed screens and high-speed X-ray films has contributed greatly to the decrease in radiation dosage to the population. All diagnostic X-ray equipment now being produced is provided with good collimating systems allowing the operator to collimate the primary beam so that it exposes only that area of the body which is being examined. The use of grids to eliminate the fogging effects of scattered radiation has led to decreased dosage, since better films obtained in this manner minimize the need to repeat films. Image intensifier systems in fluoroscopic units have led to considerable dose reductions for patients undergoing fluoroscopic examinations. The advent of television monitoring, the image intensifier units, and video tape recording has greatly decreased time required for fluoroscopic examinations and hence radiation dosage to patients undergoing such examinations.

The equipment manufacturer can only go so far in decreasing radiation dosage to patients. The intelligent utilization of this equipment by the radiologist and by well-trained radiologic technologists is mandatory. This implies that proper choice of grids, collimators, screens, technique selection, etc., will be made by the radiologist or X-ray technologist.

There must be protection to the unborn population. This requires that shielding be available to reduce exposure to the gonads of patients who are in, or below, the reproductive age. Female patients in the child-bearing age should be selectively scheduled for examinations to avoid irradiating the early pregnant woman. This implies that any elective procedure would be scheduled only during the first 10 days after the onset of the menstrual cycle. Where there is any possible question of pregnancy, and where the medical problem requiring radiologic examination is not acute, the radiologic examination should be delayed until the onset of the menstrual cycle.

14.6 FALLOUT

The source and characteristics of fallout radiation are dependent on the type of weapon and the location of detonation, i.e., in the air, on the earth's surface, below the surface, or below the sea. Radiation from a fission-type weapon is predominantly due to fission products and to the small amount of uranium or plutonium not utilized in the fission reaction. In the fusion-type weapon, i.e., the hydrogen bomb, there is a combination of fission products originating from the atomic weapon used to detonate the hydrogen weapon, and the neutron-induced radiation from the large number of high-energy neutrons which are produced in the fusion weapon.

One of the main hazards from such weapons is the fallout of the residual radioactive particles that are created by the fission or fusion process. The induced radioactivity comes from neutron interaction with components of the bomb and with surface material, i.e., earth or sea water. The intense heat generated by these weapons causes vaporization of many of the induced radioactive surface elements which rise along with the fission products in the fireball to very high altitudes. These radioactive products are distributed over wide areas, dependent upon the wind direction and velocity and upon particle sizes. Another factor determining the extent of the residual radioactivity is the design of the weapon involved, i.e., whether it is a "clean" weapon, designed to minimize the amount of residual radioactivity, or whether it is a "dirty" weapon, salted with special materials in order to deliberately create a high level of radioactivity. For instance, the so-called cobalt bomb utilizes a fusion bomb with a component of stable cobalt material which, on interacting with the neutrons of the fusion weapon, convert to radioactive cobalt. Upon detonation this radioactive matter is spread by fallout over a wide area. In this manner large areas of earth would be rendered no man's land by the fallout.

The radiation dosage being delivered by the fallout from atomic or hydrogen weapons depends upon the distance from ground zero, wind velocity, and wind direction. The magnitude of a radiation dosage at distances as far as 100 miles downwind from ground zero (one-megaton weapon, 15-mph wind) could be lethal for a person remaining outdoors without any shielding. Under these conditions, radiation symptoms would be seen in persons located as far as 140 miles downwind. This fallout radiation would be a mixture of beta- and gamma-radiation. With these factors to consider, proper personnel protection should be obtained to protect atomic energy workers from radiation exposures. In addition, the civil defense agencies have sponsored the development of fallout shelter programs throughout the United States. Many communities already have such programs in existence.

A second facet of the fallout problem is the long-term effect of the long half-life radioactive fallout products. These would contribute to an increase in the background radiation. In addition, the possibility of the concentration of many of these radioactive products in the ecologic cycle poses an important problem. For example, radioactive strontium could create a significant problem in the dairy industry by contamination of its products and consequent bone problems in growing children. Similarly, there could be concentration of radioactive iodine in fish and other water organisms which are subject to consumption by humans. For these reasons, fallout not only is an acute problem associated with the detonation of nuclear weapons but also is a long-term problem that may be related to an increase in background levels of radiation and problems in ecosystems.

There are programs which continuously monitor specific facets of the fallout problem, e.g., radioactive strontium in milk and bones and other radionuclides that may be involved in ecologic cycles. Such monitoring programs are carried out by both the Atomic Energy Commission and the United States Public Health Service throughout the United States and the world.

It is particularly important that the community radiologist acquaint himself with the concerns of radioactive fallout from nuclear warfare, since the practicing radiologist is generally recognized as the radiation authority in most communities. It is therefore recommended that references pertaining to fallout and associated problems be obtained by the radiologist for his personal reference.

Rerences

1. King, I. E. R. (ed.): *Survival in Nuclear Warfare.* CIBA Chemical Symposia, *14*(1), 1962.
2. Morgan, K. Z., and Turner, J. E. (eds.): *Principals of Radiation Protection: A Text Book of Health Physics.* New York, John Wiley, 1967.
3. Stanton, L.: *Basic Medical Radiation Physics.* New York, Appleton-Century-Crofts, 1969.

Regulation of Radiation Usage

James Vandergrift, M.S.

14.7   INTRODUCTION

This section considers how knowledge of radiation injury becomes translated into human precautionary activities. Previous (and following) chapters clearly point out that radiation in biologic systems represents a two-edged sword. It is at once both a powerful tool and a formidable enemy. While radiation provides a means to gain insight, to bring about desirable change, and to provide human comforts, it also is a potential threat to health, life, and future well-being. Consequently, this dual character of radiation requires that human applications involve a deliberate and continuous effort to balance the risks against the benefits.

Unfortunately, the potential benefits seem so great that the threatening aspects may be ignored. This could result in unnecessary danger to the user, to his fellow workers, to his patient, to innocent people in the vicinity, or even to future generations. By not recognizing the hazards and not taking the appropriate precautions, the user becomes negligent.

These realities of radiation and of man make it imperative that safety standards be established, enforced, and maintained "up-to-date." It is not enough to simply charge radiation workers with the responsibility of safety (although the responsibility for proper use is inherent in any clinical setting). Early in the history of radiation usage, it became apparent that scientists, physicians, and men of law must establish a point of reference around which they could make judgments regarding the safe use of radiation. The continuing pursuit of these

TABLE 14–3 MEDICALLY IMPORTANT
RADIATION SOURCES

Radiation-Producing Device	Use
1. X-ray generators	Diagnosis and therapy
2. Teleradioisotope units	Radiotherapy
3. Accelerators (these include cyclotrons, linear accelerators, Van de Graaff accelerators, etc.)	Generation of particles (electrons, protons, neutrons, etc.) for radiotherapy
	Generation of X-rays for radiotherapy
	Production of radionuclides
4. Radionuclides (includes natural, by-product, and accelerator-produced)	Diagnosis and therapy
5. Microwave generators	Physical therapy, radar, diathermy therapy
6. Lasers	Surgical applications, ophthalmology

objectives is what is referred to as "regulation of radiation usage."

14.8 MEDICAL USES OF RADIATION SOURCES

The term radiation, unless otherwise specifically indicated, refers to all particulate as well as electromagnetic forms of radiation.

Table 14–3 summarizes the sources of radiation of medical significance along with the areas of application. X-rays, teleradioisotope therapy units, internally administered radionuclides, and brachytherapy are

TABLE 14–4 MEDICAL RADIATION EXPOSURE
IN THE UNITED STATES

Radiation Source	Application	Patients/Year	Year
X-rays (medical)	Diagnostic	92,936,000	1964
X-rays (dental)	Diagnostic	50,053,000	1964
X-rays (medical)	Therapeutic	597,000	1964
	Subtotal	143,586,000	
Radioisotopes	Diagnostic	1,525,823	1966
Radioisotopes*	Therapeutic	3,445,354	1966
	Subtotal	4,971,177	
	Total	148,557,177	

*Does not include radium therapy, but does include teletherapy and brachytherapy with ^{60}Co, ^{137}Cs, and other sealed radioisotopic sources.

currently of greatest interest because of the number of patients who are exposed to these sources. With time, however, more and more patients will be irradiated by accelerator-produced radiation. Table 14–4 summarizes the number of patients exposed to radiation. The data are the most recent available (note that some information is dated as far back as 1964). In addition, this table does not include more than a million patients on whom *in vitro* radioisotopic studies were done. With the growth of radiology and nuclear medicine, these numbers are increasing at a rapid rate.

One would conclude that a large fraction of patients are exposed to radiation for medical reasons and that a relatively large fraction of the total population receives medical radiation exposure. Another fact which can be inferred from Table 14–4 is that a large number of physicians and paramedical personnel are occupationally exposed to X-rays and radionuclides. As a result, factors such as those indicated previously point out that regulation and control of radiation is an important endeavor in the field of medicine.

14.9 AUTHORITIES AND THEIR JURISDICTION

The authorities in the field of radiation regulations are considered as such by virtue of their expertise in matters of radiation protection, their legal responsibilities in setting and enforcing radiation standards, or both. As a general rule, the "experts" are called upon to convene and make recommendations regarding some aspect of radiation protection or measurement. These deliberations are then used in the formulation and promulgation of rules and regulations by duly authorized agencies of federal, state, or local governments.

An effort will be made to indicate the status of each group with respect to a) geographical jurisdiction; b) compliance requirements—voluntary or regulatory; and c) specific radiation source(s) over which the agency has authority.

A. International Authorities

As one might assume, international groups are strictly advisory; their aim is to establish continuity between nations. Two such international radiation-oriented groups are the International Commission on Radiological Protection (ICRP) and the International Atomic Energy Agency (IAEA). There are others, but these two are most frequently referenced by national and state regulatory agencies.

The recommendations made by the ICRP and IAEA deal primarily with those safety problems of basic but general interest. Permissible radiation doses to occupational and general population groups, permissible concentrations of radioactive materials in air, water, and food, and permissible gonadal doses to the general population are examples of the areas covered in recommendations put forth by these groups.

B. National Authorities

At the national level, the groups providing input for the regulatory machinery are many and diversified. They range from professional groups with very limited interest in the utilization of radiation (e.g., the American Society of Civil Engineers, whose primary concern is in reactor design) to groups with broad interests (such as the American National Standards Institute, (ANSI) and the National Council on Radiation Protection and Measurement (NCRP).)

The authorities in this category are advisory. Compliance with the recommendations from these organizations and agencies is a matter of voluntary choice on the part of the user. Even though their recommendations are sound and their standards and competence widely accepted, these agencies lack the legal power to enforce their recommendations. Their "power" of control rests in their influence upon regulatory authorities. The collaborating group may make recommendations as a body; more often its contribution will be in the form of an individual spokesman meeting with others to develop formal reports.

In virtually all cases, the recommendations of these advisory groups are not only accepted by the regulatory authorities but are actively sought. Therefore, the advice and recommendations from these groups have an excellent chance of appearing in the form of national, state, or local regulations which carry the force of law.

C. State Authorities

State and local authorities will differ somewhat from state to state. They are most often an integral part of a state's public health agency. In two states (Arizona and Louisiana) radiation control authority lies with special state agencies. Massachusetts has made its Department of Labor and Industries responsible for radiation protection. In North Dakota, the responsible agency is the Water Conservation Commission.

The scope and type of control activities also vary from state to state. Compliance may be mandatory or voluntary. Regulations may cover only specific radiation sources or they may be all-inclusive. Approval or permission may require registration or licensing. The registration or licensing may be of the radiation source or of its user.

No attempt will be made here to cover specific state requirements. A general view will, however, indicate specific areas of concern with regard to regulatory activities.

14.10   X-RAYS

The establishment of standards or regulations with respect to X-rays is basically a three-pronged effort with concerns in the following: a) the manufacture, distribution, and repair of X-ray generators and their associated equipment; b) facility design; and c) personnel qualifications and procedural policies.

There are two national bodies who set standards or write regulations regarding medical radiography. They are the NCRP and the Department of Health, Education, and Welfare (HEW).

The NCRP, as mentioned earlier, is an advisory group that makes recommendations on safety standards. Previously their recommendations were published by the U.S. Department of Commerce in the form of National Bureau of Standards handbooks. At the present time, however, the NCRP is publishing its own booklets, and recommendations are in the form of NCRP reports.

One aspect of these reports which makes them extremely useful is the fact that they generally provide two sets of recommendations. These are distinguished from one another by the use of the terms shall and should. "Shall" indicates a recommendation that is necessary to meet the currently accepted standards of radiation protection. "Should" indicates an advisory recommendation that is to be applied when practicable.

To illustrate the fact that the NCRP recommendations are not the result of "outsiders" imposing their wishes upon the medical community, the following is a list of some professional organizations who collaborate with the NCRP in the development of recommendations.

American Academy of Dermatology
American Association of Physicists in Medicine
American College of Radiology
American Dental Association
American Medical Association
American Roentgen Ray Society
Radiation Research Society
Radiological Society of North America
Society of Nuclear Medicine

Federal control of X-ray sources at the present time focuses upon the establishment of rules and regulations regarding the manufacture, import, distribution, repair, and performance of generators and their related devices. This control was made possible under Public Law 90–602 (Radiation Control for Health and Safety Act of 1968). This law directs the Secretary of HEW to establish radiation control standards for electronic products including medical X-rays.

The first of these is found among the Food and Drug Administration's (FDA) regulations in the Code of Federal Regulations (42CFR78).

This set of performance standards in terms of its impact upon the user, stipulates the following:

a) The supplier must provide equipment or components which meet specific performance and safety standards. New X-ray equipment purchased one year after regulations are published in the Federal register must, for example, provide for positive beam limiting devices to restrict the useful beam to the size of the image receptor.

b) The supplier or installer is responsible for insuring that the equipment, after installation, complies with relevant standards when manufacturer's instructions are followed.

c) State and local standards must be identical to those of the FDA when applicable to the same equipment. They cannot be more or less restrictive than the Federal regulations.

Facility design and personnel qualifications for medical use of X-rays have not come under Federal control.

Physician or paramedical personnel qualifications are established and voluntarily followed by the various professional organizations. Although there have been constant efforts under way by individual states to enact legislation to license radiologic technologists, in 1970 only four of the 50 states had such laws (Arizona, California, New Jersey, and New York).

14.11 RADIOACTIVE MATERIALS

Medically important radionuclides and their associated radiopharmaceuticals are controlled at the Federal level by three different agencies. That is to say, there are three different agencies that have primary responsibility over radioactive materials. Again, this responsibility is expressed in the form of recommendations and regulatory authority.

14.12 THE ATOMIC ENERGY COMMISSION

The Atomic Energy Act of 1954 (68 Stat. 919) authorized the AEC to set standards and to establish regulations for the control of by-product, source, and special nuclear materials. It does *not* include natural or accelerator-produced radionuclides. Under this act, physicians desiring to use radioactive materials are required to obtain a specific license or general license number before suppliers are authorized to ship them the material.

Regulations pertaining to the licensing and use of by-product materials in medicine are to be found in the following parts of Title 10 of the Code of Federal Regulations:

10CFR20 Standards of Protection Against Radiation

10CFR30 Rules of General Applicability to Licensing of By-Product Material

10CFR35 Human Use of By-Product Materials

Extremely useful publications for anyone concerned with making application for an AEC license are "AEC Licensing Guide—Medical Programs" and "AEC Licensing Guide—Teletherapy Programs." Persons directing a program of training for physicians who expect to use radionuclides in their practice should refer to these publications. The required training and experience for licensing purposes can be planned into the curriculum and the relevant individual records kept. These publications may be obtained from the Division of Materials Licensing, United States Atomic Energy Commission, Washington, D.C. 20545.

The AEC issues two classes of licenses: general and specific. A *general* license is provided to virtually anyone for small (microcurie) quantities of each by-product nuclide. The medical use of radionuclides on humans, however small, is not included under the general license.

The *specific* license is by far the most common one for medical uses. This license is issued to an individual or institution and the use is specifically limited by (a) nuclide and chemical form, (b) total possession limit, and (c) specific approved diagnostic therapeutic procedures.

The primary advantage of an institutional specific license is that it allows for the physicians, not meeting the training and experience requirements, to work under the direction and supervision of "qualified" physicians. An individual specific license is solely for the use of the physician named on the license.

The third type of specific license is one of broad scope issued to an institution having experience in operating under a specific institutional license and engaged in medical research. This license authorizes multiple quantities and types of by-product materials for unspecified uses; it is imperative for the smooth and productive operation of a large teaching hospital or medical center.

The primary difference between the specific institutional license and the specific license of broad scope is in terms of the user's responsibility and freedom of action. Within certain limits the ultimate regulatory activities are delegated to the medical radioisotopes committee within the institution. This committee is charged with the responsibility of screening individual users and their proposed use of radionuclides. This mechanism allows the freedom required for research and development while maintaining informed peer group control.

14.13 DEPARTMENT OF HEALTH, EDUCATION, AND WELFARE

A. Federal Food and Drug Administration (FDA)

Until very recently the AEC had total authority over by-product radiopharmaceuticals which were not classed as biologicals. Normally the FDA has the responsibility of evaluating the safety and effectiveness of new drugs. The AEC is now in the process of turning this responsibility with respect to radiopharmaceuticals over to the FDA. This change is not expected to cause great changes in the current practice of nuclear medicine. Very likely the greatest impact will be on the radiopharmaceutical companies.

B. National Institutes of Health (NIH)

The sale of biologic material tagged with radioisotopes is under the control of the Division of Biologic Standards of the National Institutes of Health. This occurs because of the rather unique sterility and compatability requirements of these materials. Biologicals in nuclear medicine are primarily in the form of tagged blood fractions.

C. Bureau of Radiological Health

This agency of HEW conducts a wide variety of activities, among which are surveys, research, and recommendations relative to the safe use of radium.

Even with the availability of ^{137}Cs, ^{60}Co, and ^{252}Cf, radium is still in wide use in radiotherapy. Radium, however, does not fall under the jurisdiction of the AEC because it is a *naturally* occurring radionuclide.

14.14 DEPARTMENT OF LABOR (DOL)

The passage of the Occupational Safety and Health Act of 1970 gives the Secretary of Labor the responsibility and authority to set mandatory safety standards. This will mean that all occupational hazards are subject to Federal control. Therefore, any source of radiation not specifically controlled by other agencies will come under the jurisdiction of the DOL.

Medical applications of all radiation sources come under this law with respect to safe working conditions of all personnel employed by a hospital, private physician's office, or such facility. This does not mean that there is a duplication of control; radiation sources regulated under the Atomic Energy Act of 1954 by Federal agencies or agreement states will remain as they have been for the past 17 years. Sources other than by-product (reactor-produced radionuclides), source, and special nuclear materials not covered by Federal law can come under the control of the DOL for purposes of occupational safety.

14.15 ACCELERATORS

Accelerators present an unique set of radiation safety problems. Both the accelerator-produced radiations and the accelerator radionuclides create unusual hazards and require special safety standards. At the present, no Federal agency has tackled the problem of regulatory control of accelerators. The Department of Health, Education, and Welfare, through its various bureaus and agencies, has made recommendations regarding accelerator safety, however. The National Bureau of Standards Handbook 107 is the best single reference available at this time. Consequently, to obtain safety standards for the operation of an accelerator, one must "borrow" standards already in existence for other radiation sources. For example, shielding against heavy charged particles, gamma-radiation, and neutrons is a safety problem associated with nuclear reactors, X-ray machines, and teletherapy machines. The shielding requirements developed for these various individual radiation sources can, without too much difficulty, be applied to the corresponding radiations from a particular accelerator facility. The safe personnel dose level will, of course, be the same but special care is required regarding the dose unit. Due to the wide range in the LET (and conse-

quently the RBE) of accelerator radiations, one should use the rem exclusively in dose determinations.

The establishment of national safety standards relative to the operation of accelerators, it seems, will be developed in the very near future.

14.16 MICROWAVES, LASERS, AND OTHER RADIATIONS

The Radiation Control for Health and Safety Act of 1968 and the Occupational Safety and Health Act of 1970 are the Federal laws under which microwave, laser, ultrasonic, or other forms of radiation are controlled by regulations. The Bureau of Radiological Health, under the Secretary of the Department of Health, Education, and Welfare, is the group with primary responsibility of establishing safety standards for these sources of radiation under the act of 1968.

It would seem that a division of labor is developing between HEW and DOL, with the former body becoming responsible for safety standards for the protection of patients and the latter taking responsibility for the safe use of radiation sources with respect to occupational exposures.

The Bureau of Radiological Health has made surveys to estimate the scope of the problems in these areas. It has also made some recommendations regarding type and magnitude of biologic injury associated with the non-ionizing radiation and in a few cases recommended safe limits for occupational exposure. It seems that our understanding of the effects of non-ionizing radiation is limited to the early effects resulting from extremely high exposures. Information about delayed and late effects is minimal.

14.17 STATE AUTHORITIES

The similarity of hazards and means of avoiding injury from one source of radiation as compared to another is obvious to all. The network of regulatory and advisory agencies at the Federal level does not reflect this consistency, and this is unfortunate. Although consistency does exist to a very high degree as far as specific safety limits are concerned, the fact that these

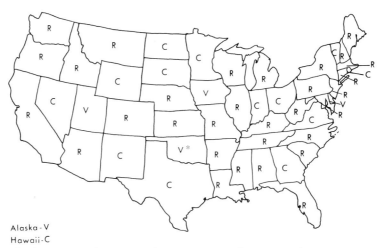

FIGURE 14–1   Medical X-ray regulations as of 1969. *R*, states having regulatory programs; *V*, states having voluntary programs; *C*, states having combination programs. An asterisk (*) indicates that the program is regulatory with respect to Medicare hospitals only.

limits are issued in the form of regulations by at least three agencies or sub-agencies does leave the "consumer" with a feeling that much effort is being duplicated. This would probably never occur to an industry such as the nuclear power industry. Medicine, on the other hand, with its adoption of such a wide sprectrum of radiation devices and sources, is caught in a virtual crossfire of regulatory activities.

In about one-half of the states, this dilemma has been solved as far as the physician is concerned. Laws have been passed, agencies have been empowered, and standards have been promulgated as regulations or voluntary standards. The physician prac-

ticing in these states need look no further than his state health department or similar agency for registration or licensing his radiation source. The same state agency maintains and enforces the regulations. Generally speaking, state control of medical radiation sources for the safety of workers and the general public has been more effective than has Federal control.

Radiation control at the state level is not an ideal solution for the industrial support that health care requires. The manufacture, marketing, and shipping of radiation-emitting equipment and radiopharmaceuticals involves many interstate agreements and controls. Interstate commerce involving

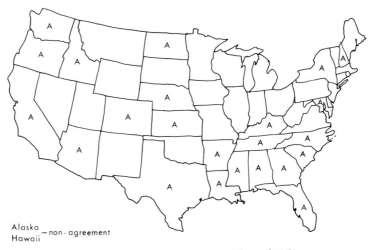

FIGURE 14–2   Agreement states (A) as of 1971.

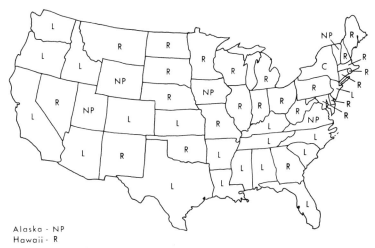

FIGURE 14–3 Radium and radon regulations: *L,* users are licensed; *R,* requires registration of sources; *C,* combination; *NP,* no program.

radiation devices and sources is legitimately and logically the responsibility of Federal agencies.

Many of the states now have comprehensive programs for control of radiation sources. In these instances, control is not restricted to radiation from a specific type of source. Consequently, states with such programs very often will control X-rays, radionuclides (by-product, natural, and accelerator-produced), microwaves, lasers, and accelerators.

Figure 14–1 shows status of each state with respect to how it regulates medical use of X-rays. As of 1969, 31 states had regulatory control, i.e., the compulsory registration of the X-ray machine. Failure to comply with these requirements can result in fines or imprisonment. The voluntary program being carried out in five states implies that some effort to control radiation uses is being made, but its implementation is at the discretion of the user. The combination program, used by 14 of the states, is one which controls some uses or some specific radiation sources while not controlling others.

Figure 14–2 shows 23 states which have entered into agreement with the AEC under Section 274 of the Atomic Energy Act of 1954. Within these states the regulation of by-product, source, and special nuclear materials is by an agency of the state government. The use of these materials in Federal installations or when used to constitute a "critical mass" (nuclear reactor) still falls under the control of the AEC.

As indicated previously, most of these agreement states do not restrict their control over radioactive materials to reactor-produced sources.

Radium and radon represent a relatively unique source of radiation with respect to regulatory activities. The usage and regulatory control of these sources have evolved quite independently of other radioactive materials. There are six states (Fig. 14–3) that have not yet developed regulatory programs covering these naturally occurring sources. Twenty-five of the states require registration of the sources; 18 of the states require licensure of users. New York is the only state with a combination of registration and licensure with respect to radium and radon.

14.18 PRACTICAL CONSIDERATIONS IN THE OPERATION OF A MEDICAL RADIATION FACILITY

There are many problems with the establishment and operation of a medical radiation facility. Since factors such as occupational safety and regulatory requirements seem alien, many physicians obtain the services of a radiologic physicist or a health physicist in the initial phases. Frequently, staff members in the regulatory agencies can assist in making this selection.

In the interest of economy, the owner-user of the radiation sources should become familiar with standard practices, registry, and licensing requirements, record-keeping practices, and limitations associated with his particular scope of operations.

A. Development of a Radiation Facility

The following check list will be helpful in setting up radiographic, radiotherapeutic, and nuclear medicine facilities.

1. General requirements for any radiation facility to determine shielding requirements
  a) Floor plan of the facility including all environs (adjacent areas, floor above and below)
  b) Space designations by occupancy, radiation-sensitive equipment, storage, etc.
  c) Location of radiation source(s), as well as its "output" during duty cycle and during non-use
  d) Existing or proposed structural materials in walls, floors, doors, etc.
2. Requirements for X-ray facility shielding determinations
  a) Types and energies of the radiation to be used (i.e., maximum energizing tube potential—kVp or kVcp)
  b) Maximum possible work load in ma·min/wk or R/wk at 1 meter
  c) All possible tube angulations during exposure
  d) Type of equipment (radiographic, fluoroscopic, therapy, etc.)
3. Requirements for evaluation of a radioisotope facility design
  a) Storage area
    1) Maximum activity for design purposes
    2) Nuclides and their chemical forms
    3) Air duct or ventilation system
  b) Areas for handling open sources
    1) Materials used for surfacing
    2) Shields, mirrors, glove boxes, etc.
  c) Radiation detection equipment
    1) Measuring equipment location and type
    2) Monitoring equipment type and provisions for calibration
  d) Radioactive waste disposal
    1) Storage facilities for liquid and solid waste and reclaimable equipment

    2) "In-house" or outside disposal arrangements
  e) Administrative
    1) Institutional radiation safety committee to insure long range safety through policy-making, remedial, and training activities. This committee is the key to long term success of radiation safety activities
    2) A qualified radiation safety officer to be personally responsible for carrying out the policies of the radiation safety committee
    3) Central record-keeping on orders, deliveries, inventory, and disposal

B. Operation of a Radiation Facility

The ultimate determining factor in establishing adequacy in the design and operation of a radiation facility will be the complexity of handling the radiation sources. A nuclear medicine facility can range from one in which are performed the most simple *in vitro* procedures (involving fractions of microcuries) to one in which there are "in-house" preparations involving many millicuries of activity for *in vivo* studies.

Beyond the planning stage of a facility one must establish and execute procedures for the continuous appraisal of radiation safety. Some of these procedures include:

1. Personnel monitoring—this will commonly take the form of a film badge, but thermoluminescent dosimetry (TLD) is being used more and more.

2. Area monitoring or surveying—this should be on a routine basis and should immediately follow any change which could affect radiation exposures.

3. Contamination control—this is extremely important in a nuclear medicine facility. The control of contamination may include wipe test, whole body counts, thyroid counts, blood or urine counts, and so forth. The critical areas will be personnel exposures and data validity.

4. Radioactive disposal records—this is required by the license. Both the amounts disposed and methods of disposal are of importance. This is one of the more difficult factors to control in large facilities.

5. Source calibration and integrity—this

applies to diagnostic and therapeutic X-rays, teletherapy, radium, or any source of radiation.

14.19 SUMMARY

While these practical considerations have been limited to X- and gamma-rays and radionuclide applications, they do point out safety problems common to all sources of radiation. There is a continuing responsibility by all medical radiation users to reduce the hazards to radiation workers, the patient, the community, and the environment.

The assumption that radiation can safely be used to benefit man rests upon the premise that it will remain under the control of informed, reasonable, and dedicated individuals.

As the user confronts problems he is encouraged to seek the guidance and assistance of his local regulatory body, be it Federal, state, or municipal. Staff members of these organizations are very much interested in the development and maintenance of properly operating radiation facilities.

15 MEDICO-LEGAL CONSIDERATIONS

Vincent P. Collins, M.D.

15.0 INTRODUCTION

The medico-legal aspects of radiologic practice are of two general types, administrative or regulatory law, and civil law.

Under administrative law the radiologist is subject to a wide variety of federal, state, and municipal regulations. The proximate authority governing the use of radiation is, in most instances, vested in a division of the state department of public health. State regulations define the area of control, set standards of radiation protection, and set forth the rules governing licensing and registration, record keeping, and reports. The scope and detail of state regulations do not lend themselves to summary. Much of the content touches on the daily activity and responsibility of the radiologist, and failure to observe could not be excused for lack of familiarity. Such regulations will contain a provision to the effect that, "Any person who violates any provision of the act may be guilty of a misdemeanor and, upon conviction, may be punished by fine, imprisonment or both, as provided by the law." Obviously, state regulations for the control of radiation merit close reading.

Such controls are not static. HEW has published an annual review, "State Radiation Control Legislation," covering major state legislation enacted, defeated, or pending throughout the country. About 50 per cent of radiation bills fail to pass but the remainder may be of vital significance to the practicing radiologist.

Public Law 90–602, formally cited as The Radiation Control for Health and Safety Act of 1968, controls all electronic product radiation, ionizing or non-ionizing, electromagnetic or particulate, sonic, infrasonic and ultrasonic. One provision is the requirement for an annual report to the Congress on the administration of the act. This is an available document containing a very valuable review of activities and problems affecting many aspects of the practice of radiology.

The reports of the National Council on Radiation Protection and Measurements should be part of the library of every department of radiology (available reports can be obtained from NCRP Publications, P.O. Box 4867, Washington, D.C. 20008).

Environmental Health Studies and Radiological Health are technical reports issued by the Bureau of Radiological Health. They provide essential information to the radiologist who often finds himself called upon as the community expert in radiation matters. These are available through the Office of Public Information and Education, Environmental Control Administration, Consumer Protection and Environmental Health Service, U.S. Department of Health, Education and Welfare, Rockville, Maryland 20852.

Familiarity with, and observance of, regulations governing the use of radiation is a minimum requirement, and the concerned and informed radiologist should go further. Administrative and technical aspects of legislation and regulation governing radiation shape the medical usages. The radiologist should familiarize himself with the established mechanisms for communication with legislative committees and regulatory agencies so that he may be aware of, and participate in, current developments at the point where medical expertise can be brought to bear on formulation.

Under the heading of civil law, the radiologist may come to court as an expert witness or as a participant in a civil suit. Most representatives of the medical or scientific communities have little knowledge or patience for civil procedure, yet controversies will come to court; the outcome, with the precedents engendered, can be no better than the quality of effort brought to bear on scientific as well as social and legal arguments. Considerations presented here are presented in a legal context. Training and practice provide the radiologist with medical and scientific background, but this background requires adaptation to serve social and legal purposes in court.

A. Torts

A capsule outline of torts and malpractice will allow a more succinct discussion of specific medico-legal problems of the radiologist. If the physician has some grasp of the nature of the area of law known as *torts,* he is in the best position to practice defensive medicine. This area is defined as the study of the extent to which the individual's rights, wants, and desires are so far recognized by the law, such that a duty arises in all or perhaps only certain individuals to observe these or be liable for interference with their realization. It is inherent in the definition that recognized rights, wants, and desires change with developing legal, social, and scientific concepts and that the past is not necessarily a sure guide to careful conduct.

A *tort* is an injury caused by the act of another, in violation of a duty that exists between the parties, and it may be intentional or unintentional. The intentional torts are assault (threat without contact), battery (contact injury), interference with peace of mind (causing anxiety neurosis), and false imprisonment (restriction of freedom). The unintentional tort involves negligence and a distinction between danger and risk. Danger is the possibility of injury; danger is not created by the actor, and conduct that involves danger may still be careful. Risk is the probability of injury; risk may be increased or decreased by the actor, and conduct that involves unreasonable risk is negligence. The usual criterion of reasonableness is the standard of care in the community.

B. Areas of Malpractice

Based on the law of torts, there are four areas of malpractice:

1. Where the physician's act produced an intended result but the patient claims the act was unauthorized and the result unwanted. The charge is battery. The defense is to show the act had the consent of the patient. A gross example would be an extension of a surgical operation beyond the patient's original contemplation. The minimal example could be drawing blood or taking an X-ray of the chest on the wrong patient.

2. Where an unintended result of the physician's act occurs and the patient claims injury. The charge is negligence. The patient must prove his injury, that it was caused by the physician's act, that it was a foreseeable danger, and that there was unreasonable risk violating the physician's duty of care toward the patient. The defense would be to show that the act was in keeping with the standards of medical practice in the community. Examples might be found in complications such as hemorrhage, following surgery, or radiation injury due to miscalculation of dose.

3. Where a patient has not given his informed consent. It is held that a patient cannot consent without adequate knowledge of what he is consenting to. He should know the reason for treatment, the alternative forms of treatment, and the possible complications of treatment. This category of malpractice is a recent development with some elements of battery and negligence, but differing from both. The act would be an intended one, but failure to inform might be negligent. The procedure might be skillful and successful with no physical injury but a failure to observe a patient's right to know.

4. When a patient has accepted treatment based on a promised result, and this result has not been realized. This is a breach of warranty rather than a tort.

It will be of importance to any who attempt to bridge the gap between law and medicine to realize the distinction between medical or scientific injury and proof, and legal injury and proof.

Injury in medical usage connotes trauma or physical damage. In law, injury has a much broader definition: "a wrong or damage done to another, either in his person, rights, reputation, or property." Injury to an individual's rights should particularly concern us because of increasing assertion and recognition throughout society. A right not to be exposed to unwanted radiation could readily be found, and an infringement on this right would not require a showing of any radiobiologic damage. Right is correlative of duty; one does not exist without the other. Thus, a right of an individual not to be exposed to radiation coexists with a duty on the part of another individual not to subject the first to exposure. Violation of this duty is not dependent on causing physical damage and would be independent of any application of a threshold dose concept.

Proof in medical and scientific circles is a process of investigation, accumulation, and analysis of evidence, that knows no deadline for final conclusion, is never beyond re-examination and re-assessment, and is never achieved by persuasion. Proof in legal usage is "the conviction or persuasion of the mind of a judge or jury, by exhibition of evidence, of the reality of a fact alleged." More succinctly, whatever the judge or the jury come to believe is considered proven. It is to be expected, therefore, that it is easier to recognize a radiation injury or to prove the cause of cancer in the courtroom than in the medical examining room or laboratory.

With this brief background, some recurring medico-legal problems can be discussed. It should be remembered that radiobiology is an invited guest in court and may be of secondary importance to social and legal considerations, in the same fashion that legal considerations may be of secondary importance in the face of need to control hemorrhage in the operating room.

C. The Maximum Permissible Dose

The validity of this concept depends on its intended purpose.

As a medical or scientific decision of biologic import, it would be unacceptable as an arbitrary and artificial value. No biologically informed individual could propose a level beyond which injury would with certainty occur and below which safety would with equal certainty obtain, or even the probabilities of either of these. No one informed in dosimetry could consider the single number obtained from film badge or dosimeter to be a meaningful description of the amount and bodily distribution of absorbed energy that could relate to injury produced.

As a standard for legal purposes, the maximum permissible dose is a very useful number. A regulatory body is entitled to set such standards, and a good standard should be objective. It may be arbitrary within limits, but it must be reasonable for the purpose intended. A highway speed of 70 miles per hour is an arbitrary limit but is reasonable for its purpose. When autos, highways, and drivers are judged adequate for higher speeds, the speed limit may be adjusted. When conditions permit the required usages of radiation to be carried out with a lower environmental level of radiation dose, the maximum permissible dose will be lowered. In this case a maximum permissible dose is essentially a monitor of the radiation environment. It is set as low as is deemed practical to permit the continued necessary uses of an essential tool of medicine and industry.

When biologic consequences are inferred from the maximum permissible dose, its usefulness is impaired. A highway speed limit is not derived from identified parameters of human physiology or the vulnerability of human anatomy to injury. No more is the maximum permissible dose derived from careful quantitation of biologic consequences of radiation exposure except most indirectly. The maximum permissible dose does not imply, and one may not infer, safety below or danger above the arbitrary number set as the maximum permissible dose.

If the film badge or dosimeter reads below the maximum permissible dose, it is evidence of operation within recommended limits for environmental exposure, but if it reads above, it is evidence of a break in radiation control and a possible violation of safety regulations.

D. Liability for Radiation Injury

The rules for establishing liability for personal injury are long-established. When the exposure is documented, the injury obvious, and the causal relation not in doubt, the process of establishing liability and assessing damages is the same for radiation as for any other agent. The unique features of litigation involving radiation arise when the injury is equivocal, non-specific, or greatly delayed, or where the exposure is unattended by any immediate or observable effect, where it is below that consistently causing observable injury, or where there have been repeated exposures at different times, in different places, and under different circumstances (such as occupational exposure plus medical exposure for diagnostic or therapeutic purpose). Now the court is asked to believe the injury and find the cause, based on evidence that science could not interpret or that would, at best, produce conflicting opinions by expert witnesses. The court can find an answer in rules of law, in legal precedent and in statutes specifically designed to achieve a solution that may satisfy social demands if not scientific criteria.

E. Radiotherapy and Radiation Injury

The simplest situation occurs when injury results in the course of radiation treatment. This was the case in *Ferrara* v. *Galluchio*, where in the course of treatment for bursitis a radiation burn of the shoulder region occurred. Damages were awarded for the radiation injury, but this became a landmark case for another reason. The patient consulted a dermatologist who advised continued observation because of the possibility that cancer might develop. This so alarmed the patient that she developed an anxiety neurosis, which the court found believable as an additional injury for which additional damages were specifically awarded. Note that, for this kind of injury, there is clearly no threshold dose and neither radiation physics or radiobiology would be relevant considerations. Anxiety

neurosis following exposure to unwanted radiation would appear to be a likely area for exploitation in malpractice litigation.

Another landmark case involving clear-cut radiation injury in the course of radiotherapy is that of *Natanson* v. *Kline*. Mrs. Natanson was referred for radiation following a radical mastectomy and as a result of this treatment suffered an injury, colorfully described in the record in these words: "The skin, flesh, and muscles beneath her left arm sloughed away and the ribs of her left chest were so burned that they became necrotic, or dead." Postoperative radiation was administered to the chest wall by a type of rotation therapy where dosimetry might well be difficult to evaluate, and some difference of opinion is expressed in the record by the expert witnesses. A plausible explanation for the injury is found in the record, but it appears to have been overlooked. It is recorded that there was a drainage from the region of the axilla when treatment was undertaken. There is commonly persistent fluid below the skin flaps following a radical mastectomy, and unless this is drained it induces a sterile inflammatory process. The attendant increase in blood supply would provide a biologic basis for an accelerated and excessive reaction even though the accurately determined dose might be within the usual tolerance limits. The court accepted the physical injury as an inherent danger of radiation treatment and found no conduct on the part of Dr. Kline such as would have increased the risk of the injury and thus given rise to a claim of negligence. Rather the court saw here an injury to the patient's right—the right to know what danger was involved in the radiation treatment. Since the patient had not been warned of the danger, she could not give a valid consent. This case gave rise to the current concept of informed consent and the now widely recognized requirement to fully inform a patient of the possible or at least the probable sequelae.

The Texas Supreme Court has elaborated on the matter of informed consent, saying that the patient has not truly given his consent to an operation of any elective nature or to a specific treatment until he has been informed by his physician of (a) the probable results of the proposed procedure, (b) the primary collateral hazards, and (c) the alternative procedures available if any exist. In addition the patient must, of course, be given accurate and complete answers to any question. An exception may be made, however, in those cases where there is a medical reason not to inform the patient of certain facts.

In the *Brumlop* case, the duty of the physician to provide information concerning the hazards of treatment was extended to the referring physician. Here a psychiatrist referred a patient to the state hospital for shock therapy. The referring psychiatrist did not give the shock therapy and was not present at the time but, nevertheless, was held liable for failing to have informed the patient of the risk at the time her recommendation for treatment was made. Under this rule the physician who referred Mrs. Ferrera to Dr. Galluchio for treatment of bursitis might have been liable for her injury.

F. Radiation Exposure and Cancer

The spectrum of decisions as to liability for cancer following a radiation exposure ranges from a requirement for proof at the level of "reasonable medical probability" to absolute liability, which in effect admits the impossibility of proof, foregoes the need for showing causation, and shifts the burden of the injury from the victim to society by a mechanism such as insurance, where the cost of premiums is passed on to the consumer as a cost of doing business. This seems not unreasonable, but it also means that anyone would be eminently provident to seek even temporary employment in the radiation field, and thereafter the individual would be eligible for compensation if he should ever develop cancer, the second most common cause of death in the general population.

The *Parker* case is a Texas Supreme Court decision which discussed the requirement of causation for establishing the relation of radiation exposure and cancer. Plaintiff Parker was employed by a private company under contract to the United States Government. He handled radioactive materials and was an operator who assembled and disassembled nuclear weapons. Film badges, when worn, were worn beneath a leaded glove and the total recorded badge exposure was 36 millirems.

After four years of employment he developed an enlarged cervical lymph node which, on biopsy, showed metastatic carcinoma and was eventually classified as seminoma. He died some 32 months later.

Under Texas Workmen's Compensation law an employee is entitled to compensation if his disability resulted from a "diseased condition caused by exposure to X-rays or radioactive substances." The sine qua non test must be met: but for the employment would the patient have suffered the harm and developed the cancer? The court will require more than a possible causal relation; there must be a reasonable medical probability. This requirement does in some instances place extraordinary burdens of proof on claimants. Once the claimant's theory of causation leaves the realm of lay knowledge for esoteric scientific theory, however, it must be more than a possibility to the scientists who created it. For to the scientific mind, all things are possible. And with all things possible, citizens would have no reasoned protection from the speculations of courts and juries.

The *Besner* case is an example of a more liberal result in a New York State Court. The plaintiff was the widow of a 35-year-old theoretical physicist who had a diagnosis of acute myeloblastic leukemia made one year after employment with a firm. The record indicates that he worked at a desk some 200 feet from and only occasionally went to the laboratory where two Cobalt-60 sources were stored, one 201 millicuries and another one millicurie. The exposure for the year was reported to be 2250 millirems. The physicist died of his disease and his widow was awarded death benefits under New York Workmen's Compensation Law, for the acute myeloblastic leukemia was found to be due to exposure to radiation. Compensation was granted and, in affirming, the court relied upon the statutory presumption of the New York Workmen's Compensation Law dealing with disability due to ionizing radiation. "The testimony of the medical experts is emphatic that there is really no 'threshold' or 'safe' dosage of radiation because at the present stage of scientific knowledge it cannot be ascertained exactly what effects radiation has on the human body. It is also admitted that each individual reacts differently to exposure to radiation. The award is supported by substantial evidence and by the presumptions, especially so in view of decedent's good health prior to his employment."

The word presumptions refers here to a statutory mechanism for decision-making when a causal relationship is unclear and where consistency is held to be a greater virtue than a requirement for reasonable certainty. Under these circumstances, if the plaintiff has ever been exposed to radiation in less than the MPD, the cancer is presumed due to the exposure but subject to rebuttal by the defense. If the plaintiff has been exposed to more than the permissible dose, a non-rebuttable presumption arises that cancer was due to the radiation exposure. In this particular case, the expert testimony that there is no threshold or safe dosage of radiation impresses the court and, there being no proof to the contrary, causation is considered to be established. Such a use of the maximum permissible dose might be startling from the point of view of the radiobiologist, but it is a logical application for a carefully derived standard.

G. The Basis for Liability for Diagnostic Radiation Exposure

The fundamentals of tort law are being brought to bear on practices in diagnostic X-ray departments. It has been a long-established rule that a surgical operation is a technical battery, regardless of its results, and it is excusable only when there is express or implied consent of the patient. This should be no surprise, since in torts any unwanted touching is a battery, whether involving a scalpel, needle, the examining hand, or a Bardex catheter.

In *Mims* v. *Boland,* also known as the "Barium Enema Case," the question was whether the patient's piteous objections to the forcible insertion of a Bardex catheter into a colostomy constituted a withdrawal of consent. While ruling for the defendant radiologist, the court held that "an unauthorized and unprivileged contact by doctor to his patient in examination, treatment, or surgery amounts to a battery. . . . In the interest of one's right of inviolability of person, any unlawful touching is a physical injury to the person and is actionable."

This principle can readily be extended to the penetrating X-ray beam, which is an unwanted touching and a violation of one's right of inviolability of the person, unless the patient has consented. These days, the consent should be an informed one and the duty to inform may well be shared by both the referring physician and the radiologist responsible for the examination.

15.1 GENERAL AREAS

A. Physical Injury

In the course of a diagnostic X-ray examination a physical injury may result, e.g., a reaction to contrast medium. The rules are clear with regard to proving the injury to the patient, the act of the radiologist (there may be vicarious liability for the act of the technician who injected the contrast medium), and causation, i.e., that the contrast medium did in fact cause the injury. The charge may be battery, and the defense would be to show consent; implied consent may do, expressed consent would be better, but informed consent would be preferred. The charge may be negligence, and the defense would be to show conduct in keeping with the standard of the community, i.e., what is generally accepted as prudent practice under the circumstances.

Salgo v. *Stanford* is a case involving contrast media that illustrates the factor of hostility that may be injected if the court is not satisfied with medical testimony. The patient, Salgo, had undergone aortography and the procedure as described in the law report was carried out in the normal manner with no occurrence to suggest that complications might ensue. "The next morning when plaintiff awoke he noticed that his lower extremities were paralyzed. This condition is permanent. . . . None of the experts could determine the exact cause of the paraplegia." The court was not pleased and spoke of the "conspiracy of silence." The doctors could not explain the complication; the court felt they would not. The patient would be in no position to explain the injury, so, in order to equalize the situation, the court invoked the 'doctrine of res ipsa loquitur' by placing the burden on the doctor of explaining what occurred in order to overcome an inference of negligence. This inference could arise because "certain medical and surgical procedures became so common that in many of them the laymen knew that, if properly conducted, untoward results did not occur." So the injury was unexplained—the medical experts could not disprove negligence and damages were allowed. In retrospect, the record clearly describes a prematurely aged individual and a candidate for lumbar spondylosis, a condition in which prolonged prone positioning and lumbar extension, as for this procedure, may cause compression of the cauda equina with resulting paraplegia quite unrelated to the contrast material injected. Although this decision was reversed on appeal, it has significance for cases involving alleged radiation injury: the court may see a "conspiracy of silence" and draw an inference of negligence based on laymen's knowledge of radiation effects. This knowledge is apt to come from press reports of scientific papers or popular writings or scientists which may dazzle rather than inform in the areas where answers are far from final. To the degree that we come to court poorly prepared to fill the teaching role of an expert witness, or that we avoid or lightly assume responsibility for education in the public press, we must expect to be "hoist with our own petard" or, in current jargon, to be "bombed" on the witness stand.

Favalora v. *Aetna* involved a radiologist who carried out a fluoroscopic examination without requiring completion of a requisition which contained a space for entry of the patient's history. The patient fainted, fell, and was injured. The court reasoned that had the radiologist carried out the examination with the advantage of the information requested, but not supplied on the face of the requisition, he would have known of the patient's fainting spells and could have prevented the accident. The judgment was for the plaintiff and the court expressed these opinions:

The failure of the radiologist to secure a patient's history prior to commencing X-ray examination during which patient collapsed and suffered injuries was negligence which constituted proximate cause of the accident. . . . Radiologist was liable for negligence in failing to remain sufficiently alert to reasonably foreseeable expectancy that patient undergoing X-ray examination might faint and fall. . . . The

soundness of requiring a clinical history of patients scheduled to undergo such extensive radiological examination readily impresses this court considering the many factors which may affect the physical well-being of an individual subjected to the tests plaintiff was required to undergo. Not the least important of said factors is the possibility of radium poisoning [*sic*] resulting from overexposure to gamma rays [*sic*] as a result of repeated radiological tests.

The significant points here are, first, that the court finds that failure by the radiologist to take a history is negligence and, second, that despite some confusion as to terminology the court apprehends that there is hazard in the radiation exposure involved in a diagnostic X-ray examination. Had the patient claimed this exposure as an element of injury, the court might well have been receptive, and might be expected to be understanding on any future occasion.

B. Radiation Exposure During Pregnancy

There are two aspects here, one of injury to the mother and the other of injury to the unborn child.

The injury to the mother is the simplest to deal with, remembering that the legal definition of injury goes beyond damage to the person to damage to his rights. A mother's concern for damage to her unborn child is easily understood and might well be seen as an injury. The courts have been particularly lenient in the matter of injuries and motherhood, and it would be easy to apply the reasoning of the *Galluchio* decision in a mother's concern for the effects of radiation upon her unborn child. Estep and Forgotson have concisely summarized the attitudes that courts have taken.

Mental distress caused by fear of harm to their unborn children has held to be a proper item of damages in cases involving injuries to pregnant women. Recovery is for damage to the mother herself during the period of pregnancy and is not dependent upon the right of the fetus or embryo to recovery. This apprehension of a pregnant woman that her unborn child might be injured is a proper element of damages even though it is established at the trial that such apprehension was unfounded or groundless and that plaintiff in fact gave birth to a normal, uninjured child. Medical testimony to show that the feared result would probably follow from the injury is not necessary in order for the pregnant woman to recover. The existence of this mental anguish is not disproved by evidence that if the plaintiff had been thoroughly versed in medical science she would have known that her fears were groundless; recovery is allowable if the fears are based on data that is scientifically untrue if such data is commonly believed by the general public. The defendant's ignorance of the plaintiff's pregnant condition likewise will not defeat recovery.*

The tort of "interference with peace of mind" may or may not be within the sphere of radiobiology, but it is precipitated by statements of members of the scientific community and articles in the public press such as "The Death of all Children," by Ernest J. Sternglass, a professor of radiation physics, that appeared in *Esquire*, a mass circulation magazine that published his piece in record time without bothering to check whether the theory was scientifically sound.

Until recent years the unborn child was not considered a person separate from the mother, was owed no duty and had no right the courts would protect. Recent cases have allowed recovery for prenatal injury, at least in the case of a child born alive. Granting that exposure is established, the alleged injury might be any birth defect or any postnatal condition that has ever been attributed to radiation. The non-specific nature of radiation injuries and their occurrence spontaneously or in association with other exposures to radiation or with exposure to other possibly etiologic agents or accidents are certain to call forth a wide range of expert opinion. Causation must be established. Difficult as this may seem medically, it must be remembered that in court proof equates with credibility, and a stronger presentation may be made to state what caused a given defect or disorder, than what did not.

Before liability is found, there is still the matter of the nature of the charge — whether it is negligence or battery. Concerning negligence, questions could arise regarding the need for the examination, and this could involve the referring physician as well as the radiologist. It might hinge upon whether there had been any inquiry as to possible pregnancy, or whether an effort was made to avoid the post-ovulatory phase of the menstrual cycle. Hammer-Jacobsen recommended that X-ray examination be

limited to the first 10 days following cessation of menses, thus the term "ten-day rule." Technical considerations would arise concerning exposure factors, fluoroscopy filtration, shielding, and collimation, which might tend to show care or lack of it. Customary practice and the standard of care in the community would enter into the defense. This is an area of change, and unless soundly based it might be subject to very critical review. A charge of battery would arise in the absence of consent, and consent to X-ray examinations has not been considered practical. Aflidi carried out a pilot study in securing consent for angiography which entailed a rather blunt presentation of hazards including death. Two out of 228 patients refused the examination, but it appeared that the majority of patients desired the information.

Considering the interest of the referring physician, it seems advisable to develop a policy in an institution or in a practice. Apart from the broad question of consent for the array of X-ray examinations, a policy of inquiry concerning menstrual history and pregnancy could be evolved. This would protect the patient and the documented decision as to the policy would give the radiologist the protection of an evident effort to be careful.

It is not necessary at this point to discuss the biologic aspects of radiation injury. We are concerned with the circumstances where a claim of radiation exposure and a claim of radiation injury may lead to suit. The determination of liability is based on rules outlined and the determination of facts. Where reasonable men may disagree, the jury decides.

That proof of injury or causal relation is difficult or even scientifically impossible does not impair the right to sue or preclude the existence of a cause of action. The goal is to provide a remedy for every injury and, where science fails, the law has mechanisms for decision and social purpose to fulfill by determining who should bear the burden of injury.

The court may serve its purpose by shifting the burden of injury from any innocent victim to a wrongdoer where fault is detected, or even where no fault is shown, the burden may be shifted to society in general through such mechanisms as insurance and may be charged as a cost of doing business.

*Estep, S. D., and Forgotson, E. H.: Legal liabilities for genetic injuries from radiation. 24 Louisiana Law Rev., *1*:48, 1963.

Current rules may differ from one jurisdiction to another. Some may deny recovery for injury to a non-viable fetus and others may allow for injury back to the time of conception. The general trend of decisions is to assure recovery for an innocent injured party even at the risk of allowing some fictitious or fraudulent claims.

Radiation injuries generally and prenatal injuries specifically bring into play two variations of statutes of limitation. These generally limit the period following injury, when suit may be brought, for the purpose of sparing the court problems of proof made difficult by lapse of time, loss of records, missing witnesses, and failing memory. Normally the statute of limitations is said to begin to run from the time of the act that caused the injury, particularly where two are simultaneous or clearly sequential. Where the injurious effect of the act was delayed in appearance, the court may rule that statute of limitations did not begin to run until the patient knew, or could reasonably be expected to know, of the injury. This rule may be expected to be invoked in the case of alleged delayed radiation injury and under some circumstances might be called upon when the exposure was to the child *in utero*. A minor could not bring a suit in his own name, but a parent or guardian could institute suit for him. However, he could bring suit on reaching his majority, and an injury suffered *in utero* could be the basis for bringing suit more than 21 years after the exposure.

Liability for genetic damage has been explored in depth by Estep and Forgotson. Genetic damage constitutes a preconception injury rather than a prenatal injury. If other conditions of liability are met, a child afflicted with a genetic injury might, with the ever-mellowing climate of the law, be eligible for recovery. Recovery might be to the exposed individual for his concern for the injury that might surface in future progeny because of the damage his genes might transmit. Recovery might be to an existing individual for a recognizable condition attributable to genetic damage suffered by his ancestors. Such eventualities become less than a current concern when we consider the mind-boggling problem of proof of causation for generations exposed to mutagens on occasions beyond counting and when even legitimacy of ancestors could be challenged.

C. The Avoidable X-ray Examination

It oversimplifies the problem to justify the negative examination by reasoning that had we known the examination was negative it would not have been done. Many types of X-ray examination have little or no medical requirement: X-rays obtained for legal purposes in personal injury cases, pre-employment examinations such as lumbosacral series, and routine periodic health examinations. Then there are repeated examinations because of unsatisfactory technique, because of lost films, and because of overzealous duplication of orders.

The X-ray examination should be considered in the light of the patient's right and the physician's duty. The patient has reason and right to avoid unnecessary and unwanted radiation exposure. The physician has duty and growing reason—on radiobiologic and legal grounds—to spare the patient unnecessary and unwanted radiation exposure.

Radiation exposure need not produce a detectable or even suspected physical injury in the medical sense. As an unwanted touching it is a battery infringing upon the right of inviolability of the person. Exposure without knowledge or consent could arise within the customary practices of any community. The patient might be unaware of the whole body exposure if a chest film were obtained without use of a collimator. The patient could not give informed consent to fluoroscopy with a fluorescent screen, if he had not been informed of the lesser exposure with an image intensifying system.

There is a shared responsibility for the case with which an examination is ordered by the referring physician and carried out by the radiologist. Court decisions indicating the liability of the referring physician and the responsibility of the radiologist to communicate with the referring physician concerning the reason for the examination are a matter of record.

15.2 SUMMARY

In summary, the purspose of this discussion is twofold. It should alert the radiologist to his duties and to the patient's rights concerning the use of radiation for diagnostic or therapeutic purposes. It should inform him of the medico-legal risks he assumes in the practice of radiology.

The practice of medicine is the balancing of competing risks, a risk involved in disease and a risk involved in treatment. Within the limits of sound medical practice and clinical judgment the patient must be informed of both risks, but courts recognize that circumstances may exist that would make it medically inadvisable to inform a patient of every danger. Rules to guide the radiologist's conduct are to be found in the custom of accepted medical practice, from rules and opinions expressed in court decisions and from prescience that evokes from a continuing effort to maintain an informed position on scientific and social matters.

Hypothetical medical fact situations with legal implications may lead to entertaining and educational opinions, but no final answer exists until the court has acted on specific cases presented within the adversary system. Still the law is apt to find its standard in the conduct of "the reasonable man," and conduct that evolves from plausible reason is likely to appeal to the court. The basic conduct expected of the radiologist includes recognition of a danger, competence to minimize the risk and an effort the court would find reasonable to fulfill his duty to inform and meet the patient's right to know.

While custom and precedent are guides to acceptable conduct, changing views and standards must be anticipated. Whenever the court feels the need to abandon precedent or disregard custom, it is apt to recall the opinion of Judge Learned Hand in the *Hooper* case:

Indeed in most cases reasonable prudence is in fact common prudence; but strictly it is never its measure, a whole calling may have unduly lagged in the adoption of new and available devices. It never may set its own tests, however persuasive be its usages. Courts must in the end say what is required; there are precautions so imperative that even their universal disregard will not excuse their omission.

References

1. Alfidi, R. J.: Informed consent; A study of patient reaction. J.A.M.A., *216*:1325–1329, 1971.
2. Boffey, P. M., and Sternglass, E. J.: Controversial prophet of doom. Science, *166*:195–200, 1969.
3. Collins, V. P.: The medical and scientific basis for legal liability related to radiation exposure. *In* Excerpta Medica Foundation: *Diagnosis and Treatment of Deposited Radionuclides;* A symposium held at Richland, Wash. May, 1967.
4. Daves, M.: Diagnostic overkill. J.A.M.A., *200*:999, 1967.
5. Ehni, G., Clark, K., Wilson, C. B., and Alexander, E. Jr.: Significance of the small lumbar spinal canal: Cauda Equina compression syndromes due to spondylolysis; An introduction in four parts. J. Neurosurg., *31*:490–519, 1969.
6. Heller, M. B.: Infant and fetal mortality caused by ^{90}Sr?—A review. A.A.P.M. Quart. Bull., *1*:24–27, 1970.
7. Hammer-Jacobsen, E.: Therapeutic abortion on account of X-ray examination during pregnancy. Danish Med. Bull., 6:716–717, 1959.
8. Overton, P. R., and Stone, S. V., Jr.: Texas Supreme Court sets guidelines concerning patient informed consent. Texas Med., *63*:122–123, 1967.
9. Sternglass, E. J.: The death of all children. Esquire, *72* (Sept.), 1969.
10. Sternglass, E. J.: Infant mortality and nuclear testing—A reply. A.A.P.M. Quart. Bull., *4*:115–119, 1970.

APPENDIX I

Mathematical Principles

In radiobiology, we are concerned with four basic equations. They are:

$$y(x) = mx + b \qquad \text{Equation 1. Linear equation}$$

$$y(x) = y_o e^{-ax} \qquad \text{Equation 2. Exponential equation}$$

$$y(x) = \frac{e^{-a}a^x}{x!} \qquad \text{Equation 3. Poisson distribution}$$

$$y(x) = 1(1 - e^{-x/a})^b \qquad \text{Equation 4. Multitarget model}$$

A1.1 THE LINEAR EQUATION

$$y(x) = mx + b$$

At the outset, the nomenclature should be clarified. The term $y(x)$ is stated "y-of-x." It means the value of the right side of the equation, given a specific value of x. As an example,

$$y(x) = 2x + 1$$

If $x = 0$, then

$$y(0) = 2(0) + 1$$
$$= 1$$

If $x = -1$, then

$$y(-1) = 2(-1) + 1$$
$$= -2 + 1$$
$$= -1$$

etc.

In Equation 1, m and b are parameters; they are *constants*. By definition, x is called the *independent* variable, while $y(x)$ is the *dependent* variable. The key is constant vs. variable. In an experimental situation, the experimenter controls the value of x. The value of $y(x)$ is the result of the experiment at each and any given x.

For demonstration, consider the following:

You want to make a chemical analysis of a material using a chemical reaction which produces a color—the more material, the less light transmitted. You also

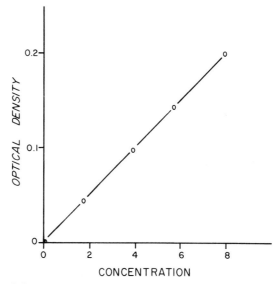

FIGURE A1–1   Optical density as a function of concentration. Data plotted on linear coordinates.

have a device (colorimeter) which can quantitate the amount of light absorbed (optical density). You set up standards having increasing concentrations of the chemical (mg/ml). The data you obtain are:

(x) Concentration in mg/ml	y(x) Optical Density
0	.005
2	.045
4	.085
6	.125
8	.165

Figure A1–1 shows the data plotted on linear coordinates. From the curve we can calculate the parameters. Initially, let $x = 0$. Then,

$$y(0) = m \cdot (0) + b$$
$$y(0) = b;$$
when $x = 0$, $b =$ the y intercept;
from the data given, $y(0) = 0.005$

To calculate m, some algebraic manipulation is necessary:

$$y(x) = mx + b$$

Subtract b from both sides:

$$y(x) - b = mx$$

Divide both sides by x (as long as x does not equal 0):

$$\frac{y(x) - b}{x} = m$$

Since we have already calculated b [it equals $y(0)$],

$$m = \frac{y(x) - y(0)}{x} = \frac{y(x) - 0.005}{x}$$

We can select any x,y(x) pair: for example, the coordinates 2,0.0405:

$$m = \frac{0.045 - 0.005}{2} = \frac{0.040}{2} = 0.020$$

The parameter m is the slope. It gives the amount of change in y(x) (optical density units) per unit change in x(mg/cc).

The final equation is

$$y(x) = 0.020x + 0.005$$

In the literature, you may find terms such as F(X), f(X), H(X), and so forth. They mean the same thing as y(x) as used above.

Before we look at Equation 2, some concepts should be remembered. The logarithm has properties that are of value in the solution of Equation 2. By definition, the logarithm, when placed on its *base* as a power gives a number — the antilogarithm. As an example, consider the following:

$$\underset{\text{base}}{\nearrow} \quad \log_{10} \underset{\text{antilog}}{(100)} \quad = 2 \underset{\text{logarithm}}{\nwarrow}$$

$$10^2 = 100$$

While logarithms commonly have a base of 10, any positive number can be used

$$\log_a(n) = b$$
$$a^b = n$$

From the numeric example above, we can see other properties of logarithms.

$$\log_{10}(100) = \log_{10}(10^2)$$
$$= 2 \log_{10}(10)$$

Anytime the form $\log_a(a)$ occurs, it equals 1. Consequently $\log_{10}(10) = \log_e(e) = \log_2(2) \dots$ etc. $= 1$. Therefore, $2 \log_{10}(10) = 2$.

Other properties of logarithms are

$$\log (a \cdot b) = \log a + \log b \qquad \text{Multiplication with logarithms}$$

The log of a product equals the sum of the logs.

$$\log \frac{a}{b} = \log a - \log b \qquad \text{Division}$$

The log of a quotient equals the difference between the logs.

$$\log a^b = b \log (a) \qquad \text{Exponentiation}$$

To raise a number to a power, multiply the log by the power.

$$\log (a^{1/b}) = \frac{1}{b} \log (a) \qquad \text{Roots}$$

To find the root of a, divide the log by the root.

A1.2 THE EXPONENTIAL EQUATION

$$y(x) = y(0) e^{-ax}$$

This is known as an exponential equation. In radioisotopes it appears as

$$a(t) = a_0 e^{-\lambda t}$$

where a(t) represents the activity of a radioisotope at time t. In radiologic physics, the equation also appears as

$$d(x) = d_0 e^{-\mu x}$$

where d(x) is the dose rate at a depth of x in an absorber. And in radiation survival studies as

$$s = e^{-D/D_0}$$

For purposes of demonstration we will use

$$a(t) = ae^{-\lambda t}$$

As an example consider the following radioisotopic data;

t (days)	a(t) (μcuries)
0	100
5	56
10	31
15	17.3

Figure A1–2 shows the data plotted on semi-logarithmic coordinates.

We can solve the equation in the following manner:

$$a(t) = a_0 e^{-\lambda t}$$

First we determine the value of the parameter a_0:

$$a(0) = a_0$$
$$\text{When } T = O, \; e^{-\lambda(0)} = 1$$
$$\text{Therefore } a(0) = a_0 e^{-\lambda(0)}$$
$$\text{Since } e^{-0} = 1,$$
$$a(0) = \alpha_0$$

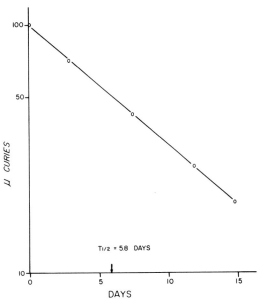

FIGURE A1–2 Radioactivity as a function of time. Data plotted on semi-logarithmic coordinates.

For the example $a_0 = 100$, to calculate the value of λ, divide both sides by a_0:

$$\frac{a(t)}{a_0} = e^{-\lambda t}$$

then take natural logarithms ($\log_e$ — or abbreviated ln) of both sides.

$$\ln\frac{(a(t))}{(a_0)} = \ln(e^{-\lambda t})$$
$$= -\lambda t \ln(e)$$
$$= -\lambda t$$

Recall that $\ln(e) = \log_e(e) = 1$.

At first the term $\ln\frac{(a(t))}{(a_0)}$ would seem to cause difficulty. We will define a specific value of t such that

$$\frac{a(t)}{a_0} = \tfrac{1}{2}$$

From the drawing, this value is seen to be the half-life of the isotope ($T_{1/2}$). Therefore, to be more correct,

$$\frac{a(T_{1/2})}{a_0} = \tfrac{1}{2}$$

where $T_{1/2}$ = the half-life. Substitution then gives

$$\ln\frac{(a(t))}{(a_0)} = \ln\left(\tfrac{1}{2}\right) = -0.693$$

but since we mean a specific value of t,

$$-0.693 = -\lambda T_{1/2}$$

Dividing both sides by $-T_{1/2}$ gives

$$-\lambda = \frac{-0.693}{T_{1/2}}$$

For the example $T_{1/2} = 5.8$, then

$$\lambda = 0.119$$

Therefore, we can calculate the values of the two parameters with ease:

$$a_0 = a(0) = \text{the y intercept (semilog paper)}$$
$$\lambda = \frac{0.693}{T_{1/2}}$$

For other forms of the equation, the solution is the same. Instead of half-life, the units would be half value layer, and so forth.

The interpretation of the parameters is

a_0 = the amount of $\dfrac{\text{(isotope)}}{\text{(beam intensity)}}$ initially present, etc.

λ = the fractional change of a(t) per unit change in t. In the example, it would equal to the fraction of the isotope decaying per day.

A1.3   THE POISSON DISTRIBUTION

$$y(x) = \frac{e^{-a}a^x}{x!}$$

where a is a constant and x assumes *only* positive integer values, 0, 1, 2, and so forth.

In the more familiar terms, this is the Poisson formula used in target theory:

$$f(n) = \frac{e^{-a}a^n}{n!}$$

where a is the *average* number of inactivating events per target, n is the number of hits on the target, and f(n) is the *fraction* of targets receiving *exactly* n hits.

The term n! means "n factorial." For example:

$$0! = 1$$
$$1! = 1$$
$$2! = 2 \cdot 1 = 2$$
$$3! = 3 \cdot 2 \cdot 1 = 6$$
$$4! = 4 \cdot 3 \cdot 2 \cdot 1 = 24$$
$$5! = 5 \cdot 4 \cdot 3 \cdot 2 \cdot 1 = 120$$

and so forth. As an example, assume that a dose of X-rays produces an average of one inactivating event per target. Consequently,

$$a = 1$$

According to target theory, if a target receives one or more hits, it is inactivated. If the target avoids a hit, it survives. From the formula, f(0) equals the fraction of targets which would receive 0 hits (and thereby survive). This is calulated by

$$f(0) = \frac{e^{-1}1^{-0}}{0!} = 0.368$$

(note: $e^{-1} = \frac{1}{e} = \frac{1}{2.72} = 0.368$)

This result states that if a dose provides an *average* of one hit per target, about 37 per cent of the targets escape hits. The remaining 63 per cent of the targets, then, receive one or more hits. Since only one hit is necessary to inactivate, the targets which get *more* than one hit have been "overkilled."

Next, we will determine what fraction of the targets receive one hit.

$$f(1) = \frac{e^{-1}1^1}{1!} = 0.368$$

The fraction receiving two hits:

$$f(2) = \frac{e^1 1^2}{2!} = 0.184$$

The fraction receiving three hits:

$$f(3) = \frac{e^{-1}1^3}{3!} = \frac{0.368}{6} = 0.061$$

The fraction receiving four hits:

$$f(4) = \frac{e^{-1}1^4}{4!} = \frac{0.368}{24} = 0.015$$

The fraction receiving five hits:

$$f(5) = \frac{e^{-1}1^5}{5!} = \frac{.368}{120} = 0.003$$

If we add the fraction of targets receiving five or fewer hits, then:

$$tf = f(0) + f(1) + f(2) + f(3) + f(4) + f(5) =$$
$$0.368 + 0.368 + 0.184 + 0.061 + 0.015 + 0.003 = 0.998$$

As the value of tf shows, a fraction of only 0.002 (= 1.000 − 0.998) of the targets receive *more* than five hits (you can't have a fraction greater than 1.000).

A1.4 THE MULTITARGET MODEL

$$y(x) = 1 - (1 - e^{-x/a})^b$$

where a and b are parameters.

In the form used in radiobiology, the equation is

$$S(D) = 1 - (1 - e^{D/D_0})^N$$

where D_0 and N are parameters and S(D) gives the fraction surviving a dose of D rads. For example, consider the following data:

Dose	S(D) (Surviving Fraction)
0	1.
100	.71
200	.38
300	.165
400	.073
500	.031
600	.0145

As Figure A1–3 shows, when the data are plotted on semilog coordinates, the curve has two components — a shoulder (non-linear) at the lower doses and a straight (log-linear) segment at the higher doses. The extrapolation number, N, is easily determined graphically. The log-linear points are connected; N is the extrapolated value. For the example, N = 2.

The other parameter, D_0, can also be computed easily. By definition, it is that dose which will reduce the survival by 0.37 along the log-linear segment. Inspection of the graph shows the extrapolated line (S) to have the formula

$$S = Ne^{-D/D_0}$$

(note: when D = 0, e^{-D/D_0} = 1;
therefore, the value of S at D = 0 is N)

Divide both sides of the equation by N.

$$\frac{S}{N} = e^{-D/D_0}$$

If we select a specific dose such that S will be reduced to a value of $\frac{N}{2}$ (this dose would then be a "half-kill" dose, or $D_{1/2}$) substitution gives

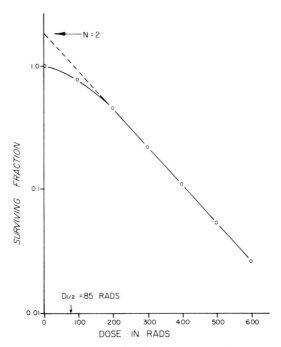

FIGURE A1–3   Typical multi-target survival curve.

$$\frac{S}{N} = \frac{1}{2} = e^{-(D_{1/2})/D_0}$$

Taking natural logarithms of both sides

$$\ln(\tfrac{1}{2}) = -0.693 = \ln(e^{-D_{1/2}/D_0})$$
$$-0.693 = -D_{1/2}/D_0$$

Dividing both sides by -0.693 while multiplying by D_0 gives

$$D_0 = D_{1/2}/0.693 = 1.44 D_{1/2}$$

To calculate D_0, then, the $D_{1/2}$ dose is determined from the extrapolated portion of the curve and is multiplied by 1.44. For the example $D_{1/2} = 85$ rads:

$$D_0 = 1.44(85) = 122 \text{ rads}$$

A second method is to multiply the extrapolation number by 0.37 and read the dose corresponding to this survival. Since $N = 2$, $0.37(2) = 0.74$. The dose corresponding to a surviving fraction of 0.74 (along the *extrapolated* curve) is 122.

APPENDIX II

Protection of Potentially Pregnant Women

Glenn V. Dalrymple, M.D. and Howard J. Barnhard, M.D.

A2.1 INTRODUCTION

As emphasized throughout this book, the 60-day period following conception represents the time of greatest radiosensitivity of the unborn child. Unfortunately, many women are unaware of possible pregnancy during a large portion of this period. Consequently, physicians using radiation should make a specific effort to learn if, indeed, female patients could be pregnant. If pregnancy cannot be ruled out by history (and in the absence of emergency conditions), the examination should be delayed until the status of pregnancy can be determined.

MEMORANDUM

SUBJECT: Radiation Exposure of Pregnant Women and Women Who May be Pregnant

FROM: Department of Radiology

TO: Clinical Faculty and Resident Staff

Background Information:

The Department of Radiology has routinely exercised all reasonable precautions to protect pregnant women from unnecessary radiation from diagnostic radiology procedures. We have done this by postponing non-urgent studies, by modifying necessary procedures to reduce radiation levels, or by adequate shielding of the fetus.

New Procedure

When a Diagnostic Radiology examination that includes the lower abdomen (Upper G. I. Series. I. V. Pyelogram, etc.) is requested on a woman of child bearing age:

a) The referring physician (or his designee) should complete and sign the new diagnostic radiology request form under "Patient is not considered pregnant because:..." OR,

b) If the examination should be done "now" regardless, the referring physician (only) should sign under the statement "Proceed with examination regardless of pregnancy or phase of menstrual cycle:"

If such authorization is not provided, each appropriate patient will have to be interviewed in Radiology. If it is determined that the possibility of pregnancy exists, the examination will be deferred until you, the referring physician, can be contacted. (Providing the authorization in advance will, of course, minimize delay and inconvenience for the patient, especially when you cannot be reached promptly.)

Regrettably, this new procedure places burdens on all of us. The Background Information given on the next page will explain why it has become necessary.

Over the years, we have repeatedly considered additional means of preventing such occurrences. But we have continued to follow the practice of the vast majority of other institutions and radiologists in "assuming" that you the referring physician had screened your female patients.

Occasionally, however, a patient is irradiated during early pregnancy, either because we were not so informed or because neither the referring doctor nor the patient herself knew of it. Unfortunately, this occurs during the most radiosensitive period for the fetus. There have already been abortions performed in Arkansas based on such occurrences.

A recent publication, "X-Ray Examinations, a Guide to Good Practice," has been prepared by the American College of Radiology with the assistance of the PHS Bureau of Radiological Health and the cooperation of the American Medical Association. It establishes and defines guidelines to follow, thereby making these the national norm. This, then, makes it ever more imperative that we take additional precautions to avoid these occasional occurrences. The new procedure has therefore been adopted with the concurrence of the heads of clinical departments and divisions.

Acceptable reasons to proceed with non-urgent examinations include:

has not yet started or has stopped menstruating
    (includes hysterectomy, oophorectomy)
tubal ligation
normal menstrual flow began less than 14 days ago
no intercourse since last period
taking "the pill" regularly
has intra-uterine contraceptive device.

FIGURE A2-1.

UNIVERSITY OF ARKANSAS
MEDICAL CENTER
UNIVERSITY HOSPITAL
Little Rock

RADIOLOGY DIAGNOSTIC REQUEST
(For THERAPY Use consultation form
For NUCL MED Use radio isotopes form)

IMPORTANT! IT MAY BE NECESSARY TO DELAY EXAM(S) IF INFORMATION IS INCOMPLETE

Requesting Service/Code
Hospital Location of Pt

UAMC XRAY Past 10 Yrs? YES ☐ NO ☐
Pt. Cannot Walk; Need WHEELCHAIR ☐ STRETCHER ☐

Examination(s) Desired:

Use Identification Plate
Name
Unit No. Race Sex
Birth-date
City

Purpose or Point of Concern (Optional)

IF FEMALE & LOWER ABDOMEN INCLUDED, COMPLETE THIS BLOCK:
Patient is not considered pregnant because:

OR (Signature of Interviewer)

Proceed with examination regardless of pregnancy or phase of menstrual cycle:
M.D.
Full Signature

Exam is Desired: Soon As Possible ☐ or Date

Date of Request

History

REQUESTED BY:
(Physician Authorization)
Initials Number

DIAGNOSIS: Provisional? Proven?

FIGURE A2–2.

In the sections that follow we describe the system in use in the Diagnostic Roentgenology Section and the Nuclear Medicine Division of the University of Arkansas Medical Center. We should point out that our current system is in a state of evolution. Very likely changes will be made over the course of the next few years.

A2.2 DIAGNOSTIC RADIOLOGY SECTION

Figure A2–1 is a facsimile of a memorandum sent to all members of the clinical staff. This memorandum set the stage for the new request form for diagnostic radiology, Figure A2–2. Note the lower right portion of the form in which the

FROM: Department of Radiology

TO: Referring Physician

RE: Diagnostic Radiology Request (attached)

☐ Please complete information in general

☐ Please complete: ______________________________

[X] This patient may be pregnant. Either defer examination, or sign the statement, "Proceed with examination regardless of pregnancy or phase of menstrual cycle."

Thank you for your cooperation.
It helps us do a better job for you and your patient.

FIGURE A2–3.

PROCEDURE BEFORE DOING DIAGNOSTIC RADIOLOGY EXAM

If <u>all</u> of the following:

- female between 11 and 50 years of age

- lower abdomen to be included in radiologic examination (e. g., Upper G. I., IVP, pelvis, lumbar spine, hysterosalpingogram, pelvic pneumogram)

- no statement from referring physician to go ahead in spite of pregnancy risk

- Patient is <u>not</u> an obvious emergency.

THEN ASK -- Is it possible that you are pregnant?

If "<u>yes</u>" - refer as follows:

        Outpatient - Attach "incomplete information" form to diagnostic
                     request and have patient return with it to clinic.

        ER - Call referring physician.

        Inpatient - Have radiologist evaluate.

If "<u>no</u>" - document* reason as:

        has not started menstruating yet

        has stopped menstruating (menopause, hysterectomy, oophorectomy)

        bilateral tubal ligation

        taking birth control pills regularly

        has intra-uterine coil

        no intercourse since last period

        normal menstrual flow began less than 14 days ago

        other?

* make note on front of request
  sign it
  proceed with examination

FIGURE A2-4.

ward personnel make an assessment of possible pregnancy—and sign the form. If the patient is an emergency, the requesting physician may so indicate by signing the lower line. If the ward personnel fail to complete their portions (and the patient is not an obvious emergency), the requisition is returned with a form (Figure A2-3) which indicates those portions to be completed (the third box refers to the question of possible pregnancy).

In addition to the screening provided by the ward personnel, additional screening is accomplished by radiology personnel. Figure A2-4 is a form provided to personnel in the diagnostic radiology section. All female patients within the child-bearing age are to be questioned, and a disposition made for patients in whom pregnancy cannot be ruled out.

A2.3 THE DIVISION OF NUCLEAR MEDICINE

Because all internally administered radionuclides present a possible danger to the unborn child, every female patient is carefully screened by a member of the nuclear medicine staff. Figure A2-5 represents a form which is completed by all sexually mature females. After the interview, the patient is asked to sign the form. In addition, the physician administering the radionuclide also signs the form.

In the event the patient cannot sign the form, the reason for the emergency is noted and the radionuclide injected.

FORM FOR PATIENT INTERVIEW

FOR FEMALE PATIENTS

YOU ARE BEING EXAMINED IN NUCLEAR MEDICINE AT THE REQUEST OF YOUR PHYSICIAN. THIS REQUIRES THE USE OF MATERIALS WHICH CONTAIN SMALL AMOUNTS OF RADIO-ACTIVITY. BECAUSE OF A POSSIBLE SMALL RISK TO UNBORN CHILDREN. IT IS NECESSARY FOR US TO DETERMINE IF YOU POSSIBLE COULD BE PREGNANT. WE WOULD APPRECIATE YOU ANSWERING THESE QUESTIONS HONESTLY SO WE MAY PROCEED SAFELY FOR YOUR BENEFIT. SOME OF THE QUESTIONS MAY NOT APPLY TO YOU, AND IF NOT, PLEASE WRITE "NO" IN THE BLANK.

DATE OF LAST MENSTRUAL PERIOD _____.

ARE YOU, OR COULD YOU BE PREGNANT NOW? YES_____ NO_____

DO YOU TAKE BIRTH CONTROL PILLS NOW? YES_____ NO_____

DO YOU USE AN INTRAUTERINE CONTRACEPTIVE DEVICE (LIKE A COIL) NOW? YES_____ NO_____

HAVE YOU HAD AN OPERATION WHICH HAS MADE YOU STERILE? YES_____ NO_____

SIGNATURE_____

RADIOISOTOPE ADMINISTERED BY _____, M. D.

INSTRUCTIONS FOR NUCLEAR MEDICINE PERSONNEL

FOR FEMALE PATIENTS 11-50 YEARS OLD

PROCEED WITH TEST IF:

(1) MENSTRUAL PERIOD BEGAN LESS THAN 14 DAYS AGO

(2) "YES" ANSWERS TO ANY OF LAST 3 QUESTIONS

CHECK WITH PHYSICIAN IF:

(1) DATE OF LAST MENSTRUAL PERIOD IS OVER 14 DAYS FROM DATE OF EXAMINATION

(2) PATIENT COULD BE PREGNANT

(3) NO "YES" ANSWERS TO LAST 3 QUESTIONS AND (1) ABOVE APPLIES

FIGURE A2–5.

A2.4 CONCLUSION

We believe that a moderate effort on the part of individuals ordering and performing diagnostic studies will prevent the inadvertent irradiation of most unborn children. Hopefully, the future will provide a rapid, and simple, test to affirm (or exclude) the diagnosis of pregnancy.

APPENDIX III

General References

1. Ackerman, L. V., and del Regato, J. A.: *Cancer Diagnosis, Treatment, and Prognosis,* ed. 4. St. Louis, C. V. Mosby, 1970.
2. Alexander, P.: *Atomic Radiation and Life.* Baltimore, Penguin Books, 1957.
3. Altman, K. I., Gerber, G. V., and Okada, S.: *Radiation Biochemistry.* New York, Academic Press, 1970.
4. Andrews, H. L.: *Radiation Biophysics.* Englewood Cliffs, N.Y., Prentice-Hall, 1961.
5. Andrews, J. R., and Moody, J. M.: The dose-time relationship in radiotherapy. Am. J. Roentgen., 75:590–596, 1956.
6. Arena, V.: *Ionizing Radiation and Life.* St. Louis, C. V. Mosby, 1971.
7. Attix, F. H., Roesch, W. C., and Tochilin, E.: *Radiation Dosimetry,* Vols. 1, 2, and 3. New York, Academic Press, 1969.
8. Augenstein, L. G., Mason, R., Quastler, H., and Zelle, M.: *Advances in Radiation Biology.* New York, Academic Press, 1964, 1966, 1969.
9. Bacq, Z. M., and Alexander, P.: *Fundamentals of Radiobiology.* London, Butterworth, 1955.
10. Bacq, Z. M., and Alexander, P.: *Fundamentals of Radiobiology,* Vol. 5, ed. 2. New York, Pergamon Press, 1961.
11. Barendsen, G. W.: In *Time and Dose Relationships in Radiation Biology as Applied to Radiotherapy.* National Cancer Institute–AEC Monograph, Brookhaven Nat'l Laboratory, Upton, N.Y., 1970.
12. Benison, D., Placer, A., and van der Elst, E.: Estudio de un caso de irradiación humana accidental. Handling of Radiation Accidents. IAEA Vienna, 415, 1970.
13. Berg, N. O., and Lindgren, M.: Time-dose relationship and morphology of delayed radiation lesions of the brain in rabbits. Acta Radiol. (suppl.), *167*:1–118, 1958.
14. Berg, N. O., and Lindgren, M.: Relation between field size and tolerance of rabbit's brain to roentgen irradiation (200 kV) via a slit-shaped field. Acta Radiol. (N. S.), *1*:147–168, 1963.
15. Bergonie, J., and Tribondeau, L.: Interpretation de quelques resultats de la radio-therapie et essai de fixation d'une technique rationelle. C. R. Acad. Sci. [D] (Paris), *143*:983–985, 1906.
16. Berry, R. J.: "Small cones" in irradiated tumor cells *in vivo.* Brit. J. Radiol., *40*:285–291, 1967.
17. *Besner* versus *Kidde* 24, A. D., 2d 1045, 1965.
18. Boag, J. W.: The action of ionizing radiation on dilute aqueous solutions. Phys. Med. Biol. *10*:457–476, 1965.
19. Bogardus, C. R.: *Clinical Applications of Physics of Radiology and Nuclear Medicine.* St. Louis, Warren H. Green, 1969.
20. Bonarigo, B., and Rubin, P.: The non-union of pathologic fracture after radiation therapy. Radiology, 88:889–904, 1967.
21. Bond, V. P., Fliedner, T. M., and Archambeau, J. O.: *Mammalian Radiation Lethality.* New York, Academic Press, 1965.

22. *Bonner* versus *Morgan*, 126 Fed. 2d 121 (1941).

23. Borsanyi, S. J., Blanchard, C. L., and Thorne, B.: The effects of ionizing radiation on the ear. Ann. Otol., *70*:255–262, 1961.

24. Braams, R., and Van Harpen, G.: The effects of ionizing radiation on some fibrous proteins. *In* Duchesne, J. (ed.): *Advances in Chemical Physics 7*:259–381. New York, Interscience, 1964.

25. Brookhaven National Laboratory Associated Universities, Inc.: *Time and Dose Relationships in Radiation Biology as Applied to Radiation Therapy;* National Cancer Institute–AEC Conference, Carmel, Calif., 1969. Springfield, Virginia, National Bureau of Standards, U.S. Department of Commerce, 1970.

26. Burton, M., Kirby-Smith, J. S., and Magee, J. L.: *Comparative Effects of Radiation.* New York, John Wiley, 1960.

27. Casarett, G. W.: Concept and criteria of radiologic aging. *In* Harris, R. J. C. (ed.): *Cellular Basis and Aetiology of Late Somatic Effects of Ionizing Radiation.* London, Academic Press, 1963.

28. Casarett, A, P.: *Radiation Biology,* Englewood Cliffs, N.Y., Prentice-Hall, 1968.

29. Christensen, E. E., Curry, Thomas S., III, and Nunnally, James, E.: *An Introduction to the Physics of Diagnostic Radiology.* Philadelphia, Lea and Febiger, 1971.

30. Claus, W.: *Radiation Biology and Medicine.* Reading, Mass., Addison-Wesley, 1959.

31. Coggle, J. E.: *Biological Effects of Radiation.* London, Wykeham Publications (Science Series No. 34), 1971.

32. Cooper, G., Jr., Guerrant, J. L., Harden, A. G., and Teates, D.: Some consequences of pulmonary irradiation. Am. J. Roentgen., 85:865–874, 1961.

33. Coutard, H.: Sur les delais d'apparition et d'evolution des reactions de la peare, et des muqueuses de la bouche et de pharynx, provoquees par les rayons X. C. R. Soc. Biol. (Paris), 86:1140–1141, 1922.

34. Coutard, H.: Roentgen therapy of epitheliomas of tonsilar regions, hypopharynx, and larynx from 1920 to 1926. Am. J. Roentgen., 28:313–331, 1932.

35. DeBryn, P. Q. H.: Lymph node and intestinal lymphatic tissues. *In* Bloom, W. (ed.): *Histopathology of Irradiation from External and Internal Sources.* New York, McGraw-Hill, 1948.

36. Dertinger, H., and Jung, H.: The action of ionizing radiation on elementary biological objects. *In* Jung, H. (ed.): *Molecular Radiation Biology* (English translation). New York, Springer-Verlag, 1970.

37. Dettman, P. M., King, E. R., and Zimberg, Y. H.: Evaluation of lymph node function following irradiation or surgery. Am. J. Roentgen., 96:711–718, 1966.

38. Diczfalusy, E., Notter, G., Edsmyr, F., and Westman, A.: Estrogen excretion in breast cancer patients before and after ovarian irradiation and oophorectomy. J. Clin. Endocr., *19*:1230–1244, 1959.

39. Doig, R. K., Funder, J. F., and Weiden, S.: Serial gastric biopsy studies in a case of duodenal ulcer treated by deep X-ray therapy. Med. J. Australia, 38:828–830, 1951.

40. Ebert, M., Keene, J. P., Swallow, A. J., and Baxendale, J. H. (eds.): *Pulse Radiolysis.* New York, Academic Press, 1965.

41. Ebert, M., and Howard, A. (eds.): *Current Topics in Radiation Research*, Vols. I–VI. New York, John Wiley, 1970.

42. Einhorn, J., Fragraeus, A., and Jonsson, J.: Thyroid antibodies after ^{131}I treatment for hyperthyroidism. J. Clin. Endocr., 25:1218–1230, 1965.

43. Elkind, M. M., and Whitmore, G. F.: *The Radiobiology of Cultured Mammalian Cells.* New York, Gordon and Breach, 1967.

44. Ellinger, F.: *Medical Radiation Biology.* Springfield, Ill., Charles C Thomas, 1957.

45. Emirgil, C., and Heinemann, H. O.: Effects of irradiation of chest on pulmonary function in man. J. Appl. Physiol., *16*:331, 1961.

46. *Employers Mutual Liability Insurance Company of Wisconsin* versus *Alton A. Parker,* 418 S. W. 2d 570, 1969.

47. Engeset, A.: Irradiation of lymph nodes and vessels: Experiments in rats, with reference to cancer therapy. Acta Radiol. (suppl.), 229:5–125, 1964.

48. Errera, M., and Forssberg, A.: *Mechanisms in Radiobiology.* New York, Academic Press, 1960, 1961 (two Vols.).

49. Estep, S. D., and Forgotson, E. H.: Legal liability for genetic injuries from radiation. Louisiana Law Review, *XXIV*:1–53, (December) 1963.

50. *Favalora* versus *Aetna* 144 So. 2d 544, 1962.

51. *Ferrara* versus *Galluchio* 152 N. E. 2d 249, 1958.

52. Friedman, M.: Calculated risks of radiation injury of normal tissue in the treatment of cancer of the testis. Proc. 2d Nat. Cancer Conference, *1*:390, 1952.

53. Garrison, W. M.: Radiation chemistry of organo-nitrogen compounds. *In* Ebert, M., and Howard, A. (eds.): *Current Topics in Radiation Research 4*:43–94. New York, Interscience, 1968.

54. Gish, J. R., Coates, E. D., DuSault, L. A., and Doub, H. P.: Pulmonary radiation reaction: A vital capacity and time-dose study. Radiology, 73:679, 1959.

55. Glassner, A., and Hart, E. J.: Basic mechanisms in the radiation chemistry of aqueous media. Radiat. Res., suppl. 4, 1964.

56. Glasstone, S.: *Sourcebook on Atomic Energy*, ed 2. Princeton, D. Van Nostrand, 1958.

57. Glasstone, S.: *The Effects of Nuclear Weapons*, rev. ed. U.S. Department of Defense. Washington, D.C., Atomic Energy Commission, 1962. Obtain from Supt. of Documents, U.S. Gov't Printing Office, Washington, 1962.

58. Gould, R. F.: *Aqueous Media, Biology, Dosimetry; Advances in Chemistry.* Washington, D.C., American Chemical Society (No. 81. Vol. I), 1968.

59. Gould, R. F.: *Gases, Solids, Organic Liquids; Advances in Chemistry.* Washington, D.C., American Chemical Society (No. 82, Vol. II), 1968.

60. Gould, R. F.: *Advances in Chemistry.* Washington, D.C., American Chemical Society (No. 50), 1968.

61. Gregersen, M. I., Pallaricini, C., and Chien, S.: Studies on the chemical composition of the central nervous system in relation to the effects of X-irradiation and of disturbances in water and salt balance. Radiat. Res., *17*:209–225, 1962.

62. Grosch, D. S.: *Biological Effects of Radiation.* New York, Blaisdell Publishing, 1965.

63. Haissinski, M.: *The Chemical and Biological Actions of Radiations*, Vol. 10. New York, Academic Press, 1966.

64. Harris, R. J. C.: *The Initial Effects of Ionizing Radiation on Cells.* New York, Academic Press, 1961.

65. Hayes, D. F.: *Summary of Accidents and Incidents Involving Radiation in Atomic Energy Activities, June 1945–December 1955.* TID-5360. Oak Ridge, Tenn. Technical Information Extension Service, 1956.

66. Hayes, D. F.: *Summary of Incidents Involving Radioactive Material in Atomic Energy Activities, January–December 1956.* TID-5366 (suppl). Oak Ridge, Tenn., Technical Information Extension Service, 1957.

67. Hewett, H. B., and Wilson, C. W.: Survival curves for tumor cells irradiated *in vivo.* Ann. N.Y. Acad. Sci., 95:818–827, 1961.

68. Hine, G. J., and Brownell, G. L.: *Radiation Dosimetry.* New York, Academic Press, 1961.

69. Hollaender, A.: *High Energy Radiation. Vol. I. Radiation Biology.* New York, McGraw-Hill, 1954.

70. Howland, J. W., and Warren, S. L.: Effects of atomic bomb irradiation on Japanese. Advances Biol. Med. Phys., *1*:387–408, 1948.

71. ICRP (International Council on Radiological Protection): *Permissible Dose for Internal Radiation.* No. 2, 1959. (All ICRP publications may be obtained from U.S. Government Printing Office, Washington, D.C.   20402.)

72. ICRP: *Protection Against Electromagnetic Radiation Above 3 MeV and Electrons, Neutrons, and Protons.* No. 4, 1963.

73. ICRP: *Principles of Environmental Monitoring Related to the Handling of Radioactive Materials.* No. 7, 1965.

74. ICRP: *The Evaluation of Risks from Radiation.* No. 8, 1965.

75. ICRP: *Recommendations.* No. 9, 1965.

76. ICRP: *Evaluation of Radiation Doses to Body Tissue from Internal Contamination Due to Occupational Exposure.* No. 10, 1968.

77. ICRP: *A Review of the Radiosensitivity of the Tissues of the Bone.* No. 11, 1967.

78. ICRP: *General Principles of Monitoring for Radiation Protection of Workers.* No. 12, 1968.

78a. ICRU (International Commission on Radiation Units and Measurements): *Radiation Dosimetry, 0.6–50 MeV.* No. 14, 1969. (All ICRU publications may be obtained from International Commission on Radiation Units and Measurements, Washington, D.C.)

78b. ICRU: *Radiation Dosimetry, 5–150 kV.* No. 17, 1970.

79. Ingold, J. A., Reed, G. B., Kaplan, H. S., and Bagshaw, M. A. Radiation hepatitis. Am. J. Roentgen., 93:200–208, 1965.

80. Jackson, K. L., and Entenman, C.: The role of bile secretion in the gastrointestinal radiation syndrome. Radiat. Res., *10*:67, 1959.

81. Johnson, G. R., and Scholes, G.: *The Chemistry of Ionization and Excitation.* London, Taylor and Francis, 1966.

82. Kashima, H. K., Kirkham, W. R., and Andrews, J. R.: Postirradiation sialadenitis; A study of the clinical features, histopathologic changes, and serum enzyme variations following irradiation of human salivary glands. Am. J. Roentgen., 94:271–291, 1965.

83. Knowlton, N. P., Leifer, E., Hogness, J. R., Hempelman, L. H., Blaney, L. F., Gill, D.C., Oakes, W. R., and Shafer, C. L.: Beta ray burns of human skin. J.A.M.A., *141*:239, 1949.

84. Lea, D. E.: *Actions of Radiations on Living Cells*, ed. 2. New York, Cambridge University Press, 1955.

85. Leach, J. E., and Sugiura, K.: The effect of high voltage roentgen rays on the heart of adult rats. Am. J. Roentgen., *41*:414–425, 1941.

85a. Lederer, C. M., Hollander, J. M., and Perlman, I.: *Table of Isotopes.* New York, John Wiley, 1967.

86. Lindgren, M.: On tolerance of brain tissue and sensitivity of brain tumors to irradiation. Acta Radiol. (suppl.), *170*:1–73, 1958.

87. Loutit, J. F.: *Irradiation of mice and men.* Chicago, University of Chicago Press, 1962.

88. Lushbaugh, C. C., and Ricks, R. C.: Radiation effect and tolerance of normal tissues (basic concepts in radiation pathology). *In* Vol. 6 of Vaeth, J. (ed.): *Frontiers in Radiation Therapy and Oncology.* New York, S. Karger, 1972.

89. Luxton, R. W.: The Clinical and Pathological Effects of Renal Irradiation. Vol. II *in* Buschke, F., (ed.): *Progression in Radiation Therapy.* New York, Grune and Stratton, 1962.

90. Matheson, M. S., and Dorfman, L. M.: *Research Monographs in Radiation Chemistry. No. I. Pulse Radiolysis.* Cambridge, Mass., M.I.T. Press, 1969.

91. Maxfield, W. S., and Porter, G. H.: Accidental radiation exposure from iridium-192 camera. Handling of radiation accidents. IAEA, Vienna, 459, 1970.

92. Merriam, G. R., Jr., and Focht, E. F.: Radiation dose to the lens in treatment of tumors of the eye and adjacent structures; Possibilities of cataract formation. Radiology, *71*:357, 1958.

93. *Mims* versus *Boland* 138 S. E. 2d 902, 1964; 110 Ga App. 477, 1964.

94. Mozumbder, A.: Charged particle tracks and their structure. *In* Burton, M., and Magee, J. L. (eds.): *Advances in Radiation Chemistry 1*:1–102. New York, Interscience, 1969.

95. NCRP (National Council on Radiation Protection): *Control and Removal of Radioactive Contamination in Laboratories.* No. 8, 1951. (All NCRP publications may be obtained from NCRP Publications, P.O. Box 4867, Washington, D.C. 20008.)

96. NCRP: *Recommendations for Waste Disposal of Phosphorous-32 and Iodine-131 for Medical Users.* No. 9, 1951.

97. NCRP: *Radiological Monitoring Methods and Instruments.* No. 10, 1952.

98. NCRP: *Protection Against Betatron-Synchroton Radiations up to 100 Million Electron Volts.* No. 14, 1954.

99. NCRP: *Permissible Dose from External Sources of Ionizing Radiation.* (Includes Addendum NBS Handbook, 59, 1958.) No. 17, 1954.

100. NCRP: *Protection Against Neutron Radiation Up to 30 Million Electron Volts.* No. 20, 1957.

101. NCRP: *Safe Handling of Bodies Containing Radioactive Isotopes.* No. 21, 1958.

102. NCRP: *Maximum Permissible Body Burdens and Maximum Permissible Concentrations of Radionuclides in Air and in Water for Occupational Exposure.*

103. NCRP: *Measurement of Neutron Flux and Spectra for Physical and Biological Applications.* No. 23, 1960.

104. NCRP: *Protection Against Radiations from Sealed Gamma Sources.* No. 24, 1960.

105. NCRP: *Measurement of Absorbed Dose of Neutrons and of Mixtures of Neutrons and Gamma Rays.* No. 25, 1961.

106. NCRP: *Medical X-Ray Protection up to Three Million Volts.*

107. NCRP: *Stopping Powers for Use with Cavity Chambers.* No. 27, 1961.

108. NCRP: *A Manual of Radioactivity Procedures.* No. 28, 1961.

109. NCRP: *Exposure to Radiation in an Emergency.* No. 29, 1962.

110. NCRP: *Safe Handling of Radioactive Materials.* No. 30, 1964.

111. NCRP: *Shielding for High-Energy Electron Accelerator Installations.* No. 31, 1964.
112. NCRP: *Radiation Protection in Educational Institutions.* No. 32, 1966.
113. NCRP: *Medical X-ray and Gamma-Ray Protection for Energies up to 10 MeV — Equipment Design and Use.* No. 33, 1968.
114. NCRP: *Medical X-Ray and Gamma-Ray Protection for Energies up to 10 MeV — Structural Shielding Design and Evaluation.* No. 34, 1970.
115. NCRP: *Dental X-Ray Protection.* No. 35, 1970.
116. NCRP: *Precautions in the Management of Patients Who Have Received Therapeutic Amounts of Radionuclides.* No. 37, 1971.
117. NCRP: *Basic Radiation Protection Criteria.* No. 39, 1971.
118. *Natanson* versus *Kline* 350 P. 2d 1093, 1960; 354 P. 2d 670, 1960.
119. NBS: *Protection Against Betatron-Synchroton Radiations up to 100 Million Electron Volts.* Handbook 55, (All NBS Handbooks may be obtained from Supt. of Documents, U.S. Government Printing Office, Washington, D.C.)
120. NBS: *Maximum Permissible Body Burdens and Maximum Permissible Concentration of Radionuclides in Air and in Water for Occupational Exposures.* Handbook 69, 1959.
121. NBS: *Protection Against Radiation from Sealed Gamma Sources.* Handbook 73, 1960.
122. NBS: *Medical X-Ray Protection Up to Three Million Volts.* Handbook 76, 1961.
123. NBS: *1959 ICRU Report.* Handbook 78, January, 1961.
124. NBS: *Radiation Quantities and Units.* Handbook 84, November, 1962.
125. NBS: *Physical Aspects of Irradiation.* Handbook 85, March, 1964.
126. NBS: *Radioactivity.* Handbook 86, November, 1963.
127. NBS: *Clinical Dosimetry.* Handbook 87, August, 1963.
128. NBS: *Radiobiological Dosimetry.* Handbook 88, April, 1963.
129. Neary, G. J., Munson, R. J., and Mole, R. H.: *Chronic Radiation Hazards.* London, Pergamon Press, 1957.
130. Neuhauser, E. B., Wittenborg, M. H., Bergman, C. Z., and Cohen, J.: Irradiation effects of roentgen therapy on growing spine. Radiology, 56:637–650, 1952.
131. *New York Workmen's Compensation Law*, Section 3, Subd. 2, 47.
132. Ng, E., Chambers, F. W., Jr., Ogden, H. S., Coggs, G. C., and Crane, J. T.: Osteomyelitis of the mandible following irradiation; An experimental study. Radiology, 72:68–74, 1959.
133. Notter, G.: A technique for destruction of the hypophysis using Y^{90}-spheres. Acta Radiol. (suppl.), 184:1–128, 1959.
134. O'Donnell, J. H., and Sangster, D. F.: *Principles of Radiation Chemistry.* New York, Elsevier, 1970.
135. *Parker* versus *Employers Mutual Liability Insurance Company of Wisconsin*, 440 S.W. 2d 43, 1969.
136. Paterson, R.: *The Treatment of Malignant Disease by Radiotherapy.* Baltimore, Williams and Wilkins, 1963.
137. Peck, W. S., and McGreer, J. T. (with Kretzschman, N. R., and Brown, W. E.): Castration of the female by irradiation; The results in 334 patients. Radiology, 34:176–186, 1940.
138. Perez-Tamayo, R., Soberon, M., and Le Vaivre, R.: Systems of Quantitative Correlation of Treatment Schedules (SQCTS): Time, Dose, Volume, Quality, NSD, EAD, and Cell-Surviving Fraction Tables.
139. Perthes, G.: Über den Einfluss der Röntgenstrahlen auf Epitheliale Gewebe, Insbesondere auf das Carcinom. Arch. Klin. Chir., 71:955–1000, 1903.
140. Pikaev, A. K.: *Pulse Radiolysis of Water and Aqueous Solutions.* Bloomington, Ind., Indiana University Press, 1967.
141. Read, J., and Gray, L. H.: *Radiation Biology of* Vicia faba *in Relation to the General Problem.* Springfield, Ill., Charles C Thomas, 1959.
142. Redd, B. L.: Radiation nephritis; Review, case report, and animal study. Am. J. Roentgen., 83:88–106, 1960.
143. Reeves, R. J., Sanders, A. P., Isely, J. K., Sharpe, K. W., and Baylin, G. J.: Fat absorption studies and small bowel X-ray studies in patients undergoing ^{60}Co teletherapy and/or radium application. Am. J. Roentgen., 94:848–851, 1965.
144. Rothberg, H., Blair, E. B., Gomez, A. C., and McNulty, W.: Observations on chimpanzees after whole body radiation and homologous bone marrow treatment. Blood, 14:1302, 1959.

145. Saenger, E. L.: Radiation accidents. Am. J. Roentgen., *84*:715, 1960.
146. *Salgo* versus *Leland Stanford Jr. of University Board of Trustees* 317 P. 2d 170, 1957; 154 Cal. App. 2d 560, 1957.
147. Schubert, J.: *Copper and Peroxides in Radiobiology and Medicine.* Springfield, Ill., Charles C Thomas, 1964.
148. Shilling, C. W.: *Atomic Energy Encyclopedia in the Life Sciences.* Philadelphia, W. B. Saunders, 1964.
149. Silini, G.: *Radiation Research.* Amsterdam, North-Holland Publishing, 1967.
150. Silverman, S., and Sheline, G. E.: Effects of radiation on exfoliated normal and malignant oral cells; A preliminary study. Cancer, *14*:587–596, 1961.
151. Slater, John C.: *Modern Physics.* New York, McGraw-Hill, 1955.
152. Sorenson, D. K., Bond, V. P., Cronkite, E. P., and Perman, V.: An effective therapeutic regimen for hemopoietic phase of the acute radiation syndrome in dogs. Radiat. Res., *13*:669, 1960.
153. Spear, F. G.: *Radiations and Living Cells.* New York, John Wiley, 1953.
154. Stanton, L.: *Basic Medical Radiation Physics.* New York, Appleton-Century-Crofts, 1969.
155. Stein, G.: *Radiation Chemistry of Aqueous Systems.* Jerusalem, Weizmann Science Press, 1968.
156. Stewart, J. R., and Fajardo, L. F.: Dose response in human and experimental radiation induced heart disease; Application of the nominal standard dose (NSD) concept. Radiology, 99:403–408, 1971.
157. Strandqvist, M.: Studien über die Kumulative Wirkung der Röntgenstrahlen bie Fraktionierung. Acta Radiol. (Stockholm) (suppl.), 55:1–293, 1944.
158. Swallow, A. J.: *Radiation Chemistry of Organic Compounds.* Oxford, Pergamon Press, 1960.
159. Sweaney, S. K., Moss, W. T., and Haddy, F. J.: The effects of chest irradiation on pulmonary function. J. Clin. Invest., *38*:587–593, 1959.
160. Sykes, M. P., Chu, F. C. H., and Wilkerson, W. G.: Local bone-marrow changes secondary to therapeutic irradiation. Radiology, 75:919–924, 1960.
161. Sykes, M. P., Chu, F. C. H., Savel, H., Bonadonna, G., and Mathis, H.: The effects of varying dosages of irradiation upon sternal-marrow regeneration. Radiology, *83*: 1084–1088, 1963.
162. Thomas, J. K.: Elementary processes and reactions in the radiolysis of matter. In Burton, M., and Magee, J. L. (eds.): *Advances in Radiation Chemistry 1*:103–198. New York, Interscience, 1969.
163. Tobias, C. A., Lawrence, J. H., Lyman, J., Born, J. L., Gottschalk, A., Linfoot, J., and McDonald, J.: Progress report on pituitary irradiation. *In* Haley, T. J., and Snider, R. S. (eds.): *Response of the Nervous System to Ionizing Radiation.* Boston, Little, Brown, and Co., 1964.
164. Umiker, W. O., Lampe, I., Rapp, R., Latourett, H., and Boblett, D. E.: Irradiation effects on malignant cells in smears from oral cancers; Preliminary report. Cancer, *12*:614–619, 1959.
165. Vatistas, S., and Hornsey, S.: Radiation-induced protein loss into the gastrointestinal tract. Brit. J. Radiol., *39*:547–550, 1966.
166. Vereschchinskii, I. V., and Pikaev, A.: *Introduction to Radiation Chemistry.* (Translated from the Russian.) New York, Daniel Davey, 1964.
167. Von Essen, C. F.: Clinical radiation tolerance of the skin and upper aerodigestive tract. In Vol. 6 of Vaeth, E. (ed.): *Frontiers in Radiation Therapy and Oncology.* New York, S. Karger. 1972.
168. Wallace, B., and Dobzhansky, T.: *Radiation, Genes, and Man.* New York, Holt, Rinehart, and Winston, 1963.
169. White, G. Sienewicz, J., and Christensen, W. R.: Improved control of advanced oral cancer with massive roentgen therapy. Radiology, *63*:37, 1954.
170. *Wilson* versus *Scott* 412 S. W. 2d 299, 1967.
171. *Woods* versus *Brumlop* 377 P. 2d 520, 1962.
172. Zirkle, R. E.: *Biological Effects of X- and Gamma Radiation.* New York, McGraw-Hill, 1954.

APPENDIX IV

Decimal Values of $(F^{-0.24} \times T^{-0.11})$

(See following page for tables)

F is number of Fractions, T is Time in days

F	T=1	2	3	4	5	6	7	8	9	10
1	1.0000									
2	0.8467	0.7845	0.7503	0.7269						
3	0.7682	0.7118	0.6807	0.6595	0.6435	0.6308				
4	0.7169	0.6643	0.6353	0.6155	0.6006	0.5887	0.5788	0.5703		
5	0.6795	0.6297	0.6022	0.5834	0.5693	0.5580	0.5486	0.5406	0.5336	0.5275
6	0.6504	0.6027	0.5764	0.5584	0.5449	0.5341	0.5251	0.5174	0.5108	0.5049
7				0.5382	0.5251	0.5147	0.5060	0.4986	0.4922	0.4866
8				0.5212	0.5085	0.4984	0.4901	0.4829	0.4767	0.4712
9					0.4944	0.4846	0.4764	0.4695	0.4634	0.4581
10					0.4820	0.4725	0.4645	0.4577	0.4518	0.4466
11						0.4618	0.4540	0.4474	0.4416	0.4365

F	T=11	12	13	14	15	16	17	18	19	20
6	0.4996	0.4949	0.4905							
7	0.4815	0.4769	0.4727	0.4689	0.4653					
8	0.4663	0.4619	0.4578	0.4541	0.4507	0.4475	0.4445			
9	0.4533	0.4490	0.4450	0.4414	0.4381	0.4350	0.4321	0.4294	0.4268	
10	0.4420	0.4378	0.4339	0.4304	0.4271	0.4241	0.4213	0.4187	0.4162	0.4138
11	0.4320	0.4279	0.4241	0.4207	0.4175	0.4145	0.4118	0.4092	0.4068	0.4045
12		0.4190	0.4153	0.4120	0.4089	0.4060	0.4033	0.4007	0.3984	0.3961
13			0.4074	0.4041	0.4011	0.3982	0.3956	0.3931	0.3908	0.3886
14				0.3970	0.3940	0.3912	0.3886	0.3862	0.3839	0.3817
15					0.3875	0.3848	0.3822	0.3798	0.3776	0.3755
16						0.3789	0.3764	0.3740	0.3718	0.3697
17							0.3709	0.3686	0.3664	0.3644
18								0.3636	0.3614	0.3594
19									0.3568	0.3548
20										0.3504

F	T=21	22	23	24	25	26	27	28	29	30
12	0.3940	0.3920	0.3901							
13	0.3865	0.3845	0.3827							
14	0.3797	0.3778	0.3759	0.3742	0.3725	0.3709				
15	0.3735	0.3715	0.3697	0.3680	0.3664	0.3648				
16	0.3677	0.3658	0.3641	0.3623	0.3607	0.3592	0.3577	0.3563	0.3549	
17	0.3624	0.3606	0.3588	0.3571	0.3555	0.3540	0.3525	0.3511	0.3498	0.3485
18	0.3575	0.3556	0.3539	0.3522	0.3507	0.3492	0.3477	0.3463	0.3450	0.3437
19	0.3529	0.3511	0.3493	0.3477	0.3461	0.3447	0.3432	0.3419	0.3405	0.3393
20	0.3485	0.3468	0.3451	0.3435	0.3419	0.3404	0.3390	0.3377	0.3364	0.3351
21	0.3445	0.3427	0.3410	0.3395	0.3379	0.3365	0.3351	0.3337	0.3325	0.3312
22			0.3373	0.3357	0.3342	0.3327	0.3314	0.3300	0.3288	0.3275
23					0.3306	0.3292	0.3278	0.3265	0.3253	0.3241
24					0.3273	0.3259	0.3245	0.3232	0.3220	0.3208
25									0.3188	0.3176
26									0.3158	0.3147

F	31	32	33	34	35	36	37	38	39	40
17	0.3472	0.3460								
18	0.3425	0.3413	0.3401	0.3390						
19	0.3381	0.3369	0.3357	0.3346						
20	0.3339	0.3328	0.3316	0.3305	0.3295	0.3285	0.3275			
21	0.3300	0.3289	0.3278	0.3267	0.3257	0.3246	0.3237			
22	0.3264	0.3252	0.3241	0.3231	0.3220	0.3210	0.3201	0.3191	0.3182	
23	0.3229	0.3218	0.3207	0.3196	0.3186	0.3176	0.3167	0.3157	0.3148	0.3140
24	0.3196	0.3185	0.3174	0.3164	0.3154	0.3144	0.3135	0.3125	0.3116	0.3108
25	0.3165	0.3154	0.3143	0.3133	0.3123	0.3113	0.3104	0.3095	0.3086	0.3077
26	0.3135	0.3124	0.3114	0.3104	0.3094	0.3084	0.3075	0.3066	0.3057	0.3049
27		0.3096	0.3086	0.3076	0.3066	0.3056	0.3047	0.3038	0.3030	0.3021
28		0.3069	0.3059	0.3049	0.3039	0.3030	0.3021	0.3012	0.3003	0.2995
29				0.3023	0.3014	0.3004	0.2995	0.2987	0.2978	0.2970
30				0.2999	0.2989	0.2980	0.2971	0.2962	0.2954	0.2946
31						0.2957	0.2948	0.2939	0.2931	0.2923
32								0.2917	0.2909	0.2900
33									0.2887	0.2879
34									0.2867	0.2859
35										0.2839
36										0.2820

F	41	42	43	44	45	46	47	48	49	50
23	0.3131									
24	0.3099	0.3091	0.3083	0.3075						
25	0.3069	0.3061	0.3053	0.3045	0.3038	0.3031				
26	0.3040	0.3032	0.3024	0.3017	0.3009	0.3002	0.2995			
27	0.3013	0.3005	0.2997	0.2990	0.2982	0.2975	0.2968	0.2961		
28	0.2987	0.2979	0.2971	0.2964	0.2956	0.2949	0.2942	0.2935	0.2929	0.2922
29	0.2962	0.2954	0.2946	0.2939	0.2932	0.2924	0.2918	0.2911	0.2904	0.2898
30	0.2938	0.2930	0.2922	0.2915	0.2908	0.2901	0.2894	0.2887	0.2881	0.2874
31	0.2915	0.2907	0.2899	0.2892	0.2885	0.2878	0.2871	0.2865	0.2858	0.2852
32	0.2893	0.2885	0.2877	0.2870	0.2863	0.2856	0.2849	0.2843	0.2836	0.2830
33	0.2871	0.2864	0.2856	0.2849	0.2842	0.2835	0.2828	0.2822	0.2816	0.2809
34	0.2851	0.2843	0.2836	0.2829	0.2822	0.2815	0.2808	0.2802	0.2795	0.2789
35	0.2831	0.2824	0.2816	0.2809	0.2802	0.2795	0.2789	0.2782	0.2776	0.2770
36	0.2812	0.2804	0.2797	0.2790	0.2783	0.2777	0.2770	0.2764	0.2757	0.2751
37		0.2786	0.2779	0.2772	0.2765	0.2758	0.2752	0.2745	0.2739	0.2733
38				0.2754	0.2747	0.2741	0.2734	0.2728	0.2722	0.2716
39				0.2737	0.2730	0.2724	0.2717	0.2711	0.2705	0.2699
40					0.2714	0.2707	0.2701	0.2695	0.2688	0.2682
41						0.2691	0.2685	0.2679	0.2673	0.2667
42								0.2663	0.2657	0.2651
43									0.2642	0.2636
44										0.2622

Table continued on following page.

F is number of Fractions, T is Time in days

F	51	52	53	54	55	56	57	58	59	60
28	0.2916									
29	0.2891	0.2885								
30	0.2868	0.2862	0.2856							
31	0.2846	0.2839	0.2834							
32	0.2824	0.2818	0.2812	0.2806	0.2801					
33	0.2803	0.2797	0.2791	0.2786	0.2780	0.2774				
34	0.2783	0.2777	0.2771	0.2766	0.2760	0.2755	0.2749	0.2744		
35	0.2764	0.2758	0.2752	0.2747	0.2741	0.2736	0.2730	0.2725		
36	0.2745	0.2739	0.2734	0.2728	0.2723	0.2717	0.2712	0.2707	0.2702	0.2697
37	0.2727	0.2721	0.2716	0.2710	0.2705	0.2699	0.2694	0.2689	0.2684	0.2679
38	0.2710	0.2704	0.2698	0.2693	0.2687	0.2682	0.2677	0.2672	0.2667	0.2662
39	0.2693	0.2687	0.2682	0.2676	0.2671	0.2665	0.2660	0.2655	0.2650	0.2645
40	0.2677	0.2671	0.2665	0.2660	0.2655	0.2649	0.2644	0.2639	0.2634	0.2629
41	0.2661	0.2655	0.2650	0.2644	0.2639	0.2634	0.2628	0.2623	0.2619	0.2614
42	0.2645	0.2640	0.2634	0.2629	0.2624	0.2618	0.2613	0.2608	0.2603	0.2599
43	0.2631	0.2625	0.2619	0.2614	0.2609	0.2604	0.2599	0.2594	0.2589	0.2584
44	0.2616	0.2611	0.2605	0.2600	0.2594	0.2589	0.2584	0.2579	0.2575	0.2570
45			0.2591	0.2586	0.2581	0.2575	0.2570	0.2565	0.2561	0.2556
46			0.2577	0.2572	0.2567	0.2562	0.2557	0.2552	0.2547	0.2542
47					0.2554	0.2549	0.2544	0.2539	0.2534	0.2529
48					0.2541	0.2536	0.2531	0.2526	0.2521	0.2517
49							0.2518	0.2514	0.2509	0.2504
50							0.2506	0.2501	0.2497	0.2492
51									0.2485	0.2480
52										

F	61	62	63	64	65	66	67	68	69	70
36	0.2692	0.2687	0.2682							
37	0.2674	0.2669	0.2665	0.2660	0.2655					
38	0.2657	0.2652	0.2648	0.2643	0.2638	0.2634	0.2630			
39	0.2640	0.2636	0.2631	0.2627	0.2622	0.2618	0.2613			
40	0.2624	0.2620	0.2615	0.2611	0.2606	0.2602	0.2597	0.2593		
41	0.2609	0.2604	0.2600	0.2595	0.2591	0.2586	0.2582	0.2578		
42	0.2594	0.2589	0.2585	0.2580	0.2576	0.2571	0.2567	0.2563	0.2559	0.2555
43	0.2579	0.2575	0.2570	0.2566	0.2561	0.2557	0.2553	0.2549	0.2545	0.2541
44	0.2565	0.2560	0.2556	0.2552	0.2547	0.2543	0.2539	0.2535	0.2531	0.2527
45	0.2551	0.2547	0.2542	0.2538	0.2534	0.2529	0.2525	0.2521	0.2517	0.2513
46	0.2538	0.2533	0.2529	0.2524	0.2520	0.2516	0.2512	0.2508	0.2504	0.2500

Table (T = 61–70):

F	61	62	63	64	65	66	67	68	69	70
47	0.2525	0.2520	0.2516	0.2511	0.2507	0.2503	0.2499	0.2495	0.2491	0.2487
48	0.2512	0.2508	0.2503	0.2499	0.2495	0.2490	0.2486	0.2482	0.2478	0.2474
49	0.2500	0.2495	0.2491	0.2486	0.2482	0.2478	0.2474	0.2470	0.2466	0.2462
50	0.2488	0.2483	0.2479	0.2474	0.2470	0.2466	0.2462	0.2458	0.2454	0.2450
51	0.2476	0.2471	0.2467	0.2463	0.2459	0.2454	0.2450	0.2446	0.2442	0.2439
52	0.2464	0.2460	0.2456	0.2451	0.2447	0.2443	0.2439	0.2435	0.2431	0.2427
53		0.2449	0.2444	0.2440	0.2436	0.2432	0.2428	0.2424	0.2420	0.2416
54		0.2438	0.2433	0.2429	0.2425	0.2421	0.2417	0.2413	0.2409	0.2405
55					0.2414	0.2410	0.2406	0.2402	0.2399	0.2395
56							0.2396	0.2392	0.2388	0.2384
57							0.2386	0.2382	0.2378	0.2374
58									0.2368	0.2364
59									0.2358	0.2355
60									0.2349	0.2345

Table (T = 71–80):

F	T = 71	72	73	74	75	76	77	78	79	80
42	0.2551	0.2547								
43	0.2537	0.2533	0.2529	0.2525	0.2521					
44	0.2523	0.2519	0.2515	0.2511	0.2507	0.2504	0.2500	0.2497		
45	0.2509	0.2505	0.2501	0.2498	0.2494	0.2490	0.2487	0.2483		
46	0.2496	0.2492	0.2488	0.2484	0.2481	0.2477	0.2474	0.2470	0.2467	0.2463
47	0.2483	0.2479	0.2475	0.2472	0.2468	0.2464	0.2461	0.2457	0.2454	0.2451
48	0.2470	0.2467	0.2463	0.2459	0.2456	0.2452	0.2448	0.2445	0.2442	0.2438
49	0.2458	0.2454	0.2451	0.2447	0.2443	0.2440	0.2436	0.2433	0.2430	0.2426
50	0.2446	0.2443	0.2439	0.2435	0.2432	0.2428	0.2425	0.2421	0.2418	0.2414
51	0.2435	0.2431	0.2427	0.2424	0.2420	0.2417	0.2413	0.2410	0.2406	0.2403
52	0.2423	0.2420	0.2416	0.2412	0.2409	0.2405	0.2402	0.2398	0.2395	0.2392
53	0.2412	0.2409	0.2405	0.2401	0.2398	0.2394	0.2391	0.2388	0.2384	0.2381
54	0.2402	0.2398	0.2394	0.2391	0.2387	0.2384	0.2380	0.2377	0.2374	0.2370
55	0.2391	0.2387	0.2384	0.2380	0.2377	0.2373	0.2370	0.2366	0.2363	0.2360
56	0.2381	0.2377	0.2373	0.2370	0.2366	0.2363	0.2360	0.2356	0.2353	0.2350
57	0.2371	0.2367	0.2363	0.2360	0.2356	0.2353	0.2350	0.2346	0.2343	0.2340
58	0.2361	0.2357	0.2354	0.2350	0.2347	0.2343	0.2340	0.2336	0.2333	0.2330
59	0.2351	0.2347	0.2344	0.2340	0.2337	0.2334	0.2330	0.2327	0.2324	0.2320
60	0.2342	0.2338	0.2334	0.2331	0.2328	0.2324	0.2321	0.2317	0.2314	0.2311
61	0.2332	0.2329	0.2325	0.2322	0.2318	0.2315	0.2312	0.2308	0.2305	0.2302

Glossary

Abscopal — A remote effect, such as tumor shrinkage in an untreated area, resulting from irradiation of another portion of the disease.

Absorbed Dose — Energy per unit mass deposited in a material as a consequence of being irradiated. The unit of absorbed dose is the rad.

Absorption — The loss of energy from a particle beam as a result of interactions of that particle beam with material.

Absorption Coefficient — The fractional energy loss from a particle beam as a result of interactions with material.

Acentric Fragment — A chromosome fragment without a centromere, and hence without a site for spindle attachment.

Actinium — Chemical element, found in uranium ore, having radioactive properties.

Adenine — Decomposition product of nuclein, found in pancreas, spleen, and urine. One of the bases of DNA and RNA.

Adenocarcinoma — A malignancy arising from glandular tissue.

Adjuvant — Any substance that when mixed with an antigen enhances antigenicity and gives superior immune response.

Alimentary Tract — That system in living organisms involved with utilization of food.

Alkaloid — A chemotherapeutic agent commonly used in the treatment of lymphomas.

Alkylating Agent — A drug which acts upon nucleic acids.

Allele — One of a series of genes at the same locus on homologous chromosomes.

Allogenic — Of disparate or foreign origin or genotype within a given species.

Alpha Particle — The nucleus of the helium atom, containing two protons and two neutrons.

Anamnestic Reaction — A rapid immunologic reaction that occurs when a previously sensitized animal is reinjected with the original antigen; it thus constitutes evidence of immunologic memory.

Anaphase — Stage in mitosis, following metaphase, in which halves of divided chromosomes move apart toward the poles of the spindle to form the diaster.

Anaplastic — Without specific morphology, a loss of identity with the parent cells.

Androgen — Male hormone.

Aneuploidy — The state of having more or less than the diploid number of chromosomes.

Annihilation Radiation — The release of 1.02 MeV, usually in the form of two photons (each 0.51 MeV) when a positron and an electron mutually annihilate each other.

Anorexia — Lack or loss of appetite for food.

Anoxia — A reduction of oxygen concentration below the level normally present in the system.

Antibiotic — A chemical substance produced by microorganisms that has a capacity to inhibit the growth of other organisms. Often used as a chemotherapeutic agent based upon its toxicity.

Antibody — A protein produced in the body in response to contact of the body with an antigen and having the specific capacity of neutralizing or reacting with the antigen.

Antigen — Any substance which, when introduced into a vertebrate elicits the production of molecules (antibodies) which bind specifically to the inducing substance.

Antimetabolite — A drug that acts by interfering with the synthesis of nucleic acid.

Ataxia — Loss of muscular coordination with impaired balance.

Atom — Any one of the ultimate particles of a molecule or of any matter. The smallest quantity of an element that can exist and still retain the chemical properties of the element.

317

Atomic Number — A part of the description of an atomic nucleus; the total number of elementary positive charges in the nucleus, sometimes said to be the number of protons in the nucleus. Denoted by the letter Z.

Attenuation — Reduction in the number of particles from a beam as a result of interactions of that particle beam with material.

Attenuation Coefficient — The fractional number of particles lost from a beam per unit of thickness of material traversed.

Auger Effect — A process by which excess energy, stored by one or more electrons in higher orbits, may be released from an atom. This process competes with fluorescence for the release of such energy. In this process, the energy which is liberated by one electron making a transition from a higher to a lower orbit is made available to another electron in a higher orbit, overcoming the binding energy of that other electron and giving to it a characterizable additional kinetic energy.

Auger Electrons — Electrons emerging from an atom as a result of the excitation by Auger effect.

Autologous — Related to self-designating components of same individual organism.

Autoradiogram — When a photographic emulsion is placed in contact with radioactive material (e.g., thin sections of a cell), the radiation exposes the film, revealing details of the location and geometry of the radioactive components.

Autosome — A chromosome which is not a sex chromosome.

Background Radiation — The radiation to which a detector is sensitive and which is a part of the environment, as contrasted with any particular sample that might be presumably under test.

Basal Cell Carcinoma — A cancer arising from the basal cell layers of the skin.

Bases — The lowest part or foundation of anything; main ingredient of a compound. Nonacid part of salt.

Benign — Not malignant, favorable for recovery, not associated with cancer.

Beta Decay — A mechanism of radioactivity, in which an atomic nucleus emits an electron, a neutrino, and in some instances one or more gamma rays. In this mechanism the mass number (A) of the nucleus is unchanged while its atomic number (Z) increases by one.

Beta Particle — Charged particle emitted from the nucleus of an atom, with a mass and charge equal in magnitude to that of the electron.

Betatron — An apparatus which accelerates electrons to millions of electron volts by means of magnetic induction.

Binding Energy — The work which must be done to liberate a particle. The liberation may be an electron from an atomic orbit or a nucleon from the nucleus.

Biologic Half-Life — In radioactive decay, the time interval during which a given chemical form, particularly one which is tagged with a radionuclide, is eliminated from a location site by physiologic processes alone, and not accounting for any physical decay.

Bivalent — Composed of two homologous chromosomes joined end to end or associated in pairs.

Bohr Atom — A mechanical model describing the internal construction of an atom. A heavy positive nucleus, said to contain neutrons and protons, is encircled by electrons in specific orbital positions. The positive charge in the nucleus is exactly balanced by the combined negative charges of the circulating electrons.

Branching Ratio — In radioactive decay, a statement of the fractional or percentage distribution among alternate pathways for the decay of a particular radionuclide.

Bremsstrahlung — Photons produced as a result of deflection interaction of an incident energetic electron with an atomic nucleus. The amount of energy transferred to the photon in the deflection process depends on the closeness of approach of the incident electron to the nucleus; there is no restriction on this closeness, whence all energies are found in the photon beam from very low values up to full energy of the incident electron. Thus, the photon spectrum has a continuous distribution against energy, this radiation is sometimes called continuous X-radiation.

Calorimeter — A device for measuring heat deposited. Specifically, the measurement of temperature changes in a particular absorber due to energy deposited in that absorber as a result of irradiation.

Centric Fragment — Fragment of chromosome containing the centromere.

Centromere — The constricted area of the chromosome evident during mitosis where attachment to the spindle fiber occurs.

Characteristic X-rays — A photon emerging from an atom with an energy in excess of a few KeV as a result of transmission of an electron from an excited state to fill a vacancy in a lower orbit. If the vacancy being filled is in the K shell, one speaks of K X-rays. The photon energies which appear are characteristic of the atomic number of the atom in which the transitions occur and also of the quantum numbers of the levels particularly involved.

Charge (Elementary)—Quantity of electricity. Total charge as a bulk transfer concept is measured in Coulombs and is usually determined by integrating electric current over a time interval. Individual charges, such as those on electrons and protons, are found to have a very specific magnitude which is invariant. The elementary charge is approximately 1.6×10^{-19} Coulombs.

Chemotherapy—The use of systemic drugs to treat neoplasia.

Chromatid—At metaphase each chromosome is seen to be split longitudinally into two pieces except in the region of the centromere. Each half chromosome is a chromatid, and it is the two chromatids of the chromosome which separate at mitosis.

Chromophore—Any chemical group whose presence gives a decided color to a compound and which unites with certain other groups to form dyes.

Chromosome—Any of the small, dark-staining bodies located in cell nuclei, composed of DNA, RNA, and basic proteins, and which result from condensation of the nuclear chromatin of cells at mitosis or meiosis. Contain genes (hereditary factors). The number of chromosomes is usually constant for each species.

Chromosome Aberration—Any abnormality in structure or number of chromosomes. Some are associated with specific disease syndromes, such as neoplasms; some are related to chemical or physical damage to somatic cells.

Chromosome Bridge—A dicentric chromosome that bridges between the diverging chromosomes in anaphase because its two centromeres are moving toward opposite poles.

Chromosome Mutation—A change in the number of whole chromosomes, which alters the amount of DNA, or one or more breaks in a chromosome, which alters the amount of DNA and/or the linear sequence of genes.

Clone—A population of cells derived from a single parent.

Codon—The triplet of nucleotides in a DNA or messenger RNA that codes for a particular amino acid (or signals the end of the message).

Coenzyme—Organic, dialyzable, thermostable compound with which an apoenzyme must unite in order to function.

Coherent Scattering—Diffusion of roentgen rays produced by a medium through which the rays pass.

Compton Effect—A photon attenuation process in which the incident photon is scattered by an atomic electron. The energy of the outgoing photon is reduced in a relationship involving the angle of scattering, and the energy loss given to that orbital electron which participated in the scattering.

Cosmic Ray—High energy particulate and electromagnetic radiation which originates outside the earth's atmosphere.

Coulomb Force—The force between charged particles directly proportional to the product of the charges of the particles involved and inversely proportionate to the square of the distance separating them.

Cyclotron—An apparatus for accelerating protons or deuterons to high energies by a combination of a constant magnet and an oscillating electrical field.

Cytokinesis—The changes that take place in the cytoplasm during mitosis, meiosis, and fertilization.

Cytosine—A base, one of the disintegration products of nucleic acid.

D_0—The dose necessary to reduce the surviving fraction from some value f to $e^{-1}f$ (approximately 0.37f) along the exponential portion of a survival curve.

Dalton—A unit of weight equal to the weight of a single hydrogen atom, approximately 1.65×10^{-24} grams.

Decay Constant—In radioactivity, the fractional decay of a particular nuclear species per unit time.

Decay Scheme—A pictorial representation showing the steps and alternate pathways by which a radionuclide emits particles and loses energy in radioactive disintegration. (See Energy Level Diagram.)

Decay Series—A situation in which a radioactive parent nucleus decays to a daughter nucleus which is also radioactive; ultimately a stable daughter is produced. Some decay series are known to have at least 30 members before the terminal stable nuclide is reached.

De-excitation—The prompt spontaneous release of excess energy. For the orbital electrons such release is known as *Fluorescence* and *Auger Effect* (qq.v.) and for the nucleus it is *Gamma Emission* and *Internal Conversion* (q.v.). Delayed de-excitation of the orbital electrons is known as *Phosphorescence* (q.v.) and for the nuclear system is *Isomeric Transition* (q.v.).

Delta Ray — Energetic secondary electron ejected as a consequence of the ionization process of the primary radiation; a secondary electron with a substantial range of its own.

Deoxyribose — Five carbon sugar molecules characterized by absence of an oxygen moiety on second carbon.

Deuteron — The nucleus of deuterium, or heavy hydrogen, used as bombing particles for nuclear distintegration.

Differential Recovery Rate — A distinct difference in recovery between two cell systems under study.

Diffusion — Process of becoming widely spread. Dialysis through a membrane.

Diploid — Having two sets of chromosomes (2n), as normally found in the somatic cells of higher organisms.

Direct Action — Changes produced by the direct absorption of radiation by a target molecule; that is, changes produced by the direct dissociation, excitation, or ionization of the target molecule.

DNA (Deoxyribonucleic Acid) — An organic acid originally isolated from fish sperm and present in all living cells that contain nuclear material. Composed of a deoxyribose phosphate backbone formed into a double helix by pairs of bases which are bound to each other in specific complementary fashion to maintain the spatial relationships of the two strands of the helix. Hereditary molecule in all replicating organisms, with the exception of certain viruses.

DNA Ligase — An enzyme which rejoins certain single strand DNA breaks (those characterized by $5'PO_4$, $3'OH$ termini).

DNA Polymerase — An enzyme that synthesizes DNA in the presence of a DNA template and appropriate precursor (i.e., deoxyribonucleoside triphosphates).

Dominant — Capable of expression when carried by only one of a set of homologous chromosomes.

Dose — See *Absorbed Dose*.

Dose-Modifying Factor — A constant (dose-independent) factor which relates two survival curves.

Dosimetry — Strictly, the measurement of energy deposited in a material as a result of irradiation. Loosely, any quantitative measurement of effect resulting from irradiation.

Doubling Time — The average time taken for the cell number in a population to double. (See *Generation Time*.)

Down's Syndrome — Gain of one entire autosome in man; mongolism.

Effective Half-Life — In radioactive decay, the time interval during which a given activity of a radionuclide disappears from a localization site as a result of the combined processes of physical decay and biologic elimination.

Efficiency — A counting situation refers to the relative ability of a system to count the number of events at risk. It may be expressed as a fraction or a percentage. The number of disintegrations in relation to the number of particles incident on the detecting system.

Elective Booking Method — Subject to choice or decision of patient; applied to procedures that are only advantageous to patient, but not necessary to save life.

Electron — The unit, or "atom," of negative electricity.

Electron Capture — A mechanism of radioactivity in which an orbital electron (most frequently from K shell) disappears and a neutrino and one or more gamma rays are emitted from an atomic nucleus. The mass number (A) of the nucleus is unchanged, while its atomic number (Z) decreases by one.

Element — A substance which cannot be broken down by ordinary chemical means into parts having different chemical properties.

Elementary Charge — 1.601×10^{-19} Coulomb. (See *Charge*.)

Emesis — Vomiting.

Endocrine — Applied to organs whose function is to secrete into blood or lymph a substance that has a specific effect on another organ or part (internal secretion).

Endoreplication — A duplication of the chromosomes that is not followed by mitosis and cell division.

Energy — The ability to do work. In the context of dosimetry, the changes which may be observed in a detector are expected to bear a recognizable (possibly linear) relationship to the energy deposited.

Energy Level Diagram — A graphic display for energy considerations; used both for atomic and nuclear situations.

Estrogen — Female hormone.

Euploidy — A term referring to a cell which has the normal set of chromosomes corresponding to its ploidy.

Excitation — An act of irritation or stimulation; a condition of being excited.

Excited Molecule — A molecular species (or atomic species as a special case) in which a bonding or nonbonding electron has been promoted by the absorption of radiant energy into an anti-bonding orbital. It is thus energy-rich, short-lived, and will decay back to the ground state with concurrent emission of the absorbed energy as heat or light.

Excited State — A system not in its lowest energy configuration. In an atom, when one or more electrons are in orbits farther out than they would be normally, the situation is called an excited state. In a nucleus, an excited state is also reached by a rearrangement by the protons and neutrons comprising the nucleus.

Exposure — The act of irradiating any test object. Also, the unit for quantitation of an X- or gamma ray beam in terms of the ability of such beam to ionize air (the unit of quantitation is called a roentgen).

Exposure Dose — The exposure dose of X- or gamma radiation at a certain place is a measure of the radiation that is based upon its ability to produce ionization in air. The unit of the exposure dose is the roentgen.

Exposure Rate — Especially for ionizing radiation, the accumulation per unit time of quantity of X- or gamma rays. Frequently expressed in roentgens per minute.

Extrapolation Number — The intercept of the exponential portion of a survival curve extrapolated back to zero dose.

Faraday Cup — A devise for detecting charged particle beams.

Far-Ultraviolet — That portion of the UV spectrum below 300 nanometers.

Fluorescence — Prompt de-excitation of energy stored in electronic excitation levels resulting in the production of photons, usually in the visible region, but also include characteristic X-rays as a special case.

Fractionation — The breaking up of a treatment course into two or more components.

Frameshift Mutation — Alteration of linear sequence of nucleotides caused by insertion or deletion of a base. The "frame" of reading is shifted so that the triplets are different and may code for nonsense codons.

Free Radicals — An atomic or molecular species which contains one or more unpaired electrons and is thus unusually reactive chemically.

Gamma Emission — Release of a gamma ray.

Gamma Ray — A form of electromagnetic radiation, highly penetrating of nuclear origin.

Gastrointestinal Syndrome — Pertaining to stomach and intestine.

Geiger-Mueller Counter — A radiation detector producing an output voltage pulse each time it is triggered by a radiation absorption event.

Gene — A locus on the chromosome responsible for directing the synthesis of a specific enzyme, protein, or peptide.

Gene Mutation — A permanent change in the primary structure of the DNA.

Generation Time — The average time taken for a cell to complete one growth cycle. The generation time is shorter than the doubling time, when some of the population is not in the proliferative pool.

Genetic Code — The mathematical aspect of the system by which information is transferred from genetic material to proteins, the pattern of the nucleotides in the nucleic acids is thought to determine each amino acid in the chain making up each protein.

Genetic Polymorphism — Appearing in different forms at different stages of development.

Genetic Recombination — The reunion, in same or different arrangement, of formerly united elements which have become separated.

Genetically Significant Dose (GSD) — Estimated radiation dose theoretically received by every potential parent in the population.

Genome — The complete set of hereditary factors contained in the genetic constitution of an organism.

Genotype — The fundamental hereditary constitution (or assortment of genes) of an individual. Referring to the hereditary potential of an organism.

Glial Cell — Pertaining to a cell of the neuroglia.

Gonial Cells — Stem cells: precursors to germ cells.

Guanine — A white crystalline base, one of decomposition products of nuclein.

G-Value — The yield of a radiolysis product, or of loss of the target molecule expressed in terms of molecules of product produced per 100 electron volts absorbed in the system. It corresponds to the term quantum yield used in photochemistry.

Half-Life — In radioactive decay, the time interval during which a given sample of a particular radionuclide decays to half of its initial activity. (See *Physical Half-Life.*)

Half-Value Layer (HLV) — The thickness of material which will attenuate a given photon beam to half its initial value. The unit which is usually halved is the roentgen. Used to indicate X-ray quality.

Haploid — Having a single set of chromosomes as normally carried by a gamete(n).

Hemizygous — Possessing only one of a pair of genes that influence the determination of a particular trait.

Hemolysin Response — A substance which liberates hemoglobin from red corpuscles.

Hemopoietic Stem Cell — A progenitor cell which continuously produces cells that differentiate into hemopoietic cells.

Hemopoietic Syndrome — That portion of the acute radiation syndrome associated with the blood-forming organs. Appears at 8 to 14 days after exposure and is the primary cause of death in low to intermediate exposures.

Heterozygous — Possessing different alleles in regard to a given character.

Histone — A basic protein soluble in water and insoluble in dilute ammonia (e.g., globin). The protein material that surrounds the nucleic acid of chromosomes is made up of histones.

Homologus — Derived from an animal of the same species, but of different genotype. Corresponding in structure and position.

Homozygous — Possessing an identical pair of alleles in regard to a given character or to all characters.

Hormone — A chemical substance produced in the body which has a specific effect on the activity of certain organs.

Hydrated Electron — Water molecule with extra unpaired electron. A charged, free radical.

Hydrogen Bond — A direct ionic bond involving a shared proton.

Hyperbaric — The addition of oxygen to a system under study at greater than atmospheric pressure.

Hyperdiploid — An individual or cell with more than two sets of chromsomes.

Hypersensitivity — Body reacts to a foreign substance more strongly than normal.

Hypocenter — The spot immediately beneath the exact site of explosion of an atomic bomb.

Hypodiploid — An individual or cell with less than the diploid number of chromosomes.

Hypoxia — A reduction of oxygen concentration below the level normally present in the system.

Immunity — Security against any particular disease or poison.

Immunity, Acquired — Specific immunity attributable to presence of an antibody.

Immunity, Innate — Inborn, not acquired immunity.

Immunity, Humoral — Acquired immunity, in which the role of circulating antibody is predominant.

Immunosupressive — That which will depress immunologic reactions by interference with cellular or humoral antibody synthesis.

Indirect Action — Changes which are produced by reaction of target molecules with ions, radicals, or excited molecules resulting from absorption of radiation by some other molecule in the system; usually used for aqueous systems in which the water molecule is the one which absorbs the radiation.

Indirect Photoreactivation — Photoreactivating light (300 to 380 mm) is applied before irradiation. Similar to photoprotection.

Induction Phase — Period of time that elapses between the administration of an antigen and the appearance of a detectable immune response.

Internal Conversion — A radioactive decay situation in which excess energy in the nucleus is released by overcoming the binding energy of an orbital electron and expelling this electron with a kinetic energy equal to the excess nuclear energy less the binding energy. Some consider this as an internal photoelectric effect: a gamma ray carrying the excess nuclear energy is emitted by the nucleus, and some fraction of these are then said to interact with an orbital electron with identical energy consequence.

Internal Conversion Electron — Electrons from atomic orbits released as a result of nuclear de-excitation. These electrons appear with specific energies which are characteristic of the nuclear energy levels involved, as well as the binding energy for each orbit.

Inversion — The inverted reunion of the intervening segment after breakage of one chromosome at two points.

Ionization — The process of producing ions; that is, atoms or molecules which are not electrically neutral.

Ionization Chamber — A well defined volume of gas, usually air, with electrodes exposed to the gas for the purpose of collecting ions produced in the gas as a result of irradiation.

Ions — An atom or group of atoms having a charge of positive (cation) or negative (anion) electricity.

Isoprenoid Quinones — Composed of carbon-hydrogen-oxygen molecular arrangement; component of cellular respiratory chain.

Isochromatid Break — Chromosome break that occurs when both chromatids are broken at the same locus.

Isologous — Characterized by an identical genotype.

Isologous Cell Line — Cell line derived from identical twins or from highly inbred animals.

Isomer — Any compound capable of exhibiting isomerism (each molecule possessing identical number of atoms of each element, but in different arrangement).

Isomeric Transition — A mechanism of radioactivity in which an atomic nucleus exhibits a delayed emission of a gamma ray. A half-life may be determined to characterize the delay. Neither the mass number (A) nor the atomic number (Z) of the nucleus is changed by this decay.

Isotone — One of a group of nuclear species all characterized by having the same mass number (A).

Isotope — A chemical element having same atomic number as another (i.e., same number of nuclear protons) but possessing a different atomic mass (i.e., different number of nuclear neutrons).

Karyotype — A systemized arrangement of chromosomes of a single cell, typical of an individual or species.

Kilovoltage — Accelerating voltage behind a specific radiation, measured in thousands of volts.

Kinetic Energy — Pertaining to or producing motion.

Klinefelter's Syndrome — Associated with an abnormality of the sex chromosomes. A disease of males characterized by gynecomastia, aspermatogenesis, and increased levels of follicle-stimulating hormone.

Latent Period — Period between initial onset of disease and appearance of most symptoms.

LD$_{50/30}$ — A dose which is lethal to 50 per cent of the population in 30 days.

Leakage Radiation — All radiation coming from the source except the useful beam.

Lesion — Any pathologic or traumatic discontinuity of tissue or loss of function of a part.

Ligase, DNA — An enzyme which rejoins certain single strand DNA breaks (those characterized by $5'PO_4 - 3'OH$ termini).

Linear Accelerator — An instrument for producing positive ions of high energy, used for the acceleration of heavy ions.

Linear Attenuation Coefficient — See *Attenuation Coefficient.*

Linear Energy Transfer (LET or L.E.T.) — A measure of the rate of energy loss along the track of an ionizing particle, expressed in units of energy per unit track length (e.g., KeV per micron). Also, the average energy released per unit of radiation ionization track length, expressed in KeV per micron.

Liquid-Holding Recovery — Higher survival of bacteria after holding them in a liquid for a few hours. Appears to enhance excision-resynthesis repair.

Liquid Scintillation Counter — A radiation detector for charged particle beams.

Locus — In genetics, the specific site of a gene in a chromosome.

Lymphoepithelioma — A malignancy composed of epithelial cancer interspersed with lymphocytes.

Lymphoid-Macrophage System — Cell systems of lymphoid and myeloid origin that participate in the initiation and maintenance of immune responses.

Lymphosarcoma — A malignancy arising from lymphatic tissue.

Macrophage — Name for a large mononuclear wandering phagocytic cell which originates in the tissues and probably takes an active part in formation of antibody.

Malignancy — A tendency to progress in virulence, commonly associated with cancer.

Marker Chromosome — A gene of known function and known location on the chromosome.

Mass — The inertial property of matter. The proportionality coefficient between a force exerted on an object and the acceleration experienced by that object.

Mass Number — A partial description of an atomic nucleus; the sum of the number of protons and neutrons which together form the nucleus. Denoted by letter A.

Maximal Tolerance Dose — The largest quantity of an agent, such as X-ray energy, that may be administered without harm.

Maximum Permissible Dose Equivalent (MPD) — For radiation protection purposes the maximum permissible dose equivalent which a person or specified parts thereof shall be allowed to receive in a stated period of time.

Mean Free Path — The average distance that particles of a specified type travel before a given type (or types) of interaction in a specific medium.

Mean Life — In radioactive decay, the reciprocal of the decay constant. Also, the time interval in which the whole amount of a given sample of a particular radionuclide would decay if the initial rate of decay were maintained. Also, the average lifetime of all of the nuclei accounting for the individual times of decay for the whole of an initial sample of a particular radionuclide.

Megavoltage — Accelerating voltage behind a specific radiation measured in millions of volts.

Meiosis — A special method of cell division, occurring in maturation of the sex cells, by means of which each daughter nucleus receives half the number of chromosomes characteristic of the somatic cells of the species.

Mendelian Genetic Analysis — Classic method of study of gene action, involving description of the end product, the phenotype.

Metaphase — The middle stage of mitosis during which the chromosomes separate lengthwise in the equatorial plane.

Metastasis — The ability of cells or groups of cells to be disseminated from the parent malignancy and create satellite growth centers.

Microcephaly — Abnormal smallness of the head.

Microwave Radiation — That portion of the electromagnetic spectrum covering the approximate frequencies of 300 to 300,000 megahertz, with the corresponding wavelengths of one meter to one millimeter.

Mitochondria — Organelles responsible for the conversion of chemical energy in pyruvic acid to ATP via the citric acid cycle.

Mitosis — A method of indirect division of a cell, consisting of a complex of various processes, by means of which the two daughter nuclei normally receive identical complements of the number of chromosomes characteristic of the somatic cells of the species. Divided into four phases: prophase, metaphase, anaphase, and telophase.

Mitotic Curve — The fraction of cells in a population which is in mitosis at any particular time.

Moiety — An equal part; a half; a part or portion.

Molecule — The smallest particle of any substance, element, or compound as it normally exists.

Monosomic — Characterized by monosomy (absence of one chromosome from the complement of an otherwise diploid cell [2n−1]).

Mosaic — The occurrence in an individual of two or more cell populations derived from a single zygote, each population having a different chromosome complement.

Multiplier Phototube — An electronic device which converts a light signal to a voltage output signal. This device has a number of internal electrodes called dynodes, which function to multiply the number of electrons generated initially from the incoming light signal. This tube is also sometimes called a photomultiplier.

Mutant — An inheritable variation in the genome.

Mutation — An inheritable change in chromosomes.

Myoclonus — Shocklike contractions of a portion of a muscle, restricted to one area of the body or appearing synchronously or asynchronously in several areas.

Nanometer — 10^{-9} meter, abbreviated nm.

Near-Ultraviolet — Lying just beyond the violet end of the visible spectrum (infrared), 300 to 380 nm.

Necrosis — Death of tissue, usually as individual cells.

Neoplastic Cell Populations — Defined as new cell growth, generally considered synonymous with malignancy.

Nephrectomy — The removal of a kidney.

Neural — Pertaining to a nerve or nerves.

Neutrino — A hypothetical elementary particle with an extremely small mass and carrying no electric charge.

Neutron — Neutral or uncharged particle of matter existing in atoms of all elements except mass = 1 isotope of hydrogen.

Nominal Single Dose — The effects produced by a given treatment course as related to the same effects that would be produced by a single dose.

Nonconservative DNA Replication — The mode of replication in which there is no net increase in amount of DNA, but only a replacement of parental DNA with newly synthesized DNA.

Nondisjunction—Failure of a pair of chromosomes to separate at meiosis, so that both members of the pair are carried to the same daughter nucleus and the other daughter cell is lacking that particular chromosome.

Nuclear Reactor—An atomic pile in which there is control of the atomic energy produced.

Nuclear Transmutation—Nuclear reactions involving a simple rearrangement of protons and neutrons among the nucleic concerned.

Nucleic Acid—A nucleotide polymer. Any of a group of acids occurring in organic nuclear material and consisting of a combination of phosphoric acid with a carbohydrate and a base.

Nucleoprotein—A substance composed of a simple basic protein, usually a histone or protamine, combined with a nucleic acid.

Nucleotide—A compound consisting of a purine or pyrimidine base attached to a sugar-phosphate moiety (i.e., a phosphorylated nucleoside).

Nucleus—The combination of atoms forming a central element or basic framework of the molecule of a specific compound. A spheroid body within a cell consisting of a number of characteristic organelles.

Nullisomic—Lacking one pair of chromosomes.

Nystagmus—An involuntary rapid movement of eyeball; it may be horizontal, vertical, rotatory or a combination.

Occupancy Factor—The factor by which the work loads should be multiplied to correct the degree or type of occupancy of the area in question.

One-Hit Aberration—Chromosome damage produced by a single ionization, or "hit."

One-Hit Kinetics—Linear dose-effect relation explicable on the theory that one effective ionization in or very close to the target (gene, chromosome, or cell) produces an effect (mutation or death).

Orchiectomy—Removal of the testes.

Oxygen Effect—The effects produced by either the addition or deletion of oxygen from a system under study.

Oxygen Enhancement Ratio—The ratio of the radiation dose under anoxic conditions to the dose under fully oxygenated conditions required to produce an equivalent effect.

Pair Production—A photon attenuation process in which the photon entirely disappears and is replaced by an electron and a positron as a pair. In order to create the pair, the photon energy must be at least that of the mass of the two particles, 1.02 MeV, which is therefore a threshold for the reaction to occur.

Parabiosis (dialytic)—The circulation of the blood of two animals through a dialyzer, separated by a membrane which permits the removal of harmful material from the recipient's blood and the contribution of essential factors from the donor's blood.

Paramagnetic—A substance that enhances the magnetic flux density when placed in a magnetic field. Oxygen is paramagnetic, nitrogen is not.

Particle—An entity which is described in terms of observable properties, such as mass, charge, or spin.

Peak Titer—Quantity of a substance required to produce a reaction with a given volume of another substance, or amount of one substance required to correspond with a given amount of another substance.

Phenotype—Referring to the observable properties of an organism produced by the interaction of its genotype with the environment. The outward, visible expression of the hereditary constitution of an organism.

Phosphodiester Backbone—Sugar-phosphate portion of DNA molecule, to which bases are attached.

Phosphorescence—A delayed de-excitation of energy stored in electronic excitation levels.

Photoelectric Effect—The emisssion of electrons from a substance in response to the impingement of photons of sufficient energy (M/P). One of the attenuation processes for photons. In this, incident photon entirely disappears, its energy is consumed in overcoming the binding energy of an atomic orbital electron, and any remainder is given to that electron as kinetic energy.

Photomultiplier—See *Multiplier Phototube.*

Photon—A quantum of electromagnetic radiation; the frequency of the radiation (and thus its energy) may range over the entire electromagnetic spectrum, but the most commonly discussed range is from hard gamma rays to the far infrared.

Photoproduct—A substance synthesized in the body by the action of light.

Photoprotection—A phenomenon in which irradiation by near ultraviolet radiation decreases the sensitivity of certain cells to subsequent far ultraviolet radiation.

Photoreactivation — A light-requiring process whereby part of the damage produced by radiation (usually ultraviolet) is reduced.

Physical Half-Life — In radioactive decay, the time interval during which a particular radionuclide decays to half of its initial activity owing to the physical decay processes alone.

Planck's Constant — A constant, h, which represents the ratio of the energy of any quantum of radiation to its frequency; value of h is 6.55×10^{-27} erg seconds.

Plating Efficiency (P.E.) — The fraction of single cells in an *in vitro* control population which can reproduce a sufficient number of times to produce a visible colony.

Plasma Cells (protoplasm) — Fluid part of blood as distinguished from corpuscles.

Polygenic — Pertaining to, or influenced by, several different genes.

Polymerase, DNA — An enzyme that synthesizes DNA in the presence of a DNA template and appropriate precursor (i.e., deoxyribonucleoside triphosphates).

Polyploidy — Having each chromosome (except sex chromosomes) represented more than twice.

Positron — A free positive electron; a particle having the mass of an electron, but a net positive charge.

Potentially Lethal Damage — Damage which may be reparable to a nonlethal level if suitable conditions are obtained. If repair does not occur, the damage is lethal.

Primary Radiation — Radiation coming directly from the source.

Primary Immune Response — The response of the animal body to an antigen on the first occasion that it encounters it.

Primary Response — The antibody response to the first injection of an antigen.

Prodromal — Indicating the approach of a disease or other morbid state.

Prophase — The first state in the mitotic cycle in which the chromosomes condense and begin to move toward the equatorial plane. DNA synthesis and duplication of the chromosomal material has been completed by this state.

Protraction — The extension of a course of treatment over a period of time.

Pulse Height Analysis — The determination of a distribution of voltage pulses according to the magnitude of the highest point of the pulse. The significance relates to voltage pulses from multiplier phototubes (q.v.). A directly proportional relationship exists between the energy deposited in a scintillation detector (See *Solid Scintillation Counter*) and the amplitude of the output voltage pulse.

Pulse Radiolysis — Exposure of the target substance to a burst of radiation delivered in such a short time (nanoseconds to microseconds) that transient species with lifetimes longer than the irradiation time can be observed.

Purine — Heterocyclic organic compound. The fundamental form of a group of bases, some of which are constituents of nucleic acid.

Purkinje Cells — Large branching neurons in the middle layer of the cortex cerebelli.

Pyrimidine — An organic compound, a metadiazine. The fundamental form of a group of bases, some of which are constituents of nucleic acid.

Pyrimidine Dimer — Photoproduct (q.v.) of UV irradiation of pyrimidines. Two adjacent pyrimidines are converted to a pyrimidine dimer, with consequent loss of the 5,6 double bonds and formation of a four-carbon cyclobutane ring.

Rad — A unit of absorbed dose; corresponds to an energy absorption of 100 ergs per gram of irradiated material.

Radiation — Energy propagated through space. As commonly employed in radiology, the term refers to two kinds of ionizing radiation: (1) electromagnetic waves (X- and gamma rays) and (2) corpuscular emissions from radioactive substances or other sources (alpha and beta particles, etc.).

Radiation Nephritis — An acute reaction often followed by destruction of the substance of the kidney as a direct result of irradiation.

Radiation Therapy — The use of radiant energy, either particulate or photon, to treat neoplastic tissue.

Radical Ion — An atomic or molecular species which carries a formal negative or positive charge; also contains an unpaired electron.

Radioactivity — The quality of emitting or emission of corpuscular or electromagnetic radiations consequent to nuclear disintegration. A natural property of all chemical elements of atomic number above 83, and possible of induction in all other known elements.

Radiocurability — The ability to completely destroy a neoplastic cell system by radiations.

Radionuclide — An atomic nucleus which will decay spontaneously into some other nuclear species, accompanied by the liberation of energy. A nuclear species that is radioactive.

Radiosensitivity — Responsiveness of cells to radiations.

Range — The difference between the upper and lower limits of a variable or a series of values.

Rapid Renewal Populations — Cells that are replaced at an extremely high rate.

Recessive — Incapable of expression unless carried by both members of a set of homologous chromosomes.

Recombination — The appearance together in offspring of traits found separately in each of their parents.

Re-irradiation — The use of radiation therapy to treat an area that has been previously treated with radiation.

Relative Biologic Effectiveness (RBE) — Is used to compare the effectiveness of absorbed doses of radiation of different types. The ratio of the absorbed doses of two radiations required to produce the same biologic effect. In most determinations of RBE it is customary to use orthovoltage X-rays (200 kVp) as the standard.

Rem — The unit of dose equivalent. For radiation protection purposes, the number of rems may be considered to equal the number of rads multiplied by the RBE (q.v.).

Renewing Cell Population — A cell system that undergoes a continuous renewal and replacement process.

Repair Replication — A non-conservative form of DNA replication in which DNA precursors are taken up into already synthesized DNA strands. Repair synthesis.

Restitution — In chromosome studies, restitution refers to the reuniting of the broken parts of a chromosome to a form which is morphologically indistinguishable from the original.

Ribose — Five-carbon sugar component of RNA.

Ring Chromosomes — Formed when the two broken ends of an interstitial fragment join with each other.

RNA Polymerase — The enzyme that copies the DNA nucleotide sequence in the synthesis of complementary RNA strands.

RNA (Ribonucleic acid) — A polymer of ribonucleotides. This material, contained both in the nucleus and cytoplasm of a cell, is believed to be needed mainly for the expression of genetic determinants (i.e., protein synthesis).

Roentgen (R) — The unit of exposure dose of X- or gamma radiation. One roentgen is an exposure dose of X- or gamma radiation such that the associated corpuscular emission per 0.001293 grams of air produces in air ions carrying one electrostatic unit of quantity of electrical charge of either sign.

Sarcoma — A malignancy arising from connective tissue.

Scattered Radiation — Radiation which, by passing through matter, has deviated in direction and whose energy has usually diminished.

Scintillation — A flash of light. Particularly in reference to multiplier phototubes (q.v.), the scintillating materials are chosen to provide photons in an energy (color) range for which a multiplier phototube will be particularly sensitive. This is blue and near untraviolet.

Secondary Disease — A wasting syndrome caused by the reaction of foreign transplanted immunocompetent cells against the host.

Secondary Immune Response — The antibody response to a re-injection of antigen given sometime after the primary response has passed its peak and has dropped to a low level.

Single-Strand Chain Breaks — A break in one of the two strands of the DNA molecule.

Slope — In rectangular coordinants, the ratio of the change of the ordinate to the corresponding change of the abscissa of a point moving along a line.

Solar Flare — A sudden and temporary outburst of energy from a small area of sun's surface that is usually directly observable only in increased emission of a few spectral wavelengths (as in hydrogen line and lines of ionized calcium), but sometimes seen in white light.

Solid Scintillation Counter — A radiation detector producing a scintillation in a solid material for each radiation absorption event.

Solvated Electron — A thermalized secondary electron which has been stabilized by formation of a cage of polarized water molecules; in the absence of reactive solutes, it has a lifetime of milliseconds.

Specific Locus Method — In genetics, the method of locating the specific site on a chromosome of a gene or groups of genes.

Spectrum — The frequency distribution of the existence of particles of various energies for all valid energies in a given situation. Especially useful to display the distribution of beta rays in beta decay and also the photon energies in Bremsstrahl ung (q.v.).

Spin — The designation of angular momentum which a particle carries, in units of $h/2\pi$, h being Planck's constant.

Split Course Therapy—The breaking up of a course of radiation therapy into two or more components with a rest interval interposed.

Spontaneous Mutation—Mutations for which there is no "observable" cause.

Spur—The volume element containing the immediate dissociation products produced by a ray of ionizing radiation passing through a liquid; a track is the series of spurs remaining after passage of the radiation ray.

Squamous Cell Carcinoma—A malignancy arising from the squamous cells of the skin or mucus membranes.

Static Cell Population—A population that is not able to replace destroyed members.

Stem Cells (Primitive cell)—A cell which is not only capable of a degree of proliferation but which during proliferation may give rise to differentiated cells exhibiting a variety of characteristics.

Sublethal Damage—Damage which must be accumulated before a lethal effect can be produced. This type of damage is not lethal regardless of whether or not it is repaired.

Sublethal Injury—A type of damage which must be accumulated for lethal effect.

Suicide Experiments—Cell death resulting from the radiation emitted by incorporated radioactive isotopes.

Superficial Orthovoltage—Medial voltage 250 kVp.

Supervoltage—Very high voltage; said of roentgen ray therapy.

Survival Curve—A curve of the fractional or per cent survival of the particular organism versus the amount of stress or treatment applied (usually radiation).

Surviving Fraction—The probability of the persistence of a viability end point sometime after a given stress or treatment compared to the effect of no treatment. For example, the persistence of the colony-forming ability of irradiated versus unirradiated cells.

Synchrotron—A machine for generating high speed electrons or protons, combining features of cyclotron and betatron; will produce 70 million electron volts.

Syngeneic—Isogenic, of the same origin. Used in contrast to allogenic to denote the immunologic relationship between individuals of the same genotype. The term isologous is sometimes used in this context.

Teratoma—A tumor of embryologic origin composed of many histologically separate elements. May be benign or malignant, depending upon the elements present.

Tetraploidy—The state of having four sets of chromosomes (4n).

Tetrasomic—Characterized by presence of two additional chromosomes of one type in an otherwise diploid cell (2n+2).

Terminal Deletion—Results when two ends of a chromosome break and heal separately, a centric and acentric fragment being produced.

Thermal and Blast Injury—The injury produced by thermal (heat) and blast (air concussion) detonation of high explosive bombs.

Thermoluminescent Dosimeter (TLD)—A solid state material (frequently lithium fluoride) which stores energy which has been deposited in it as a result of irradiation. The energy stored at least in part may be released in the form of visible light following heating of the detector.

Thorium—Radioactive metal with a half-life of order of 10^{10} years; used to facilitate visualization in roentgenography.

Threshold Value—That value at which a stimulus just produces a sensation.

Threshold Hypothesis—A theory of responses to radiation which suggests that radiation must be accumulated to a threshold value before injury is expressed.

Thymine—A pyrimidine base. One of the component bases of DNA.

Total Nodal Irradiation—A relatively new concept of radiation therapy of lymphomas. The use of radiation therapy to treat all the major lymph node areas of the body.

Transcription—A process involving base pairing, whereby the genetic information contained in DNA is used to order a complementary sequence of bases in an RNA chain.

Transforming DNA—DNA purified from a strain of bacteria that carries some genetic trait (such as resistance to a given antibiotic) which, when mixed with a culture of the same type of bacteria that does not carry this trait, can be taken up by a certain fraction of the cells (the "competent" cells) and integrated into their genome. Some of the cells acquire the trait carried by the purified DNA as a result. Thus, streptomycin sensitive cells can be transformed to streptomycin-resistant, and all future progeny of these transformed cells will be streptomycin-resistant.

Translocation—The shifting of a segment of one chromosome into another part of a homologous chromosome, or into a nonhomologous chromosome.

Transmutation — The artificial transformation of one nuclear species into another by the bombardment of some kind of particle; normally involves the emission of a particle.

Triage — A collection of three things having something in common.

Triplet Production — Interaction with an orbital electron of high energy electromagnetic radiation greater than 2.04 MeV. The electron is ejected along with an electron-positron pair.

Triplet State — An excited state in which an orbital electron has an unpaired spin.

Triploidy — The state of having three sets of chromosomes (3n).

Trisomy — The presence of an additional (3d) chromosome of one type in an otherwise diploid cell (2n+1).

Tumor — A swelling; a neoplasm; a mass of new tissue which grows independently of its surrounding structures; may be either benign or malignant.

Tumoricidal Doses — Destructive to cancer cells.

Turner's Syndrome — Retarded growth and sexual development associated with abnormality of sex chromosomes.

Two-Hit Aberrations — Chromosome damage that is the result of two single hits which must occur close together in time and space.

UNSCEAR — United Nations Scientific Committee on the Effects of Atomic Radiation.

Unscheduled DNA Synthesis — DNA synthesis occurring at a time when DNA synthesis normally does not occur (i.e., other than during S phase).

Uracil — A ureide dihydroxypyrimidine obtained from nuclenic acid; a pyrimidine base of RNA.

Uranium — Hard heavy radioactive metallic element (U); atomic number 92.

Use Factor — Fraction of the work load during which the useful beam is pointed in the direction under consideration.

Van Allen Belts — Either of two zones of high intensity radiation trapped in the earth's magnetic field, beginning at an altitude of approximately 800 kilometers, and extending thousands of kilometers into space.

Viability — A term having a variety of meanings, depending upon the context. In this work the term generally refers to a cell which can carry out enough successful divisions to give rise to a visible colony of offspring.

Wild Type — The original, parental genetic type with which mutants are compared. The form of gene (allele) commonly found in nature.

Work Load — The degree of use of an X-ray or gamma ray source. For X-ray machines below 500 kVp the work load is usually expressed in milliampere minutes per week. For gamma-beam therapy sources and for X-ray equipment operating at 500 kVp or above, the work load is usually stated in terms of the weekly exposure of the useful beam at one meter from the source and is expressed in roentgens.

Xeroderma Pigmentosum — A rare, fatal disease, characterized by brown spots and ulcers of skin-muscular-cutaneous atrophy and telangiectasis; characterized by an extreme sensitivity to sunlight.

X-rays — Electromagnetic emissions of short wavelength (below 5 Å), produced when electrons moving at high velocity strike various materials, especially heavy metals. They are able to penetrate most substances to some extent, some more than others.

Zygote — Result of union of male and female sex cells.

Index

Note: Page numbers in *italics* indicate illustrations; (t) indicates table.